Cultural Variations in Psychopathology

About the Editors

Sven Barnow, PhD, is a Professor and the Chair of the Department of Clinical Psychology and Psychotherapy as well as Head of the outpatient clinic at the University of Heidelberg, Germany. Since 2010, he has been a member of the Advisory Boards for Psychotherapy as well as Personality Disorders: Theory & Practice of the Social Ministry (Treatment for Personality Disorders) Expert Group at the Ministry of Health (BMG). In addition, he serves as an expert reviewer for the German Research Foundation (DFG), the German Academic Exchange service (DAAD), the Israel Science Foundation, and the Austrian Accreditation Council. He holds the Marsilius Fellowship (2011–2012) as part of the Excellence Initiative of the University of Heidelberg. His research combines behavioral and neurophysiological measures to examine emotion regulation and its relation to psychopathology. Further research interests are social and cultural aspects of emotion regulation. He has published more than 150 articles in peer-reviewed journals and book chapters on these topics.

Nazli Balkir is currently a senior-year doctoral candidate at the Department of Clinical Psychology and Psychotherapy of the University of Heidelberg, Germany, on a 3-year full doctoral scholarship from the Excellence Initiative of the university. During this time, she has served as a member and the coordinator of the research project on "How universal is depression?" supported by the German Research Foundation. She holds a BA degree in psychology as well as an MA degree in clinical psychology and completed her training in cognitive and behavioral psychotherapy in Istanbul, Turkey. Her current research explores the role of cultural factors in dysfunctional/abnormal behavior or experience. Further research interests involve the potential relevance of indigenous explanations of distress and healing techniques for culturally tailored modalities of psychotherapy, prevention programs, and mental health service delivery.

Cultural Variations in Psychopathology

From Research to Practice

Sven Barnow
Nazli Balkir
(Editors)

HOGREFE

Library of Congress Cataloging in Publication
is available via the Library of Congress Marc Database under the
LC Control Number 2012940826

Library and Archives Canada Cataloguing in Publication

Cultural variations in psychopathology : from research to practice / Sven Barnow, Nazli Balkir, editors.

Includes bibliographical references and index.
ISBN 978-0-88937-434-8

1. Psychology, Pathological--Cross-cultural studies. 2. Cultural psychiatry. 3. Mental illness--Diagnosis. 4. Mental illness--Treatment.
I. Barnow, Sven, 1964- II. Balkir, Nazli
RC455.4.E8C84 2012 616.89'07 C2012-904425-3

PUBLISHING OFFICES
USA: Hogrefe Publishing, 875 Massachusetts Avenue, 7th Floor, Cambridge, MA 02139
Phone (866) 823-4726, Fax (617) 354-6875; E-mail customerservice@hogrefe-publishing.com
EUROPE: Hogrefe Publishing, Merkelstr. 3, 37085 Göttingen, Germany
Phone +49 551 99950-0, Fax +49 551 99950-425, E-mail publishing@hogrefe.com

SALES & DISTRIBUTION
USA: Hogrefe Publishing, Customer Services Department,
30 Amberwood Parkway, Ashland, OH 44805
Phone (800) 228-3749, Fax (419) 281-6883, E-mail customerservice@hogrefe.com
EUROPE: Hogrefe Publishing, Merkelstr. 3, 37085 Göttingen, Germany
Phone +49 551 99950-0, Fax +49 551 99950-425, E-mail publishing@hogrefe.com

OTHER OFFICES
CANADA: Hogrefe Publishing, 660 Eglinton Ave. East, Suite 119 - 514, Toronto, Ontario M4G 2K2
SWITZERLAND: Hogrefe Publishing, Länggass-Strasse 76, CH-3000 Bern 9

Hogrefe Publishing
Incorporated and registered in the Commonwealth of Massachusetts, USA, and in Göttingen, Lower Saxony, Germany

Printed and bound in the USA
ISBN: 978-0-88937-434-8

Foreword

Culture is an integral part of individual development and functioning. The impact that culture has on individuals may be acute or insidious. As the world becomes a global village as a result of globalization, it is inevitable that movement of resources, including people, will become more frequent.

We know that culture influences the way we express emotional distress, how abnormality is defined, how help is offered and from where therapeutic intervention is sought. Culture dictates expressions of illness as well as our understanding. The debate between cultural universalism and relativism is critical in psychiatry. As our patients migrate, mental health professionals move around as well. Therefore, the need to attempt to understand how cultures define and explain distress becomes urgent.

This book, emerging as a result of a closed workshop in Heidelberg, is a welcome addition to the ever-expanding field of our understanding of cultural variations. The reader will find stimulating topics that deserve further discussion and debate as we continue to strive towards providing better clinical care to our patients, irrespective of their ethnicities and cultures.

Dinesh Bhugra CBE, FRCP, FRCPsych, PhD
Professor of Mental Health and Cultural Diversity
Institute of Psychiatry, King's College London
Immediate Past President, Royal College of Psychiatrists

Preface & Acknowledgments

This book is based on an international closed workshop on "Cultural Variations in Emotion Regulation and the Treatment of Psychiatric Patients" organized by the research team of the Institute of Psychology at Heidelberg University, Germany, December 16–17, 2010. The workshop was organized in conjunction with and supported by grants from the Cluster of Excellence "Asia and Europe in a Global Context," of the Karl Jaspers Center for Advanced Transcultural Studies at the University of Heidelberg. Many of our colleagues assisted in the organization of the workshop and it is quite impossible to list all the people who contributed to the success of this effort. Our appreciation goes to the entire academic and nonacademic staff of the Institute od Psychology and of the Karl Jaspers Center for their help and support. Special thanks go to our colleague Elizabeth A. Arens, also the author of one of the chapters in this book, who gave her valuable assistance both for the organization of this workshop and for the editing process of the current book.

The aim of the workshop was to bring together a variety of distinguished academics and practitioners working with patients from ethnically diverse minority populations to exchange perspectives and methods for research and practice. We are grateful to all those who participated in the workshop and wish to thank them all for stimulating discussions. Our special appreciation goes to the contributors of this book, for devoting their valuable time to revising their papers for publication. The chapters included in the present book cover a wide range of subjects relating to cultural psychology – from basic issues to clinical matters from an interdisciplinary perspective. We genuinely hope that this volume will help researchers and mental health professionals working with ethnically diverse (migrant) communities in Europe and throughout the world to conduct relevant research and advance culturally sensitive practice in mental health care.

Sven Barnow & Nazli Balkir
July 2012

Table of Contents

I. Introduction

The Relevance of Culture for Mental Health and Illness

Introduction

Sven Barnow and Nazli Balkir

Department of Clinical Psychology and Psychotherapy, Institute of Psychology, University of Heidelberg, Germany

In the era of globalization there is a significant increase in population movements and contacts between societies and cultures. Presently, more people are moving further and faster than ever before. Historically, the number of immigrants in the world has more than doubled since 1975, with most immigrants living in Europe (56 million), Asia (50 million), and Northern America (41 million). The increasing inflow of immigrants has led Europe to become a growing pluralistic society. Each year, an average of 1.8 million people who are in search of work or are asylum seekers immigrate to Europe permanently (Lindert, Schouler-Ocak, Heinz, & Priebe, 2008). Migration is known to have significant effects on mental health. It is well established that immigration and its related acculturation stress are associated with higher risk for mental disorders, such as anxiety and depression (e.g., Bhugra, 2003). The increased diversity of service users for mental health constitutes a substantial challenge to service providers not only in EU countries but also in other developed countries receiving international immigrants. People from different ethno-cultural backgrounds often have different perceptions and comprehension of *mental health* and illness and are habituated to different modes of mental health care as well. This often results in a detrimental discrepancy between the needs and expectations of patients and the service providers, which attenuate the effectiveness of treatment and lead to unexplained high drop-out rates (White & Marsella, 1982). In support of this argument, it has been well demonstrated that the members of ethnic minority groups exhibit higher rates of drop out and lower rates of compliance to treatment compared to the native population (Haasen, Lambert, Yagdiran, & Krausz, 1997).

In response to these problems, one of the central contributions that mental health professionals can make to this process is the continued provision of culture sensitive, high-quality, evidence-based mental health care. A major solution to enhance the quality of the mental health care is the advancement of research on all aspects of the interplay between culture and mental health, including epidemiology, assessment, diagnosis, course, outcome treatment, and prevention of psychopathology as well as appropriateness of the workforce and health services (see Figure 0.1). Although the ethical, social, and political importance of considering cultural diversity in mental health care is formally acknowledged, cultural psychology is still in its infancy and is not yet officially considered as an approach by the majority of the institutions and providers of mental health care in most of the developed countries (Kirmayer, Rousseau, Corin, & Groleau, 2008). Correspondingly, compared to the other fields of mental health, the quantity and

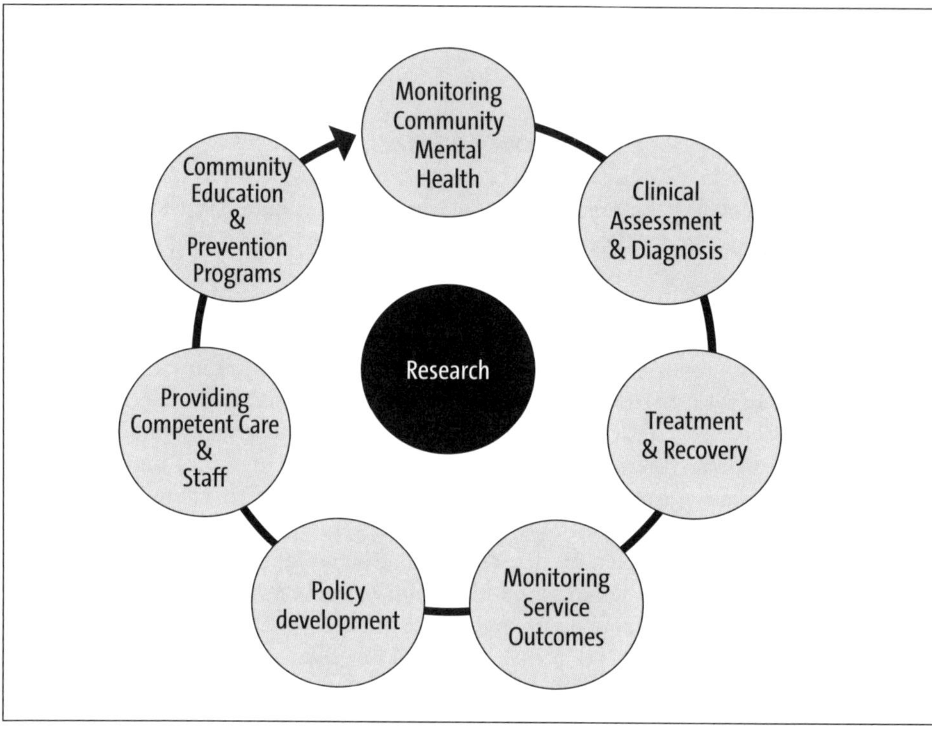

Figure 0.1. Areas of research in mental health care required for improving the quality of care provided to ethnic minority clientele.

quality of research relating to cultural psychology that is available to colleagues in and outside of Europe remains considerably limited.

In response to this limited research, with 16 chapters arranged into five sections, the objective of this book is to illuminate and understand the interplay between migration, culture, and psychopathology as well as its implications for service delivery in mental health care. We are of the opinion that an enhanced appreciation of the impact of socio-cultural factors on mental health will serve both to deepen the understanding of cultural diversity and to enhance the quality and acceptability of the mental health care provided to all. To this aim, we begin with the examination of repercussions of migration on mental health. In the first section, chapter 1 (Schouler-Ocak) provides an introductory overview of recent trends in immigration to Europe and a brief examination of epidemiology of common mental disorders prevalent among immigrants (e.g., suicidality, psychosis, affective and addictive disorders, and dementia) and thus facilitate the identification of risk and protective factors.

Subsequently, in order to obtain a better understanding of the interplay between culture and psychopathology, we provide a preliminary section that sheds light on the ways that culture shapes our brain. In chapter 2, Han provides fascinating data showing that neural substrates underlying self-related processing differ between Western and East Asian cultures. In chapter 3, Northoff and Panksepp explain how the self is related to emotion regulation and he presents data revealing that self-rated processing is related to activity in subcortical and cortical regions. Further, based on an evolutionary viewpoint he argues that self-related processing is present in different animals in different degrees. These findings can help us to understand how culture shapes self-rated processing in the brain.

Coming from this basic neurobiological research, our next focus is on the ways in which culture influences the development, course, and outcome of psychopathology. Given that emotion regulation is a transdiagnostic approach to the etiology and maintenance of psychopathology (Fairholme, Boisseau, Ellard, Ehrenreich, & Barlow, 2009), the third section starts with how cultural factors and socialization affects emotion regulation strategies, and how these strategies are associated with psychopathology. Accordingly, chapter 4 (Trommsdorff and Heikamp) discusses universal and culture-specific aspects of socialization of emotion regulation by providing some cross-cultural studies on the function of parental support, control, and sensitivity for emotion development and regulation. The authors argue that cultural models of self-other relations are transmitted through beliefs and culture-based practices, which in turn have an impact on emotion regulation. The main message from her work is that studying cultural context is important for the understanding of how emotion regulation relates to social competence and mental health.

Chapter 5 (Butler) completes the picture of the association between culture and emotion regulation by illustrating the ways in which cultural contexts modulate emotion regulatory processes and how this is related to mental health. Butler emphasizes that emotion regulation can be conceptualized in different ways. One is that the regulation of emotions is not constrained within a person; instead it is embedded in a larger cultural context. Thus, culture influences many aspects of emotional responding, which is often neglected in studies.

Chapter 6 (Arens) covers a recent study on how culture moderates the relationship between emotion regulation and mental health in the presence of psychopathology. The author asks whether or not cultural differences end where psychopathology begins. In her study she shows that healthy Turkish women less often use emotion regulation strategies such as reappraisal, but suppress their emotions more often in comparison to a healthy German control group. However, if one considers depressive patients these cultural differences disappear. These findings may indicate that although cultural differences in emotion regulation strategies exist, they are not dependent on psychopathology.

In section four, there are several chapters focusing on the cultural variations in the clinical course and manifestation of mental disorders and its implications for diagnosis and clinical assessment. For example, chapter 7 (Mezzich) aims to provide conceptual rationales for the inclusion of cultural factors in psychiatric diagnosis (i.e., cultural formulation approach) and suggestions for the content and use of this approach. Chapters 8 through 13 review the results of several studies of incidence and prevalence, patterns of clinical course, and outcome of common mental disorders prevalent among minority population. Readers are encouraged to understand the social world within mental illness and to realize the limitations of traditional constructions of illness.

The final point of consideration of this book is to shed more light on the ways in which the knowledge about the implications of cultural diversity is transferred into specific standards, policies, practices, and attitudes to eliminate ethnic disparities in mental health care. Therefore, cultural competence at individual (e.g., professionals) and systems level (mental health care organizations) was the focus of section five. In the first instance, chapter 14 (Balkir) reviews the sociocultural construction of mental illness and help-seeking behavior, in order to inform the professionals concerning the mental health care needs of ethnic minority clientele and therefore provide practical solutions for their differential service utilization. Here, we illustrate that culture is one of the major determinants of recognition of symptoms and consequently the interpretation, conceptualization, and reaction to distress, all of which determine the choice of and adherence to treatment.

Furthermore, chapter 15 (Qureshi and Eiroa Orosa) introduces cultural competence theory and practices that have the capacity to increase the mental health care professionals' proficiency in serving ethnic minority clients. This chapter presents an interpretive-relational approach to cultural competence conceptualized as a process of self-introspection rather than knowledge gathering. The final chapter (Machleidt et al.) deals with the ways in which the definition of cultural competence has been adopted by mental health care systems. By exemplifying Sonnenberg Guidelines for psychiatric-psychotherapeutic management of immigrants in Germany, the authors provide practical solutions for translating such guidelines into hands-on strategies that would renovate mental health services to make them more effective for ethnic minority populations.

To summarize, this book examines the current state of the art by exploring the broad scope of cultural psychology. It is our hope that readers' understanding of the multiple ways in which culture and human behavior can be intertwined will be enriched. We believe that an enhanced comprehension of the interplay between culture and mental health will strengthen the quality of every phase of mental health care continuum – from research to clinical practice.

References

Bhugra, D. (2003). Migration and depression. *Acta Psychiatrica Scandinavia Supplementum, 418*, 67–73.

Fairholme, C. P., Boisseau, C. L., Ellard, K. K., Ehrenreich, J. T., & Barlow, D. H. (2009). Emotions, emotion regulation, and psychological treatment: A unified perspective. In A. M. Kring & D. S. Sloan (Eds.), *Emotion regulation and psychopathology: A transdiagnostic approach to etiology and treatment* (pp. 283–309). New York: Guilford.

Haasen, C., Lambert, M., Yagdiran, O., & Krausz, M. (1997). Psychiatric disorders among migrants in Germany: Prevalence in a psychiatric clinic and implications on services and research. *European Psychiatry, 12*, 305–310.

Lindert, J., Schouler-Ocak, M., Heinz, A., & Priebe, S. (2008). Mental health and health care consumption among migrants in Europe. *European Psychiatry, 23*, 14–20.

Kirmayer, L. J, Rousseau, C., Corin, E., & Groleau, D. (2008). Training researchers in cultural psychiatry: The McGill-CIHR strategic training program. *Academic Psychiatry, 32*, 320–326.

White, G. M., & Marsella, A. J. (1982). Introduction: Cultural conceptions in mental health research and practice. In A. J. Marsella & G. M. White (Eds), *Cultural conceptions of mental health and therapy* (pp. 3–38). Dordrecht, The Netherlands: Reidel.

Chapter 1

Migration and Mental Health

An Overview from Europe

Meryam Schouler-Ocak

Charité Psychiatric University Clinic at St. Hedwig's Hospital, Berlin, Germany

Abstract

The total number of immigrants living in Europe in 2010 was 32.5 million, representing 6.5 % of the EU-27's population. Given that migration is strongly associated with higher risk for mental disorders, multiethnic societies in Europe are faced with a multiplicity of challenges, including meeting the diverse mental health care needs of ethnic-minority groups. These days, mental health specialists have regular contact with patients from different cultural backgrounds, whose health conditions also differ due to their immigration history and the social conditions in which they live in the receiving country. In this chapter an overview on risk and protective factors associated with migration and acculturation with special emphasis on suicidality, psychosis, affective and addictive disorders, and dementia are given. In order to promote mental health and its care among immigrant groups, clinicians, policymakers, and service providers need to be aware of specific needs of these immigrants.

Keywords: migration, mental disorders, Europe

Introduction

Migration is a process in which a person moves from one cultural setting to another in order to settle semi-permanently or permanently (see http://www.un.org/esa/population/publications/ReplMig). Immigrants may move en masse or singularly in many forms, including forced or voluntary movement for several reasons, such as political, economic, or educational. Although it is difficult to distinguish between forced and voluntary migration, the forms of migration often include both elements. While precise figures for the number of people moving for economic reasons remain elusive, it is estimated that over 200 million people move every year to find work and a better life. Of these, at least 30 million are so-called undocumented immigrants (Lindert, Schouler-Ocak, Heinz & Priebe, 2008). Historically, the number of immigrants in the world has more than doubled since 1975, with most immigrants living in Europe (56 million), Asia (50 million), and North America (41 million) (Lindert, Schouler-Ocak et al., 2008). In 1990, immigrants accounted for over 15% of the population in 52 countries. Most of the migration was from developing to developed countries (see http://www.eds-destatis.de/).

The total number of immigrants (people who are not citizens of their country of residence) living on the territory of the EU Member States on January 1, 2010 was 32.5 million, representing 6.5% of the EU-27's population. One year earlier, on January 1, 2009, the number of immigrants was 31.8 million, or 6.4% of the total population. More than one-third (a total of 12.3 million) of all immigrants living in the EU-27 on January 1, 2010 were citizens of another EU Member State. In absolute terms, the largest numbers of nonnationals living in the EU on January 1, 2010 were in Germany (7.1 million), Spain (5.7 million), the UK (4.4 million), Italy (4.2 million), and France (3.8 million). In relative terms, the EU Member State with the highest share of immigrants was Luxembourg, where immigrants accounted for 43.0% of the population at the beginning of 2010. The vast majority (86.3%) of nonnationals living in Luxembourg were citizens of other EU Member States (see http://epp.eurostat.ec.europa.eu/statistics_explained/index.php/Migration_and_migrant_population_statistics).

Similarly, the immigrants in Europe constitute a heterogeneous group in regard to their reasons for migration, legal status, and country of emigration as well. For instance, the majority of immigrants in Central and Eastern Europe and Scandinavian countries come from elsewhere in Europe. Germany's immigration field is also strongly European, and along with Austria and Finland receives a high proportion of its immigrants from Central and Eastern Europe. Mediterranean countries, together with the UK and The Netherlands, attract a high proportion of immigrants beyond Europe. Almost a third of the UK's and Spain's immigrants come from outside Europe (Carta, Bernal, Hardoy, & Haro-Abad, 2005). In recent years, there has been a sharp decrease in the number of asylum applicants in the EU. Having peaked in 1992 (670,000 applications in the EU-15) and again in 2001 (424,500 applications in the EU-27), there were an estimated 263,400 asylum applications received in the EU-27 in 2009. In absolute terms, the highest number of positive asylum decisions in 2009 was recorded in the UK (15,555), followed by Germany (12,060), France (10,415), Italy (9,110), and Sweden (9,085). Altogether, these latter Member States represented no less than two thirds of the total number of positive decisions issued in the EU (see http://epp.eurostat.ec.europa.eu/statistics_explained/index.php/Asylum_statistics).

Given that migration is strongly associated with higher risk for mental disorders (Bhugra, 2003), multiethnic societies in Europe are faced with a multiplicity of challenges, including meeting the diverse mental health care needs of ethnic-minority groups. These days, mental health specialists have regular contact with patients from different cultural backgrounds, whose health conditions also differ due to their immigration history and the social conditions in which they live in the receiving country. Besides, various studies demonstrated that culture plays an important role in the presentation of distress and illness, and cultural differences impact upon the diagnosis and treatment of immigrant populations in part due to linguistic, religious, and social variation from the clinician providing care (Bhugra et al., 2011). In order to achieve optimal results in diagnosing and treating mental disorders, it is important to consider the cultural and migrational background of the patients, which may have an impact on their explanatory models of mental disorders (see chapters 7, 8, and 14). Moreover, cultural competency and using cultural formulations are other important issues that should be dealt with (see chapter 15).

There is every appearance that the wider determinants of immigrants' mental health are often different from those of the settled community and require a different approach from health care professionals. Given the provision of mental health care is highly determined by the needs of its clients, an understanding of the illness experience of ethnic minority patients seems highly relevant in order to seek out and attempt to effectively address their mental health needs (Maffla, 2008). However, relevant data on immigrants' mental health concerning incidence, prevalence, and etiology of mental disorders and the utilization of mental health and psychosocial care facilities are relatively outnumbered (Lindert et al., 2008). Therefore, a major issue facing Europe is filling the current gap in the availability of high-quality data on mental health determinants, mental health status, and service utilization among immigrant populations throughout the region. As evidence-based decision making in public health and mental health care greatly depends on the availability of relevant health information, improving the collection of valid and comparable ethnic-minority health data should be regarded as a high priority (Rafnsson and Bhopal, 2008) (see chapter 14).

Risk and Protective Factors Associated with Migration and Acculturation

Migration can be a critical life event that is characterized by the processes of adaptation and readjustment, such as adjustment to a new culture, a new language, or a new religion, in which the coping strategies that were successful in the past are sometimes not suited for the new situation. This gap between the culture of origin and the host culture places immigrants at particularly high risk of social isolation, psychological distress, and reduced quality of life (e.g., unemployment, low education, poor living conditions, etc.) (van Bergen, Eikelenboom, Smit, van de Looij-Jansen, & Saharso, 2010; Berltolote, 2004). Other risk factors include loneliness, homesickness, loss of status, language problems, resident permit status, and open racism, which particularly result in higher prevalence rates of mental disorders in immigrants compared to the native population. For instance, various studies demonstrated that compared to the native population, the prevalence rates of depression, anxiety, or suicidal behavior are higher in immigrant populations (Hovey, 2000a, 2000b; Hovey & King, 1996; Kiev, 1980; Trovato, 1986; Hovey & Magaña, 2000; Merbach, Wittig, & Brähler, 2008; Bhugra, 2004; Bermejo, Mayninger, Kriston, & Härter, 2010). Bermejo et al. (2010) reported a migration-sensitive reanalysis of the supplement survey "mental disorders" of the German Health Survey 1998/1999, in which 143 immigrants were compared with 3,740 Germans. The authors pointed out that the results demonstrated significantly higher 4-week, 12-month, and lifetime prevalence rates of mental disorders for immigrants in comparison to Germans. These differences are highest regarding affective disorders (4-week prevalence: 11.7 vs. 5.8%; 12-month prevalence: 17.9 vs. 11.3%; lifetime prevalence: 24.9 vs. 18.2%) and somatoform disorders (4-week prevalence: 15.5 vs. 6.9%; 12-month prevalence: 19.9 vs. 10.3%; lifetime prevalence: 24.1 vs. 15.4%). The authors underlined that this study was a basis for further investigation of the relation between migration and mental health as well as for developing a culturally sensitive health care (Bermejo et al., 2010). On the other hand, it was also revealed that some key protective factors such as level of networking with other immigrants from the same country of origin, similarities between norms and values of the country of origin and the receiving country, and being successful after migration are associated negatively with mental disorders, which can be used in treatment planning (Porter & Haslam, 2005; Grüsser, Wölfling, Mörsen, Albrecht, & Heinz, 2005).

The following sections aim to provide an overview of some key epidemiological studies related to common psychiatric conditions prevalent in immigrants and in order to highlight potential interventions for promoting mental health among this specific patient group.

Migration and Suicidality

The major risk factors for suicide are described as potentially modifiable and nonchangeable factors. Gender, age, ethnicity, sexual orientation, and previous suicide attempts belong to the nonchangeable factors while access to methods, history or presence of a psychiatric disorder or a physical illness, social isolation, unemployment, anxiety, hopelessness, and reduced life satisfaction, most of which are associated with immigrant status as well, are placed under the rubric of potentially modifiable risk factors (Berltolote, 2004). Furthermore, it has also been revealed that suicide risk increases in the 10 years following migration (Kwan & Ip, 2007) if the age at migration was less than 12 years (Peña et al., 2008; Borges, Nock, Medina-Mora, Hwang, & Kessler, 2009) and with the frequency of residential changes (Ott, Winkler, Kyobutungi, Laki, & Becher, 2008).

Studies demonstrated substantial differences in suicidal ideation and suicidal behavior between immigrant groups. Whereas some studies have reported lower risk for suicide among some ethnic minority groups compared to majority population (Razum, Zeeb, Akgün, & Yilmaz, 1998; Razum, Zeeb, & Rohrmann, 2000; Razum & Swamy, 2001; Razum & Zeeb, 2004), other studies revealed that some ethnic groups exhibit higher suicide rates than those found in their countries of origin and in the host country into which they have immigrated (Garssen, Hoogenboezem & Kerkhof, 2006). Likewise, data of the mortality statistics from 1980 to 1997 in Germany revealed lower suicide rates in immigrants than in Germans (relative risk: 0.3). However, the group of young Turkish women shared out of line with a rate twice as high compared to same-aged native women (relative risk: 1.8) (Razum & Zeeb, 2004). In comparison to this, the suicide rates in Turkey were much lower than in immigrants of Turkish origin in Germany, which can be explained by the social coherence in the Turkish society (Sayil, 1997). Furthermore, it has been revealed that the higher rate of suicides in young Turkish immigrant woman is moderated by family conflict, which appears to be a precipitating factor. This family conflict might be due to an intergenerational culture conflict when those young women start to individuate. Likewise, another study demonstrated that the rate of suicide attempts in Turkish female immigrants who were treated in a psychiatric hospital increased by the factor 3.02 compared to the rate of German female patients (32.2% Turkish immigrants) (Grube, 2004). Another study on suicide attempts of Turkish immigrants in emergency rooms revealed that the group with the highest risk to attempt suicide is the second generation (Yilmaz & Riecher-Rössler, 2008; van Bergen, Smit, van Balkom, van Ameijden, & Saharso, 2008; Peña et al., 2008; Borges et al., 2009; Fortuna, Perez, Caninco, Sribney, & Alegria, 2007). In the Netherlands young immigrant women of South Asian, Turkish, and Moroccan origins demonstrated disproportionate rates of nonfatal suicidal behavior. For instance, van Bergen et al. (2008) collected data on suicidal behavior and ideation among female Turkish immigrants (aged 16–24), who had significantly more suicidal ideation (38.1%) compared to Dutch girls of the same age (17.9%) and compared to the same-aged Moroccan girls (12.8%). In a similar study, van Bergen et al. (2010) found that rates of attempted suicide among Turkish and South Asian-Surinamese young women were higher than that of Dutch females, while Moroccan females had lower rates than Dutch female adolescents. The authors pointed out that physical and sexual abuse and an impaired family environment, as well as parental psychopathology or parental substance abuse, contributed to nonfatal suicidal behavior of females across ethnicities. These risk factors, as well as low social economic class and level of education, did not fully explain the vulnerability of Turkish and South Asian-Surinamese females (van Bergen et al., 2008, van Bergen et al., 2010). The analysis of van Bergen et al. (2010) included a comparison of class factors as well as psychiatric and psychological risk factors. In at least half of the cases, South Asian, Turkish, and Moroccan women experienced specific stressful life events related to their family honor. Although these findings can be incorporated into strategies for prevention, the origins of ethnic disparities in suicidal behavior deserve further examination.

Migration and Psychosis

A growing body of evidence suggests that migration is a risk factor for the development of schizophrenia, although the putative mechanism remains unclear. Several European studies indicated a higher prevalence of schizophrenia and schizophrenia spectrum disorders among ethnic minority groups. For instance, in a 3–center, prospective study of first-onset psychotic syndromes over a 2–year period, Kirkbride et al. (2006) and Fearon et al. (2006) reported that psychoses were more common among ethnic minority groups, and that African Caribbeans and Black Africans in the UK were at an especially high risk of schizophrenia and mania. They described a significant and independent variation in the incidence of schizophrenia and other forms of psychoses in terms of gender, age, ethnicity, and place of residence. Further, these authors also hypothesized that environmental effects may interact with genetic and other factors in the etiology of psychosis. Likewise, Sharpley, Hutchington, McKenzie, & Murray (2001) revealed that the African Caribbean population in England is at increased risk of both schizophrenia and mania. According to the authors, these patients show more affective symptoms and a more relapsing course with greater social disruption, but fewer negative symptoms than the native English patients. Studies from the Netherlands have also demonstrated an excess of schizophrenia in immigrants, with particularly high rates in people of Surinamese, Moroccan, and Antilles origin (Selen et al., 2001; Veling et al., 2006). A Danish study also provided an evidence for high incidence of psychotic disorders among immigrants from Australia, Africa, and Greenland (Cantor-Graae, Pedersen, McNeil, & Mortensen, 2003). Likewise, Fossion et al. (2002) observed that Moroccan immigrants were significantly more likely to be diagnosed with psychoses than a Belgian comparison group. In a meta-analysis of Cantor-Graae & Selten (2005) moderate relative risk for schizophrenia 2.7 (95% CI = 2.3–3–2) was found in first-generation immigrants; however, this rate was higher in second generation 4.5 (95% CI = 1.5–13.1) immigrants. This increased risk for schizophrenia found among second-generation migrants suggests that selection hypothesis can be rejected as the sole explanation for the findings on migrants. Furthermore, the greatest relative risk for schizophrenia was seen among immigrants from developing countries (relative risk = 3.3, 95% CI = 2.8–3.9) and immigrants from countries where the majority of the population is black (relative risk = 4.8, 95% CI = 3.7–6.2), respectively. The finding concerning the greater effect size associated with black skin color may suggest that migrants whose skin color is considerably darker than the background population may share a common risk exposure, such as experience of discrimination. Similarly, Igel, Brähler, and Grande (2010) reported that discrimination determines mental and physical health of immigrants, highlighting the importance of taking experiences of discrimination into account as a psychosocial stressor. In the same sense, it was revealed that ethnic density – that is, the density of the same ethnic group around an individual – plays a significant role in genesis and maintenance of psychotic disorders among ethnic minority groups (Boydell, van Os, & McKenzie, 2001; Faris & Denham, 1960). Social support and lower rates of long-term experience of social defeat (i.e., the chronic stressful experience of outsider status in an ethnically dense environment) may act as protective factors in the beginning and relapse of psychotic disorders in individuals who have a (genetic) predisposition for the illness. Similarly, Bhugra (2005) postulated that cultural congruity, when people with similar cultural values live close to one another, might be more important in this respect. However, further work is needed to map cultural congruity and ethnic density with epidemiological data (Bhugra et al., 2011).

Finally, some researchers have argued that migrants preferentially receive schizophrenia diagnoses because of cultural misunderstanding and/or language difficulties. For instance, in a representative nationwide survey, the Psychiatry and Migration Working Group of the German Federal Conference of Psychiatric Hospital Directors (Bundesdirektorenkonferenz) examined the use of inpatient psychiatric and psychotherapeutic services in Germany by patients of immigrant origin. It was revealed that patients of immigrant origin were significantly more likely to receive an ICD-10 F2 diagnosis (Schizophrenia, schizotypal, and delusional disorders) and it was precisely patients with this diagnosis who were observed to experience difficulties in communication with caregivers (Schouler-Ocak et al., 2008). Haasen, Yagdiran, & Mass (2000) discovered discrepancies in the diagnoses made by native German-speaking and native Turkish-speaking psychiatrists for patients with paranoid symptoms. They concluded that potential misdiagnosis due to language barriers does not sufficiently explain the increased rate of schizophrenia in persons of immigrant origin. The authors pointed out that this might also be attributable to a lack of cultural familiarity, suggesting the fact that clinical judgment can be altered when practitioners are unfamiliar with the culture-specific beliefs and practices of the client.

The size of the risk for developing schizophrenia associated with migration deserves increased attention. Although the environmental risk factors that may contribute to this risk are still poorly understood, the perceptions of social inequality may be an important factor. More research is needed to elucidate the complex and interrelated biological, psychological, and social pathways to schizophrenia. Such unifying hypotheses would make a substantial contribution to the understanding of the etiology of schizophrenia among ethnically diverse immigrant populations.

Migration and Affective Disorders

The findings of prevalence rates of affective disorders among immigrants are more equivocal compared to those in the case of psychosis. In a meta-analysis of all population-based incidence studies published in peer-reviewed journals conducted from 1966 to 2005, no conclusive evidence was revealed for a large increase in the risk of mood disorders associated with migration (Swinnen & Selten, 2007). This might be due to the fact that the number of population-based incidence studies concerning mood disorders among migrants was small and the number of countries in which they had been conducted was limited. On the other hand, theoretically, it is also possible that immigrants are more likely to be depressed because of the loss events they have been exposed to such as loss of status, loss of social support, and loss of significant relationships, all of which may add to the sense of bereavement and grief. Moreover, culture shock is also regarded as one of the main risk factors associated with depression. Aspects of culture shock can be identified as strain, sense of loss and feelings of deprivation, rejection by members of the new culture, confusion in role and role expectation, values, feelings, and self-identity, as well as surprise, anxiety, disgust, indignation, and feelings of impotence (Bhugra, 2004). Additionally, some studies conducted with elderly immigrants also reported that loss of the spouse in the receiving country (Grüsser et al., 2005) and conflicts concerning remigration (Bhugra, 2005) and acculturation (Porter & Haslam, 2005) might be possible triggers to develop depressive disorders. In support of aforementioned arguments, Aichberger et al. (2010) published the data of the Survey of Health, Ageing and Retirement in Europe (SHARE), a cross-national, multidisciplinary, household-based panel survey using nationally representative probability samples (n = 28.517) of 11 European countries of the noninstitutionalized population aged 50 years and older. This study was to determine the prevalence of depression in migrants aged 50 years or older in comparison to residents without a history of migration. Depression was measured using the EURO-D scale, and odds ratios (OR) were estimated for immigrant status. Effects of sociodemographic variables, somatic comorbidities, functional impairment, cognitive functioning, geographic region, and the years of residence in the current country were assessed in multivariate logistic regression analysis. Adjusting for confounds, the OR for depression in immigrants was found to be 1.42 (95% CI, 1.28–1.59). The influence of migration status on the prevalence of depression was significantly greater in Northern (OR, 1.85; 95% CI, 1.39–2.46) and Western Europe (OR, 1.38; 95% CI, 1.22–1.57), compared to Southern Europe (OR, 1.16; 95% CI, 0.79–1.70) ($p < 0.05$ for the interaction). According to the authors, a higher prevalence of depression in first-generation immigrants aged 50 years or older, together with relevant geographical variation, was found. However, this difference was not due to other known predictors of depression at an older age (Aichberger et al., 2010).

Migration and Dementia

Although there is an increase in elderly population of ethnic minorities in most Western countries, ethnic minority patients are marginalized in the provision of dementia assessment/diagnosis and service delivery (Nielsen & Waldemar, 2010). In their comprehensive review, White and colleagues (2002) articulated several issues in dementia diagnosis and service delivery among ethnic minorities, such as differences in prevalence rates between groups; cultural deficiencies in the instruments used to assess cognitive function, especially due to language barriers, particularly in the case of first-generation migrants; differing cultural perceptions of the signs and symptoms of dementia; the stigma attached to mental illnesses; a lack of knowledge about services; and a general reticence to use health and social services, which some members of ethnic minorities may view as culturally inappropriate.

These challenges have been a topic of research and are acknowledged in studies that originated mostly from the US, Canada, and Australia. Research on dementia in elderly ethnic minority populations is, however, still limited in most European countries. In Europe, research published in English is largely restricted to studies of Indian subcontinent and African Caribbean elders in the UK (McCracken et al., 1997; Bhatnagar & Frank, 1997; Lindesay, Jagger, Hibbet, Peet, & Moledina, 1997; Shah, Lindesay,

& Jagger, 1998; Lindesay, 1998; Parker & Philp, 2004; Lawrence, Murray, Samsi, & Banjerjee, 2008). Community-based studies from both the US (Demirovic et al., 2003; Fitzpatrick et al., 2004) and the UK (McCracken et al., 1997; Livingston et al., 2001) have found a higher prevalence of dementia in some ethnic minorities compared to the majority population, while other studies have demonstrated lower rates of service utilization for dementia by ethnic minority patients and by their carers in comparison with the background population (Lindesay, Jagger, Hibbet, Peet, & Moledina, 1997; Janevic and Connell, 2001). Consistent with the aforecited studies, one notable exception from Europe, a Danish epidemiological study, has also revealed an increased frequency of dementia conditions (13.3%) in Turkish immigrants compared to the expected prevalence of 7% in the Danish population (Rosenbaum, Kristenesen, & Schmidt, 2008). The increased prevalence of dementia among minority ethnic groups can be attributed to the lack of medical health care in country of origin, physically hard labor in the receiving country, high risk of disintegration of social networks, and little or no utilization of the health care system. There is also evidence that factors such as poor education and low socioeconomic status initiate a rapid progress in developing dementia. Alternatively, these high rates may in part be due to a possible diagnostic bias. As it is concerned with dementia literature, it appears that the most important issue for minority ethnic groups is the effect that language ability has on cognitive assessment and, thus, on dementia diagnosis. It has been claimed that the fundamental issue is the language ability of the patients rather than ethnicity per se (White et al., 2002). Likewise, in a European survey evaluating the status and practice of assessing dementia in ethnic minority patients, it was reported that the majority of the practitioners generally considered diagnostic evaluation of the patients to be challenging because of communication problems and lack of adequate assessment tools (Nielsen, Andersen, Kastrup, Phung, & Waldemar, 2011), The use of the mini-mental state examination (MMSE), the most widely used cognitive screening, as a guideline instrument of screening was shown to be applicable only with modifications to persons who were illiterate and without any education, and to those first-generation immigrants who were to a limited degree integrated as citizens (Rosenbaum et al., 2008). In the same vein, several other studies have also reported the MMSE to be highly influenced by ethnicity and educational level (Parker & Philip, 2004). Consequently, it seems highly necessary to validate existing assessment tools or to develop cognitive screening instruments that are less affected by culture and language. Moreover, since evaluation of dementia mainly relies on verbal communication and observation of behavior, dementia assessments can also be undertaken by staff with the specific language skills or cultural awareness or with interpreters in order to achieve an accurate diagnosis. Numerous studies have shown that patients' satisfaction and outcomes are positively affected by the use of professional interpreters (Flores, 2005). In conclusion, there is a general need to increase health professionals' awareness concerning the implications regarding cross-cultural assessment of dementia as well as to develop appropriate assessment methods for patients from the ethnic minority populations in Europe.

Immigrants and Addictive Disorders

There is still limited knowledge and data concerning addictive disorders among immigrants in Europe. Until the mid-1990s, experts in addictive disorders paid little attention to the subject of addiction in immigrants. Van de Wijngaart (1997) reports that there are hardly any systematic data available about substance or alcohol use among ethnic minorities. Research so far has shown that immigrant groups vary greatly in their drinking practices, but the specific contributions of social, cultural, and genetic influences to these variations are not yet known. Data from Germany suggest that immigrants with addictive disorders correspond to, or even exceed, their percentage of the general population (Lindert, Priebe et al., 2008). Furthermore, in a nationwide epidemiological study, the risk of alcohol-related disorders in first- and second-generation immigrants in Sweden were compared with the Swedish majority population. The results have revealed that first- and second-generation immigrants from Finland had higher relative risks (RRs) for hospital admission because of an alcohol-related disorder compared to the Swedish background population (socioeconomic adjusted RRs of 2.1 and 1.9, respectively), whereas first-generation immigrants born in southern Europe, the Middle East, and other non-European countries had lower risks. Second-generation immigrants with origins of southern Europe, the Middle East, and other non-European countries had (socioeconomic adjusted) RRs that were higher in comparison with the first-generation immigrants but lower relative to the Swedish majority population (Hjern & Allebeck, 2004). In general, population-based studies of the risk of alcohol or drug use disorders among immigrants in Europe are scarce, thus additional research is needed to address the gaps that currently exist in the literature. The existing body of literature demonstrates that much variation exists in alcohol/drug consumption, alcohol/drug–related problems, and other issues among and within specific ethnic groups. An awareness of these differences can assist in identifying the subpopulations most at risk for developing alcohol or drug use problems.

On the other hand, it has been claimed that the public system of addiction treatment is used less by migrants with addictive disorders than by their nonmigrant counterparts (Penka, Krieg, Hunner, & Heinz, 2003). A number of barriers to access to the centers for information, counseling, and treatment of addictive disorders, such as language difficulties, lack of knowledge about the public system of addiction treatment, mistrust of government institutions (Czycholl, 1999), and fear of losing residence rights (Grüsser & Becker, 1999) or even of imprisonment (Osterloh, 2002) were acknowledged. However, access barriers can also result from a culturally different understanding of the causes and treatment of addictive behavior (Penka, et al., 2003). For instance, an examination of cultural differences in the explanatory models (i.e., an understanding of illness and disease shaped by culture and lay beliefs, see Kleinman, 1980) of addictive behavior among Turkish and German youths in Germany has revealed relevant differences between the illness concepts of Turkish and German youth with regard to addictive behaviors. Concerning substance abuse, German youth clearly differentiated between illegal drug abuse and the abuse of alcohol and nicotine. However, this finding was not evident in Turkish youth. Nearly half of the Turkish sample rejected central medical concepts such as "physical dependence" or "reduced control of substance intake" as completely inadequate to characterize problems of addictive behavior (Penka et al., 2003). These findings highlight the importance of translating medical concepts of disease and treatment properly into different languages by considering the possible connotations and implications of each term with respect to the culture in particular. Such information about ethnic group differences can be used to develop treatment programs that are culturally sensitive (Caetano & Galvan, 2001). However, further research is needed to show whether culturally sensitive programs in fact yield better treatment outcomes than generic treatment programs and whether treatment outcomes for these different types of programs vary by ethnic group. Moreover, these findings also underline the importance of the adaptation of the information materials according to the explanatory models used by each target group. Preventive information programs must consider these differences and use concepts that are accepted and clearly associated with addictive behavior by immigrant populations. Otherwise, the terms that are central to Western medical models of disease can be misunderstood, misinterpreted, or even rejected by particular ethnic groups (Penka et al., 2003) (see chapter 12).

Conclusion: Implications for Research, Policy, and Practice

Although immigrant groups were identified as a vulnerable population with respect to mental health problems, they are widely underrepresented in the existing mental health care and social services in many European countries. This is particularly true for asylum seekers and undocumented immigrants (Penka et al., 2003; Carta et al., 2005; Lindert, Schouler-Ocak et al., 2008; Lindert, Priebe et al., 2008; Bhugra et al., 2011). In order to address this treatment gap, it seems highly necessary to provide adequate financing for the continuity of research on multicultural health demands. It also seems crucial to highlight the importance of adopting an integrated approach to mental health care and implementing multidisciplinary research with cross-departmental collaboration on research projects that move away from psychiatric care only (Carta et al., 2005).

In the "World Psychiatric Association (WPA) guidance on mental health and mental health care in immigrants" Bhugra et al. (2011, p. 7) highlighted a series of recommendations to policymakers, service providers, and clinicians aimed at improving mental health care in immigrants, which are shown in Table 1.1.

In order to promote mental health and its care among immigrant groups, clinicians, policymakers, and service providers need to be aware of specific needs of immigrants. Adhering to the World Psychiatric Association (WPA) guidance on mental health and mental health care in immigrants would result in a substantial enhancement of mental health outcomes of immigrant populations (Bhugra et al., 2011, p. 7).

Table 1.1. Recommendations for improving mental health care services for migrants (from Bhugra et al., 2011, used with the permission of Dinesh Bhugra and Mario Maj)

Policymakers

- Clear policies taking into account human rights of immigrants, refugees, and asylum seekers should be developed.
- Adequate resources should be made available according to the needs.
- Adequate resources for training, including cultural competency training, should be available.
- Different parts of the government (e.g., health, education, justice, home, external affairs) should be involved.
- Changes in admission criteria should be discussed with stakeholders, rather than being imposed arbitrarily.
- Public education and public mental health messages for refugees, asylum seekers, and immigrants should be carried out.

Service providers

- Separate or joined up services should be made available, but it is essential that there are no barriers to seeking help.
- Services should be culturally sensitive, geographically accessible, and emotionally appropriate.
- Cultural competence training must be provided and mandatory measures to achieve this should be considered.
- Other models, such as culture broker or cultural liaison, should be employed where indicated.
- Regular research into epidemiological factors, along with qualitative approaches, should be carried out in order to assess and monitor pathology.
- Regular audits into treatment accessibility, acceptability, and usage must be conducted.

Clinicians

- Clinicians must have access to resources informing them of specific cultural issues.
- Cultural awareness and competence training must be mandated and regular updates must form a part of this.
- Clinicians must provide culturally appropriate services related to language and other needs of immigrants, refugees, and asylum seekers. Children, the elderly, and other special groups must have their needs met.
- Clinicians may wish to discuss and develop specific services, either condition based (e.g., trauma) or gender based.
- Wherever possible, mental health issues of immigrants, refugees, and asylum seekers should be part of the curriculum and training of clinicians.
- Cultural training is everyone's business and must be a part of training other health professionals, including primary care professionals.

References

Aichberger, M. C., Schouler-Ocak, M., Busch, M., Mundt, A., Nickels, E., Heimann, H. M., . . . Rapp, M. A. (2010). Depression in middle-aged and older first generation migrants in Europe: Results from the Survey of Health, Aging and Retirement in Europe (SHARE). *European Psychiatry, 25*(8), 468–475.

Berltolote, J. M. (2004). Suicide prevention: At what level does it work? *World Psychiatry, 3*(3), 147–151.

Bermejo, I., Mayninger, E., Kriston, L., & Härter, M. (2010). [Mental disorders in people with migration background compared with German general population.] *Psychiatrische Praxis, 37*(5), 225–232.

Bhugra, D. (2003) Migration and depression. *Acta Psychiatrica Scandinavia Supplementum, 418*, 67–73.

Bhugra, D. (2004). Migration and mental health. *Acta Psychiatrica Scandinavica, 109*(4), 243–258.

Bhugra, D. (2005). Cultural identities and cultural congruency: A new model for evaluating mental distress in immigrants. *Acta Psychiatrica Scandinavica, 111*, 84–93.

Bhugra, D., Gupta, S., Bhui, K., Craig, T., Dogra, N., Ingleby, J.D., . . . Tribe, R. (2011). WPA guidance on mental health and mental health care in migrants. *World Psychiatry, 10*(1), 2–10.

Borges, G., Nock, M. K., Medina-Mora, M. E., Hwang, I., & Kessler, R. C. (2009). Psychiatric disorders, comorbidity, and suicidality in Mexico *Journal of Affective Disorders, 124*(1–2), 98–107.

Boydell, J., van Os, J., & McKenzie, K. (2001). Incidence of schizophrenia in ethnic minorities in London: Ecological study into interactions with environment. *British Medical Journal, 323*, 1336–1336.

Caetano, R., & Galvan, F. H. (2001). Alcohol use and alcohol related problems among Latinos in the United States. In M. Aguirre-Molina, C. W. Molina, & R. E. Zambrana, (Eds.), *The Latino community* (pp.383–412). San Franciso: Jossey-Bass.

Cantor-Graae, E., Pedersen, C. B., McNeil, T. F., & Mortensen, P.B. (2003). Migration as a risk factor for schizophrenia: A Danish population-based cohort study. *The British Journal of Psychiatry, 182*, 117–122.

Cantor-Graae, E., & Selten, J. P. (2005). Schizophrenia and migration: A meta-analysis and review. *American Journal of Psychiatry, 162*(1), 12–24.

Carta, M. G., Bernal, M., Hardoy, M. C., & Haro-Abad, J. M. (2005). Report on the Mental Health in Europe Working Group. Migration and mental health in Europe (the state of the mental health in Europe working group: appendix 1). *Clinical Practice and Epidemiology in Mental Health,* 1, 13.

Czycholl, D. (1999). Migration, Suchtrisiken und Versorgungsdefizite am Beispiel von Aussiedlern in Deutschland [Migration, addiction risks, and deficits in care provision: The example of ethnic German immigrants in Germany]. In R. Salman, S. Tuna, A. Lessing, (Eds.), *Handbuch interkulturelle Suchthilfe. Modelle, Konzepte und Ansätze der Prävention, Beratung und Therapie* (pp. 222–227). Gießen, Germany: Psychosozial-Verlag.

Demirovic, J., Prineas, R., Loewenstein, D., Dean, J., Duara, R., Sevush, S., & Szapocznik, J. (2003). Prevalence of dementia in three ethnic groups: The South Florida program on aging and health. *Annals of Epidemiology, 13*, 472–478.

Faris, R., & Denham, W. (1960). *Mental disorders in urban areas*. New York: Hafner.

Fearon, P., Kirkbride, J. B., Morgan, C., Dazzan, P., Morgan, K., & Lloyd, T., . . . Murray, R. M. (2006). AESOP Study Group. Incidence of schizophrenia and other psychoses in ethnic minority groups: Results from the MRC AESOP Study. *Psychological Medicine, 36*(11), 1541–1550.

Fitzpatrick, A. L., Kuller, L. H., Ives, D. G., Lopez, O. L., Jagust, W., Breitner, J. C., . . . Dulberg, C. (2004). *Journal of the American Geriatrics Society, 52*(2), 195–204.

Flores, G. (2005). The impact of medical interpreter services on the quality of health care: A systematic review. *Medical Care Research and Review*, *62*(3), 255–299.

Fortuna, L. R., Perez, D. J., Canino G., Sribney, W., & Alegria, M. (2007). Prevalence and correlates of lifetime suicidal ideation and suicide attempts among Latino subgroups in the United States. *Journal of Clinical Psychiatry, 68*(4), 572–581.

Fossion, P., Servais, L., Rejas, M. C., Ledoux, Y., Pelc, I., & Minner, P. (2002). Psychosis, migration and social environment: An age- and gender controlled study. *European Psychiatry*, *19*, 338–343.

Garssen, M. J., Hoogenboezem, J., & Kerkhof, A. J. (2006). Zelfdoding onder migrantengroepen en autochtonen in Nederland [Suicide among migrant populations and native Dutch in The Netherlands]. *Nederlands Tijdschrift voor Geneeskunde, 30;150*, 2143–2149.

Grube, M. (2004). Suizidversuche von Migranten in der Akutpsychiatrie [Suicide attempts by migrants in acute psychiatric care]. *Der Nervenarzt, 75*, 681–687.

Grüsser, S. M., & Becker, K. (1999). Drogenabhängigkeit und Migration innerhalb der Europäischen Union (EU) [Drug addiction and migration within the European Union (EU)]. In J. Gölz (Ed.), *Moderne Suchtmedizin, 5*, 1–7.

Grüsser, S. M., Wölfling, K., Mörsen, C. P., Albrecht, U., & Heinz, A. (2005). Immigration-associated variables and substance dependence. *Journal of Studies on Alcohol and Drugs*, *66*(1), 98–104.

Haasen, C., Yagdiran, O., & Mass, R. (2000). Differenzen zwischen der psychopathologischer Evaluation in deutscher und türkischer Sprache bei türkischen Migranten [Differences observed in the psychopathological evaluation of Turkish immigrants associated with the use of the German or Turkish language]. *Nervenarzt*, *71*(11), 901–905.

Hjern, A., & Allebeck, P. (2004). Alcohol-related disorders in first and second generation immigrants in Sweden: A national cohort study. *Addiction*, *99*(2), 229–236.

Hovey, J. D. (2000a). Acculturative stress, depression, and suicidal ideation among Central American immigrants. *Suicide and Life-Threatening Behavior, 30*, 125–139.

Hovey, J. D. (2000b). Acculturative stress, depression, and suicidal ideation in Mexican immigrants. *Cultural Diversity and Ethnic Minority Psychology, 6*, 134–151.

Hovey, J. D. & King, C. A. (1996). Acculturative stress, depression, and suicidal ideation among immigrant and second-generation Latino adolescents. *Journal of the American Academy of Child and Adolescent Psychiatry, 35*, 1183–1192.

Hovey, J. D., & Magaña, C. (2000). Acculturative stress, anxiety, and depression among Mexican immigrant farmworkers in the midwest United States. *Journal of Immigrant and Minority Health, 2*(3), 119–131.

Igel, U., Brähler, E., & Grande, G. (2010). Der Einfluss von Diskriminierungserfahrungen auf die Gesundheit von Migrantinnen [The influence of perceived discrimination on health in female migrants] [Article in German]. *Psychiatrische Praxis, 37*, 183–190.

Janevic, M. R., & Connel, C. M. (2001). Racial, ethnic, and cultural differences in the dementia caregiving experience: Recent findings. *Gerontologist*, *41*, 334–347.

Kiev, A. (1980). Suizidhandlungen in transkultureller Sicht [Suicide acts from a transcultural perspective]. In W. M. Pfeiffer & W. Schoene (Eds.), *Psychopathologie im Kulturvergleich* (pp. 146–155). Stuttgart, Germany: Enke.

Kirkbride, J. B., Fearon, P., Morgan, C., Dazzan, P., Morgan, K., Tarrant, J., . . . Jones, .P. B. (2006). Heterogeneity in incidence rates of schizophrenia and other psychotic syndromes: Findings from the 3–center AESOP study. *Archives of General Psychiatry*, *63*(3), 250–258.

Kleinman, A. (1980). *Patients and healers in the context of culture: An exploration of the borderland between anthropology, medicine, and psychiatry*. Berkeley: University of California Press.

Kwan, Y. K., & Ip, W. C. (2007).Suicidality and migration among adolescents in Hong Kong. *Death Studies, 31*(1), 45–66.

Lawrence, V., Murray, J., Samsi, K., & Banjerjee, S. (2008). Attitudes and support need of Black Caribbean, south Asian and White British carers of people with dementia in the UK. *British Journal Psychiatry, 193*, 240–246

Lindert, J., Priebe, S., Penka, S., Napo, F., Schouler-Ocak, M., & Heinz, A. (2008). Versorgung psychisch kranker Patienten mit Migrationshintergrund [Providing care for mentally ill patients with a migration background]. *Psychotherapie Psychosomatik Medizinische Psychologie, 58*, 123–129.

Lindert, J., Schouler-Ocak, M., Heinz, A., & Priebe, S. (2008). Mental health and health care consumption among migrants in Europe. *European Psychiatry,* 23,14–20.

Lindesay. J. (1998). The dignosis of mental illness in elderly people from ethnic minorities. *Advances in Psychiatric Treatment, 4*, 219–226.

Lindesay, J., Jagger, C., Hibbet, M. J., Peet, S. M., & Moledina, F. (1997). Knowledge, uptake and availability of health and social services among Asian Gujarati and white elderly persons. *Ethnicity and Health, 2*(1/2), 59–69.

Livingston, G., Leavey, G., Kitchen, G., Manela, M., Sembhi, S., & Katona, C. (2001). Mental health of migrant elders – the Islington study. *British Journal of Psychiatry, 179*, 361–366.

Maffla, C. (2008). Health in the age of migration, migration and health in the EU. *Journal of Community Practice, 81*(8), 32–35.

McCracken, C. F., Boneham, M. A., Copeland, J. R., Williams, K. E., Wilson, K., Scott, A., . . . Cleave, N. (1997). Prevalence of dementia and depression among elderly people in black and ethnic minorities. *The British Journal of Psychiatry, 171*, 269–273.

Merbach, M., Wittig, U., & Brähler, E. (2008). Angst und Depression polnischer und vietnamesischer MigrantInnen in Leipzig unter besonderer Berücksichtigung ihres Eingliederungsprozesses [Anxiety and depression in Polish and Vietnamese migrants in Leipzig taking into consideration their integration process]. *Psychotherapie Psychosomatik Medizinische Psychologie, 58*(3–4), 146–54.

Nielsen, T. R., Andersen, B., Kastrup, M., Phung, T. K., & Waldemar, G. (2011). Quality of dementia diagnostic evaluation for ethnic minority patients: A nationwide study. *Dementia & Geriatric Cognitive Disoders, 31*(5), 388–396.

Nielsen, T. R., & Waldemar, G. (2010). Demens hos etniske minoriteter [Dementia in ethnic minorities]]. *Ugeskrift for Læger, 172*, 1527–1531.

Osterloh, K. (2002). Arbeit mit illegale Suchtmittel konsumierenden Migranten und Migrantinnen aus der GUS am Beispiel der Mudra Drogenhilfe Nürnberg [Working with illegal substances-consuming migrants from the former Soviet Union: The example of the Mudra drug addiction help center Nuremberg]. In W. Barth & C. Schubert (Eds.), *Migration – Sucht – Hilfe. Junge Migranten und Migrantinnen aus der GUS in den Systemen Suchthilfe und Migrationsberatung* (pp. 43–58). Nürnberg, Germany: Emwe-Verlag.

Ott, J. J., Winkler, V., Kyobutungi, C., Laki, J., & Becher, H. (2008). Effects of residential changes and time patterns on external-cause mortality in migrants: Results of a German cohort study. *Scandinavian Journal of Public Health, 36*(5), 524–531.

Parker, C., & Philip, I. (2004). Screening for cognitive impairment among older people in black minority ethnic groups. *Age and Ageing, 33*, 447–452.

Peña, J. B., Wyman, P. A., Brown, C. H,, Matthieu, M. M., Olivares, T. E., Hartel, D., & Zayas, L. H. (2008). Immigration generation status and its association with suicide attempts, substance use, and depressive symptoms among Latino adolescents in the USA. *Prevention Science, 9*(4), 299–310.

Penka, S., Krieg, S., Hunner, Ch., & Heinz, A. (2003). Unterschiedliche Erklärungsmodelle für abhängiges Verhalten bei türkischen und deutschen Jugendlichen – Bedeutung für Prävention und Behandlungsangebote [Different explanatory models for addictive behavior in Turkish and German youths in Germany: Significance for prevention and treatment]. *Nervenarzt, 74*, 581–586.

Porter, M., & Haslam, N. (2005). Predisplacement and postdisplacement factors associated with mental health of refugees and internally displaced persons. A Meta-analysis. *Journal of the American Medical Association, 294*(5), 602–612.

Rafnsson, S. B., & Bhopal, R. S. (2008). Migrant and ethnic health research: Report on the European Public Health Association Conference 2007. *Public Health, 122*(5), 532–534.

Razum, O., & Swamy, L. (2001). Direct association between social status and risk of suicide was not found in Germany. *British Medical Journal, 323*, 232–233.

Razum, O., & Zeeb, H. (2004). Suizidsterblichkeit unter Türkinnen und Türken in Deutschland [Suicide mortality among Turkish migrants in Germany]. *Nervenarzt, 75*, 1092–1098.

Razum, O., Zeeb, H., Akgün, H. S., & Yilmaz, S. (1998). Low overall mortality of Turkish residents in Germany persists and extends into second generation: Merely a healthy migrant effect? *Tropical Medicine International Health, 3*, 297–303.

Razum, O., Zeeb, H., & Rohrmann, S. (2000). The "healthy migrant effect" – not merely a fallacy of inaccurate denominator figures [letter]. *International Journal of Epidemiology, 29*, 191–192.

Rosenbaum, B., Kristensen, M., & Schmidt, J. (2008). Demenslidelser hos ældre tyrkiske indvandrere [Dementia in elderly Turkish immigrants] [Article in Danish]. *Ugeskrift for Læger, 170*(50), 4109–4113.

Sayil, I. (1997). Review of suicide studies in Turkey. *Crisis, 18*, 124–127.

Schouler-Ocak, M., Bretz, H. J., Penka, S., Koch, E., Hartkamp, N., Siefen, R. G., . . . Heinz, A. (2008). Patients of immigrant origin in inpatient psychiatric facilities –A representative national survey by the Psychiatry and Migration Working Group of the German Federal Conference of Psychiatric Hospital Directors. *European Psychiatry, 23*, 21–27.

Selen, J. P., Veen, N., Feller, W., Blom, J.D., Schols, D., Camoenië, W., . . . Kahn, R. (2001). Incidence of psychotic disorders in immigrant groups to The Netherlands. *British Journal of Psychiatry, 178*, 367–372.

Shah, A., Lindesay, J., & Jagger, C. (1998). Is the diagnosis of dementia stable over time among elderly immigrant Gujaratis in the United Kingdom (Leicester)? *International Journal of Geriatric Psychiatry, 13*(7), 440–444.

Sharpley, M., Hutchington, G., McKenzie, K., & Murray, R. M. (2001). Understanding the excess of psychosis among the African-Caribbean population in England. Review of current hypotheses. *British Journal of Psychiatry, 40*, 60–68.

Swinnen, S. G., & Selten, J. P. (2007). Mood disorders and migration: Meta-analysis. *British Journal of Psychiatry, 190*, 6–10.

Trovato, F. (1986). Suicide and ethnic factors in Canada. *International Journal of Social Psychiatry, 32*, 55–64.

Van Bergen, D. D., Eikelenboom, M., Smit, J. H., van de Looij-Jansen, P. M., & Saharso, S. (2010). Suicidal behavior and ethnicity of young females in Rotterdam, The Netherlands: Rates and risk factors. *Ethnicity & Health, 15*(5), 515–530.

Van Bergen, D. D., Smit, J. H., van Balkom, A. J., van Ameijden, E., & Saharso, S. (2008). Suicidal ideation in ethnic minority and majority adolescents in Utrecht, the Netherlands. *Crisis, 29*, 202–208.

Van de Wijngaart, G. F. (1997). Drug problems among immigrants and refugees in the Netherlands and the Dutch health care and treatment system. *Substance Use & Misuse, 32*, 909–938.

Veling, W., Selten, J. P., Veen, N., Laan, W., Blom, J. D., & Hoek, H. W. (2006). Incidence of schizophrenia among ethnic minorities in the Netherlands: A four-year first-contact study. *Schizophr Res., 86*(1–3), 189–193.

White, N., Scott, A., Woods, R. T., Wenger, G. C., Keady, J. D., & Devakumar, M. (2002). The limited utility of the Mini-Mental State Examination in screening people over the age of 75 years for dementia in primary care. *The British Journal of General Practice, 52*(485), 1002–1003.

Yilmaz, A. T., & Riecher-Rössler, A. (2008). Suizidversuche in der ersten und zweiten Generation der ImmigrantInnen aus der Türkei [Suicide attempts by first- and second-generation Turkish immigrants]. *Neuropsychiatrie, 22*, 261–267.

Meryam Schouler-Ocak
Charité Psychiatric University Clinic at St. Hedwig's Hospital in Berlin
Große Hamburger Straße 5–11
10115 Berlin
Germany
E-mail: meryam.schouler-ocak@charite.de

II. How Culture Shapes Our Brain

Chapter 2

Understanding the Self

A Cultural Neuroscience Perspective

Shihui Han

Department of Psychology, Peking University, Beijing, China

Abstract

What is the nature of mental representation of the self? While this question has been addressed extensively by philosophers and psychologists, recent brain imaging studies have investigated neural correlates of the processing of self-related information. In addition, given the psychological evidence for differences in self-construals between Western and East Asian cultures, recent brain imaging studies have investigated potential neural mechanisms that mediate cultural specific self-related processing. This chapter reviews recent brain imaging findings of Western/East Asian cultural differences in neural substrates underlying self-related processing in the perceptual and mental domains. The findings of transcultural and cultural priming imaging studies help to understand the neural basis of cultural differences in self-representation and promote the development of cultural neuroscience.

Keywords: culture, self, brain imaging, cultural neuroscience

---

Introduction

One of the central questions addressed in philosophy, sociology, and psychology is the nature of mental representation of the self. This question has induced persistent debate. What is the self? How is the self represented in the human brain? Interestingly, answers to these questions are quite different across Western and East Asian cultures.

Some philosophers in Western cultures emphasize self-identity independent of social contexts, whereas some philosophers in East Asian cultures hold different views and emphasize the key role of the relationship between self and others (Zhu & Han, 2008). The self in Western cultures – a bounded, impermeable free agent – can move from group to group and from setting to setting without significant alteration. The self in East Asian cultures, however, is connected, fluid, and conditional, and can be understood only in his or her relation to others (Nisbett, 2003). The cultural disparity in philosophic thinking of the self exerts enormous influences on psychological studies that aim to address human social behaviors and the underlying psychological processes.

Markus and Kitayama (1991, 2010) put forward a well-known theory on culture and self that has promoted searching after cultural variation rather than searching after universal laws in social psychology. They argued that Western cultures, with their emphasis onf self-identity, lead to the independent self, who is inclined to attend to self-focused information and attends to the self more than others (including intimate others such as mothers). By contrast, emphasis of fundamental social connection in East Asian cultures results in the interdependent self, who is generally sensitive to information related to significant others and attends to intimate others as much as to the self. In addition, different self-concepts shape all processes that implicate the self (Markus and Kitayama, 2003). Markus and Kitayama's theory not only promoted behavioral studies of differences in human cognition between Western and East Asian cultures but also stimulated brain imaging investigation of cultural differences in neural substrates underlying social cognition such as self-representation (e.g., Zhu, Zang, Fan, & Han, 2007; Han et al., 2008; Sui & Han, 2007; Sui, Liu, & Han, 2009; Heatherton et al., 2006; Wang et al., in press; Chiao et al., 2009a, 2009b). The brain imaging findings in turn contribute to the emergence of a new discipline – cultural neuroscience (Chiao & Ambady, 2007; Han & Northoff, 2008).

This chapter reviews two major parts of cultural neuroscience studies of the processing of self-related information. Self-face recognition represents self-related processing in the perceptual domain. Reflection on one's own traits engages the processing of self-related information in the mental domain (see chapter 3). There have been both behavioral and brain imaging studies of self-face recognition and self-reflection on traits across different cultural groups. The findings of these studies add to our knowledge of how self-representation is realized in the human brain and how neural representations of the self are shaped by individuals' cultural experience.

Culture and Neural Mechanisms of Self-Related Processing in the Perceptual Domain

Since William James (1890), psychologists have realized that the self can be divided into different constituents that emphasize the material, social, and spiritual attributes of a person. Self-identity may vary greatly across different social contexts in which the self may be recognized by others in different ways. A salient distinctiveness between the self and others in the perceptual domain is face recognition. The competence of recognizing one's own face has been confirmed at an early age of human development. Children at the second year of life show self-oriented actions in front of a mirror (Amsterdam,

1972; Asendorpf, Warkentin, & Baudonniere, 1996), suggesting early development of the ability of self-face recognition in humans. The ability of self-face recognition has been suggested to be an important component of self-awareness (Keenan, Weehler, Gallup, & Pascual-Leone, 2000).

Self-face recognition in human adults is characterized by faster behavioral responses to self-face than to faces of familiar/unfamiliar others in a visual search task (Tong and Nakayama, 1999) and tasks that require explicit (Keenan et al., 1999) or implicit (Sui, Zhu, & Han, 2006) face identification judgments. Multiple perceptual and cognitive mechanisms may contribute to the self-advantage in face recognition. For instance, Tong and Nakayama (1999) suggested that self-face advantage reflects robust representations for highly overlearned faces. Furthermore, Ma and Han (2010) proposed that a social cognitive mechanism also contributes to the self-face advantage. They hypothesized that self-face recognition and the concomitant self-awareness activate positive attribute in self-concept, which facilitates behavioral responses to self-face and thus results in self-advantage in face recognition. This implicit positive association theory of self-face recognition was supported by the findings that self-concept threat priming (i.e., a task in which the participants were asked to judge whether a number of negative personal traits were appropriate to describe themselves in order to render access of negative association of the self to participants' awareness) weakened the implicit positive association with the self and hence reduced the self-face advantage in behavioral performances. Thus, high-level social cognitive mechanisms also contribute to self-face recognition.

However, self-advantage during face recognition is highly sensitive to social contexts. To test whether social threats to one's positive associations confronted in real social situations reduce self-face advantage, Ma and Han (2009) asked Chinese graduate students to identify orientations of self-face that were intermixed with either their faculty advisor's face (high threat condition) or with the face of another faculty member who was not in their own lab (low threat condition). As negative evaluations from advisors constitute higher threats to self-esteem compared to those from other faculty members, they predicted that the self-face advantage would be reduced in the high compared to low threat conditions. Indeed, the results showed a self-face advantage in the low-threat context (i.e., faster responses to self-face than to the faculty member's face) but a self-face disadvantage in the high-threat context (i.e., slower responses to self-face compared to the advisor's face). In addition, Ma and Han found that differential responses to self-face and advisor's face were correlated with individuals' subjective ratings of fear of negative evaluations from the advisor. The findings suggest that social contexts strongly influence behavioral performances in association with self-face recognition and the presence of influential superiors modulates self-face recognition by shaping self-concept.

Given that the social contexts differ tremendously between the Western and East Asian societies, one may ask whether or not self-face recognition may be underlain by distinct mechanisms in individuals who grew up in the Western and East Asian cultural contexts. According to Markus and Kitayama's (1991) theory, the Western (North

American in particular) cultures with the emphasis on self-identity lead to the independent self who is inclined to pay much more attention to the self than to others. In contrast, the emphasis of fundamental social connection in East Asian cultures results in the interdependent self who is generally sensitive to information related to significant others and attends to intimate others as much as to the self. Such a viewpoint of cultural differences in self-construals may predict distinct self-face recognition in the Western and East Asian cultures. Specifically, the Western independent self may assign greater social salience or stronger positive association with one's own face than to others' faces, resulting in stronger attention to one's own face when presented among others' faces and inducing enhanced processing of self-face. In contrast, as the East Asian interdependent self emphasizes the significance of others in social interactions, enhanced processing of self-face in East Asians may not be as strong as that observed in Westerners.

This was tested in a recent cross-cultural event-related brain potential (ERP) study. Sui et al. (2009) recorded both behavioral performance and ERPs from two cultural groups using similar stimuli and the same paradigm. Both British and Chinese students were presented with self-face and a friend's face. They were asked to judge head orientations of the face stimuli (Figure 2.1a). Both cultural groups responded faster to self-face than friends' faces. However, the self-face advantage in reaction times was much

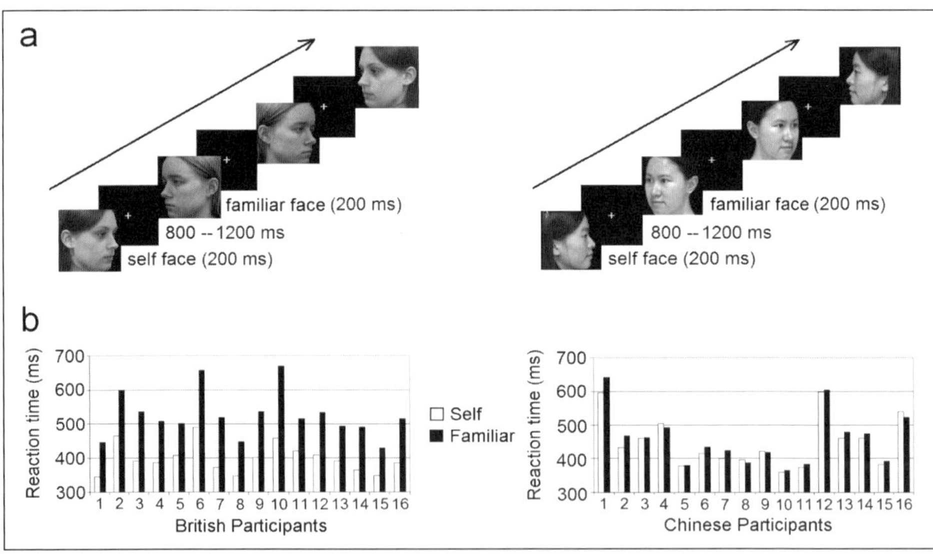

Figure 2.1. Experimental procedure and behavioral results in Sui et al. (2009). (a) Illustration of the stimuli and procedure for the British and Chinese subjects, respectively. The task was to decide whether the self or the familiar face was shown in a left or right profile. The decision was made by a button press to target faces (own face or the familiar face) using the left or right index finger and ignoring the other faces. (b) Reaction times to self and familiar faces.

greater in British than in Chinese participants (Figure 2.1b). In addition, the reaction time difference between the two cultural groups was associated with distinct underlying neural mechanisms in British but not in Chinese participants. Specifically, ERPs to self-face in British participants showed a larger negative activity at 280–340 ms over the frontal-central area (N2) relative to the familiar face. Nevertheless, a reverse effect was observed in Chinese participants, i.e., self-face elicited an anterior N2 with smaller amplitude compared to friends' faces (Figure 2.2). As the anterior N2 is associated with deeper processing of faces to benefit individuating (Kubota & Ito, 2007), the cultural specific N2 modulation supports the view that, relative to Chinese subjects, British subjects with the independent self-construal pay more attention to the information about the self than others. Thus the independent self-construals may give rise to enhanced social salience of self-face over the faces of familiar others, which results in a dissociation between self and others in behavioral performance and the underlying neural mechanisms in Western participants. In contrast, the interdependent self-construals in East Asian cultures may evolve the neurocognitive processes that assign the faces of familiar others with greater social salience over self-face.

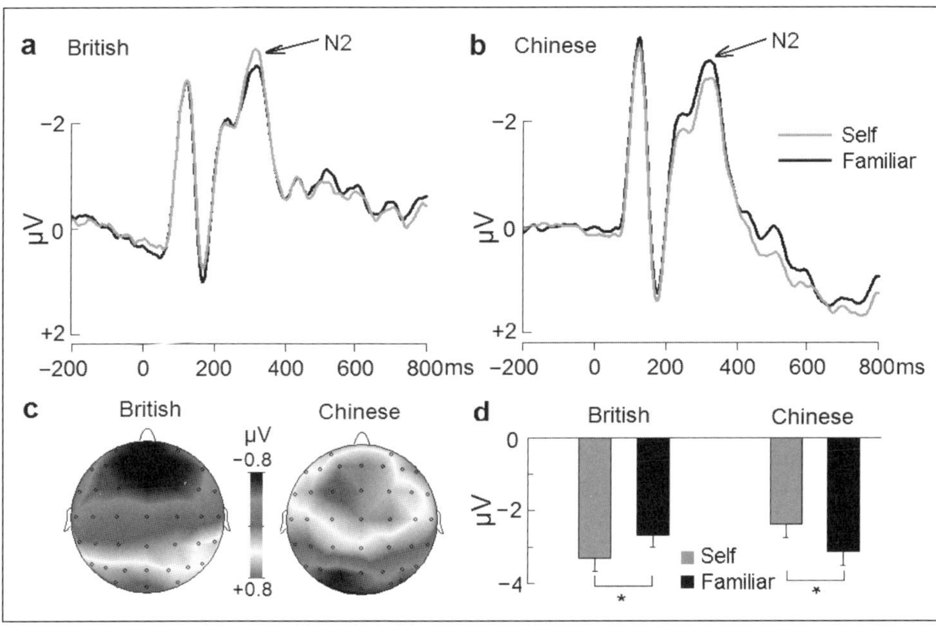

Figure 2.2. The ERP results in Sui et al. (2009). The N2 amplitudes were enlarged to own face relative to familiar face in British subjects (a), but were of smaller amplitudes to own face than familiar faces for Chinese participants (b). Top views of voltage topographies of N2 difference between self and familiar faces from the British and Chinese are shown separately in (c). Difference waves between self and familiar faces were computed at all electrode positions. The mean amplitude of N2 from the British and Chinese at Fz is shown in (d). Error bars represent standard errors.

The relation between self-construals and the neurocognitive processes of self-face was further addressed in brain imaging studies. An early positron emission tomography (PET) study found that, relative to viewing unfamiliar faces, passively viewing ones' own face or performing an explicit self-face recognition task induced increased activations in the fusiform gyrus in the left hemisphere and in the supramarginal gurys and hypothalamus in the right hemisphere (Sugiura et al., 2000). The explicit self-face recognition task was characterized with activations in the right middle and inferior frontal cortex, the right anterior cingulate gyrus, the left middle frontal gyrus, and the left anterior insula. The following functional magnetic resonance imaging (fMRI) studies also identified activation in the right frontal cortex, the right occipito-temporo-parietal junction, and the fusiform gyrus (Sugiura et al., 2005; Platek, Keenan, Gallup, & Mohamed, 2004; Platek et al., 2006; Uddin, Kaplan, Molnar-Szakaea, Zaidel, & Iacoboni, 2005; Ma and Han, in press). These findings identify neural substrates underlying self-face recognition and meanwhile raise an interesting issue of whether the brain activity involved in self-face recognition is modulated by culture-specific self-construals.

To examine the cause-effect relation between self-construals and the different patterns of neurocognitive processes involved in self-face recognition, Sui and Han (2007) used a psychological priming procedure that may activate specific cultural knowledge in individuals to clarify the contribution of self-construals to culture-specific neural mechanisms involved in self-face recognition. The self-construal priming is based on the hypothesis that an individual may have two cultural systems in knowledge and either set of the knowledge can become activated in the mind by certain contextual cues (Hong, 2009). Gardner, Gabriel, and Lee (1999) showed that one's self-construal formed chronically in one sociocultural context can be shifted by tasks of searching independent or interdependent pronouns (e.g., "I" or "We") in essays. Sui and Han (2007) investigated if the independent self-construal priming would result in neurocognitive processes of self-face recognition similar to those observed in Western cultures (e.g., large self-face advantage in behavioral performances), whereas the interdependent self-construal priming would lead to neurocognitive processes of self-face recognition similar to those observed in East Asian cultures (e.g., weak self-face advantage in behavioral performances). Moreover, by scanning participants using fMRI during judgments of head orientations of self-face or a personally familiar face after different self-construal priming procedures, they assessed whether self-construal priming may result in modulations of neurocognitive processes of self-face recognition.

Interestingly, the results revealed a significant effect of self-construal priming on reaction times to self-face and familiar faces. Participants responded faster to self-face compared to familiar faces after the independent self-construal priming. However, they showed slower responses to self-face compared to familiar faces after the interdependent self-construal priming (Figure 2.3). These results are consistent with the idea that the independent self intends to pay more attention to the self than to others and the interdependent self is sensitive to information related to significant others (Markus and Kitayama, 1991). In addition, the self-construal priming in a short time (e.g., 3 minutes in

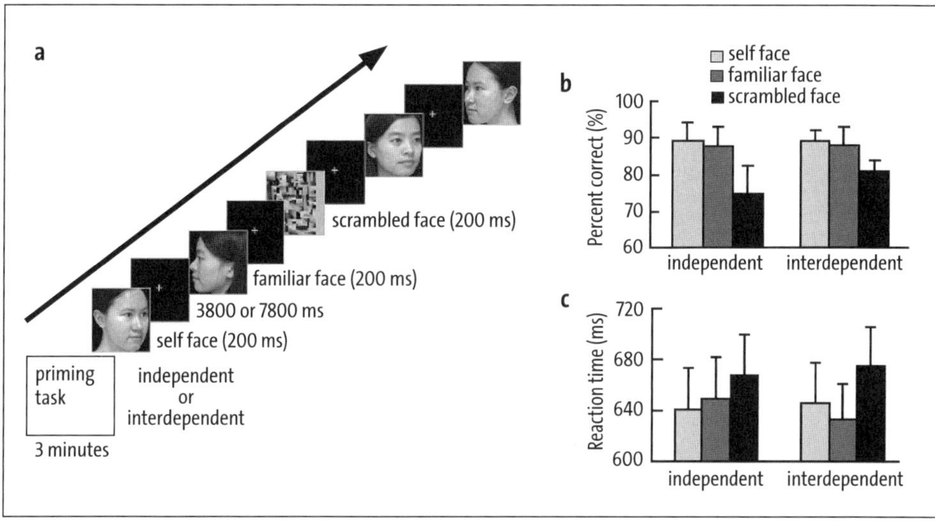

Figure 2.3. Experimental procedure and behavioral results in Sui and Han (2007). (a) Illustration of the stimuli and procedure used in the current study. After the self-construal priming task, subjects were scanned while being presented with a self face, a familiar face, and scrambled faces. They responded to head orientations of the face stimuli or the locations of the gray bars in the scrambled faces by a button press using the right index or middle finger. The order of the independent and interdependent self-construal priming tasks was counterbalanced across the subjects. (b) The response accuracy for the identification of head orientations or gray-bar locations in the scramble faces. Error bars represent standard deviations. (c) Reaction times for the identification of head orientations or gray-bar locations in the scramble faces. Informed written consent was obtained from all participants.

this study) modulated the neural activity in association with self-face recognition. It was found that, relative to familiar faces, self-face activated the right middle and inferior frontal cortex after the independent self-construal priming. However, the right frontal activity was significantly reduced after the interdependent self-construal priming (Figure 2.4). The brain imaging results indicated a cause-effect relation between cultural specific self-construals and cultural specific styles of neurocognitive processes involved in self-face recognition. Self-awareness, which was induced during face perception, was augmented by independent relative to interdependent self-construal priming.

Taken together, both behavioral and brain results suggest that cultures influence the neurocognitive processes involved in self-face recognition. These findings are consistent with the idea that the interdependent self of East Asian cultures is more sensitive to social contexts and social connections between the self and others whereas the independent self-construal in Western cultures enhances the self-other distinction in face perception.

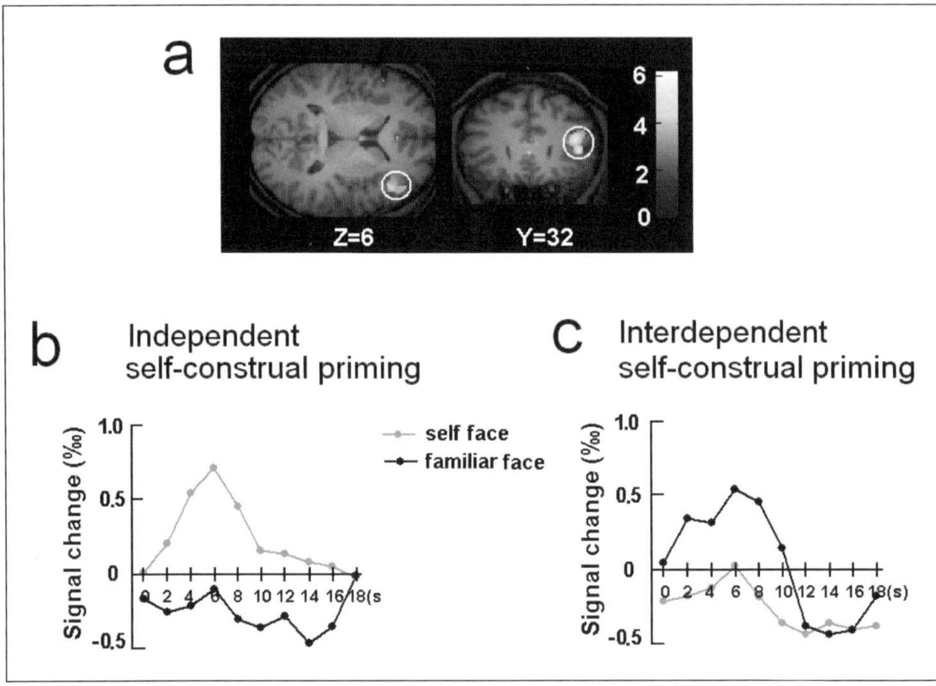

Figure 2.4. Neural activations associated with identification of the faces and scrambled faces in Sui and Han (2007). (a) Stronger activation in the right frontal cortex induced by the self relative to familiar faces after the independent self-construal priming. The time courses of the blood-oxygen-level-dependent (BOLD) signals in the right middle frontal cortex after the independent (b) and interdependent (c) self-construal priming.

Culture and Neural Mechanisms of Self-Related Processing in Mental Domain

The way in which humans conceptualize the self strongly influences their social behaviors and mental health. How is self-concept mediated by the human brain? Recent brain imaging studies have shown an increasing interest in this question and used brain imaging to explore the neural substrates underlying processes of self-related information. One line of research investigated brain regions involved in representation of one's own personal traits. Researchers in this line employed a self-referential task (Rogers, Kuiper, & Kirper, 1977) that requires personality trait judgments of the self and a celebrity and identifies brain activations associated with self-reflection on traits by contrasting brain activity related to the self versus a celebrity. It was found that reflection on one's own personal traits induced an increased activity in several brain regions such as the medial prefrontal cortex (MPFC) and precuneus (Benoit, Gilbert, Volle & Burgess, 2010; Heatherton et al., 2006; Kelley et al., 2002; Ma and Han, 2011; Moran, Macrae, Heatherton, Wyland, & Kelly, 2006). These brain areas may underlie different functions during self-reflection. Specifically, the MPFC is supposed to encode self-relevance of stimuli (Northoff et al., 2006; Han and Northoff, 2009) as increased MPFC activity is elicited by trait words that are rated high then low in self-relevance (Moran et al., 2006) and correlated with memory performance on recall of trait words associated with the self (Macrae, Moran, Heatherton, Banfield, & Kelley, 2004; Ma and Han, 2011).

However, given that the social psychological research suggests that self-concept is socially constructed and emerges during social interactions (Hogg, 2003), it may be predicted that the neural representation of self-concept may be affected by social experiences. Indeed, it was found that the relationship between individuals affected neural representations of the self and others. For instance, Mitchell, Macrae, and Banaji (2006) first had participants read descriptions of two unfamiliar individuals who were described as having opposing liberal or conservative sociopolitical views in order to create one target whose social and political views would be similar to those of the participant and another target whose views would be dissimilar. During fMRI scanning, participants mentalized about the opinions, likes, and dislikes of each of these two targets and also indicated their own responses on the same set of opinion questions. It was found that the ventral subregion of the MPFC linked to self-referential thought was activated when mentalizing about a similar other whereas mentalizing about a dissimilar other engaged a dorsal subregion of the MPFC.

While Mitchell and colleagues' (2006) findings suggest modulations of neural correlates of mentalizing others by personal experiences, it is unclear how cultural experiences shape the representations of the self and others in the MPFC. To address this issue, Zhu et al. (2007) scanned both English-speaking Westerners and Chinese using fMRI during trait judgments of the self, mother, and a public person. The critical issue addressed in this study was whether the self and mother share neural representations in the ventral MPFC in individuals in the Chinese cultural context but are dissociated from each other in the MPFC in individuals in the Western cultural context. The results revealed that both Chinese and Westerners showed greater MPFC activity to self-judgments than public-person judgments. However, neural representations of close others seemed to be different between Chinese and Westerners. In Westerners, mother-judgments failed to activate the MPFC relative to public-person-judgments, and self-judgments increased MPFC activation compared with mother-judgments (Figure 2.5). These results suggest a dissociation between the self and mother in the MPFC in Westerners. A different pattern of neural representation of mother was evident in Chinese. The contrast of mother- versus public-person judgments showed greater MPFC activity in Chinese participants. In addition, the contrast of self- and mother-judgments did not show any activation in the MPFC, suggesting comparable neural representations of the self and mother in the MPFC. These findings provide brain imaging evidence for cross-cultural variations in neural substrates underlying representations of close others in relation to the self and provide a neuroscience account of the psychological model of

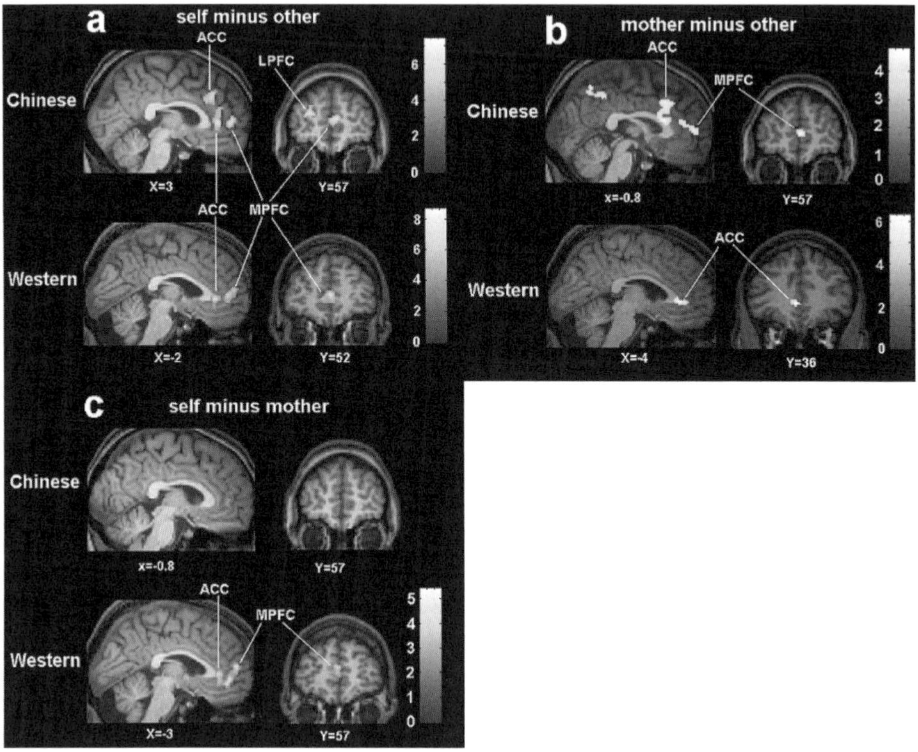

Figure 2.5. fMRI results in Zhu et al. (2007). (a) Brain activations associated with self versus a celebrity judgments. (b) Brain activations associated with mother versus a celebrity judgments. (c) Brain activations associated with self versus mother judgments.

Western versus East Asian cultural differences in self-construals (Markus & Kitayama, 1991).

The relation between self-construals and brain activity associated with reflection of personal traits of the self and close others was further assessed using self-construal priming on bicultural individuals (Ng, Han, Mao, & Lai, 2010). It was hypothesized that participants living in Hong Kong, who are exposed to both Chinese and Western cultures, may show a pattern of brain activity associated with representation of the self and close others similar to that observed in Chinese after primed with Chinese culture. After Western cultural priming, however, their neural representations of the self and close others may be similar to that observed in Westerners. Indeed, Ng et al. (2010) found that, after being primed with pictures of Chinese cultural icons, Westernized Chinese participants living in Hong Kong showed increased MPFC activity to both the self and mother during the trait judgment task. However, after being primed with pictures of Western cultural icons, MPFC activity to mother-judgments was decreased whereas

MPFC activity to self-judgments was enhanced. It seems that dynamic cognitive and neural representations of the self in relation to close others may vary as a function of cultural priming in bicultural individuals. Such temporal dynamic variations of neural representations of the self are consistent with the observed differences in self-representations in Chinese and Westerners that reflects the accumulated influences of cultural values and practice over time.

However, cultural differences in MPFC activity does not seem to be evident for all close others. For instance, Heatherton et al. (2006) found that MPFC activity associated with trait judgments differentiated self from the best friend in American participants. They found that, relative to letter judgments (uppercase vs. lower case), making judgments about the self yielded increased activation in the MPFC whereas making judgments about a friend did not. Similarly, Wang et al. (2012) asked Chinese participants to make trait judgments about the self as well as their mother, father, and best friend. They found that, while trait judgments of the self and the mother generated comparable activity in the MPFC in Chinese adults, trait judgments of the mother induced greater MPFC activity than trait judgments of the father and the best friend. However, trait judgments of the best friend did not activate MPFC compared to trait judgments of a public person. The results suggest that, while neural representations of the self and the mother overlapped in the MPFC, close others such as mother, father, and best friend are unequally represented in the MPFC in collectivistic Chinese brains.

Cultures also seem to influence neural representations of self-concept during the processing of general and contextual self-judgments. Chiao et al. (2009b) scanned Japanese and Caucasian-Americans during a general self-referential task that required responses to questions such as "in general, does this sentence describe you?" and a contextual self-referential task that required responses to questions such as "does this sentence describe you when you are talking to your mother?" They classified participants into individualist and collectivist groups, based on their self-reports on the Singelis (1994) self-construal scale, and found that individualists showed significantly greater VMPFC activation for general self-descriptions relative to contextual self-descriptions. In contrast, individuals with collectivistic cultural values showed greater activation for contextual self-descriptions compared to general self-descriptions. In addition, MPFC activity to contextual versus general self-judgments positively predicted the degree of differential collectivism versus individualism. Chiao et al. (2009a) also used self-construal priming to examine the relation between self-construals and MPFC activity related to general/contextual self trait judgments. The priming procedure consisted of a Sumerian Warrior Story task and a Similarities and Differences with Family and Friends (SDFF) task (Trafimow, Triandis, & Goto, 1991) that have been shown to influence self-construals. Asian Americans were scanned during the general or contextual self-judgment tasks. Half of the participants were primed with cultural values of individualism and half with cultural values of collectivism prior to self-judgments. It was found that the participants primed with individualistic values showed increased activation in the MPFC and posterior cingulate cortex during general relative to contextual self-judgments. In contrast, participants primed with collectivistic values showed increased responses within the MPFC and PCC during contextual relative to general self-judgments. Thus, neural correlates of a general self and a contextual self in the MPFC are shaped by cultural values of individualism and collectivism.

Neural representations of self-concept are also affected by religious cultures. Christianity emphasizes human contingency and dependence on God and advocates denial of the self, which is seen as a creature and a sinner who needs to surrender to God (Burns, 2003; Ching, 1984; Lin, 2005). In addition, in order to grow in godliness, one has to recognize one's own "nothingness" and pursue a spiritual quest for self-transcendence. A possible consequence of such a perspective on the self is to blur the boundary between the self and others. Christian beliefs about the relation between the self and God may have a strong influence on the perception of the self. For example, the mandate that "every one of us shall give account of himself to God" (Sproul, 1995, Romans 14:12) emphasizes judgment of the self from God's perspective rather than from one's own perspective.

To investigate the neural consequences of Christian belief and practice on the neurocognitive processes of the self, our research group scanned 14 nonreligious and 14 Christian Chinese participants using fMRI during personal trait judgments regarding the self or a public person (Han et al., 2008). We tested two psychological consequences of the unique spiritual quest and practice of Christianity. First, to deny oneself in order to live a spiritual life as dictated by Jesus may weaken the encoding process of stimuli as self-referential. Second, an emphasis of evaluation of the self from God's perspective may strengthen the evaluative process of self-referential stimuli and engage others' perspective during self-reflection of traits. If these hypotheses are correct, one may expect that, relative to those in nonreligious people, the ventral MPFC (VMPFC) activity related to the encoding of stimulus self-relevance is reduced in Christians. Moreover, Christian participants may recruit the brain areas involved in mentalizing others to evaluate self-related stimuli. Indeed, we found that, while the ventral MPFC was engaged during reflection of one's own traits in nonreligious participants, the same brain did not show activation in Christian participants during self-trait judgments. This is consistent with the first hypothesis as the VMPFC is supposed to encode stimulus self-relevance (Northoff et al., 2006; Han and Northoff, 2009). Interestingly, we found that the dorsal MPFC, which is activated during the processing of others' mind, was activated during self-trait judgments in Christian participants (Figure 2.6). This is consistent with the second hypothesis as the dorsal MPFC has been shown to be engaged in reappraisal and evaluation of self-related stimuli (Northoff et al., 2006) and in inference of others' mental states (Grèzes, Frith, & Passingham, 2004; Mitchell, Banaji, & Macrae, 2005). Taken together, these results indicate that Christian participants utilized the dorsal MPFC to differentiate the self from others in the trait-judgment tasks whereas nonreligious participants employed the ventral MPFC to distinguish the self from others during personal trait judgments. Thus religious cultures also modulate the neural substrates underlying representation of the self in the mental domain, although such modulations show a different pattern as the influence of Western/East Asian cultures on neural representations of the self.

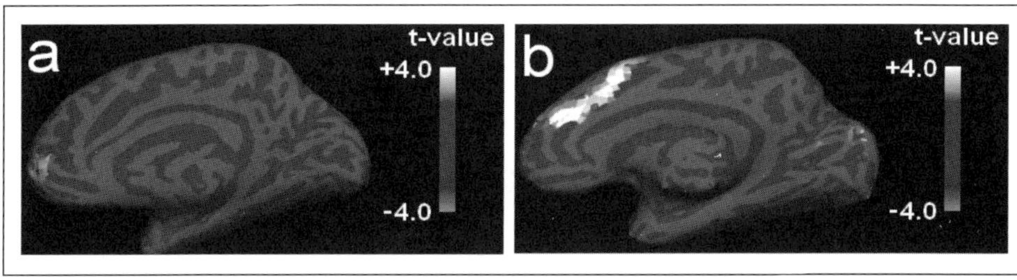

Figure 2.6. fMRI results in Han et al. (2008). (a) The ventral MPFC activity associated with self-trait judgments in nonreligious participants. (b) The dorsal VMPFC activity associated with self-trait judgments in Christian participants.

Conclusion

Remarkable cultural differences exist in self-concept in philosophical thoughts and psychological processes. Recent transcultural brain imaging studies further strengthen such a view by providing neuroscience evidence for modulation of neurocognitive processes of self-related information. The effect of cultures on self-related processing is evident in perceptual and mental domains. The heavy emphasis on interpersonal connectedness in East Asian cultures leads to the development of neural unification of the self and intimate persons such as mother. In contrast, the dominance of an independent self in Western cultures give rise to neural separation between the self and others. The brain imaging findings provide solid evidence for the view that cultures differ in how the self is conceptualized and experienced. The cultural influences on the neural mechanisms of self-related processing reflect the intrinsic nature of plasticity of the brain and context-dependence nature of social cognition.

While clinical psychological research has suggested an association between self-construals and mental problems (e.g., social anxiety disorder, Rego, 2009), the relation between the mental problems and culture-specific brain activity involved in self-representation remains unknown. However, cultural neuroscience findings suggest that sociocultural contexts result in specific patterns of brain activity related to the processing of the self and others. Mental health may require an individual to fit with a society and to enjoy the social interaction between the self and other in a specific sociocultural context. Future research should investigate how culture-specific neural representation of the self and others is related to mental health in the Western and East Asian cultures.

Acknowledgments

This work was supported by the National Natural Science Foundation of China (Project 30910103901; 91024032) and the National Basic Research Program of China (973 Program 2010CB833903).

References

Amsterdam, B. (1972). Mirror self-image reactions before age two. *Developmental Psychobiology, 5*, 297–305.

Asendorpf, J. B., Warkentin, V., & Baudonniere, P. M. (1996). Self-awareness and other-awareness II: Mirror self-recognition, social contingency awareness, and synchronic imitation. *Development Psychology, 32*, 313–321.

Benoit, R. G., Gilbert, S. J., Volle, E., & Burgess, P. W. (2010). When I think about me and simulate you: Medial rostral prefrontal cortex and self-referential processes. *NeuroImage, 50*, 1340–1349.

Burns, C. (2003). "Soul-less" Christianity and the Buddhist empirical self: Buddhist-Christian convergence? *Buddhist-Christian Studies, 23*, 87–100.

Chiao, J. Y., & Ambady, N.(2007). *Cultural neuroscience: Parsing universality and diversity across levels of analysis.* In S. Kitayama & D. Cohen (Eds.)., *Handbook of cultural psychology* (pp. 237–254). New York: Guilford.

Chiao, J. Y., Harada, T., Komeda, H., Li, Z., Mano, Y., Saito, D., . . . Iidaka, T. (2009a). Dynamic cultural influences on neural representations of the self. *Journal of Cognitive Neuroscience, 22*, 1–11.

Chiao, J. Y., Harada, T., Komeda, H., Li, Z., Mano, Y., Saito, D., . . . Iidaka, T. (2009b). Neural basis of individualistic and collectivistic views of self. *Human Brain Mapping, 30*, 2813–2820.

Ching, J. (1984). Paradigms of the self in buddhism and Christianity. *Buddist-Shistian Studies, 4*, 31–50.

Gardner, W. L., Gabriel, S., & Lee, A. Y. (1999). "I" value freedom, but "we" value relationships: Self-construal priming mirrors cultural differences in judgment. *Psychological Science, 10*, 321–326.

Grèzes, J., Frith, C. D., & Passingham, R. E. (2004). Inferring false beliefs from the actions of oneself and others: An fMRI study. *Neuroimage, 21*, 744–750.

Han, S., Mao, L., Gu, X., Zhu, Y., Ge, J., & Ma, Y. (2008). Neural consequences of religious belief on self-referential processing. *Social Neuroscience, 3*, 1–15.

Han, S., & Northoff, G. (2008). Culture-sensitive neural substrates of human cognition: A transcultural neuroimaging approach. *Nature Review Neuroscience, 9*, 646–654.

Han, S., & Northoff, G. (2009). Understanding the self: A cultural neuroscience approach. *Progress in Brain Research, 178*, 203–212.

Heatherton, T. F., Wyland, C. L., Macrae, C. N., Demos, K. E., Denny, B. T., & Kelly, W. M. (2006). Medial prefrontal activity differentiates self from close others. *Social Cognitive Affective Neuroscience, 1*, 18– 25.

Hogg, M. A. (2003). Social identity. In M. R. Leary & J. P. Tangney (Eds.), *Handbook of self and identity* (pp. 462–479). New York: Guilford.

Hong, Y. (2009). A dynamic constructivist approach to culture: Moving from describing culture to explaining culture. In R. S. Wyer, C.-y. Chiu, & Y.-y. Hong (Eds.), *Problems and solutions in cross-cultural theory, research and application* (pp 3–24). New York: Psychology Press.

James, W. (1890). *Principles of psychology.* New York: Henry Holt.

Keenan, J. P., McCutcheon, B., Sanders, G., Freund, S., Gallup, G. G., & Pascual-Leone, A. (1999). Left hand advantage in a self-face recognition task. *Neuropsychologia, 37*, 1421–1425.

Keenan, J. P., Wheeler, M. A., Gallup, G. G., & Pascual-Leone, A. (2000). Self-recognition and the right prefrontal cortex. *Trends in Cognitive Science, 4*, 338–344.

Kelly, W., Macrae, C. N., Wyland, C. L., Caglar, S., Inati, S., & Heatherton, T. F. (2002). Finding the self? An event-related fMRI study. *Journal of Cognitive Neuroscience, 14*, 785–794.

Kubota, J. T., & Ito, T. A. (2007). Multiple cues in social perception: The time course of processing race and facial expression. *Journal of Experimental Social Psychology, 43*, 738–752.

Lin, H. (2005). Religious wisdom of no-self. In Y. Wu, P. Lai, & W. Wang (Eds.) *Dialogue between Buddhism and Christianity* (pp. 317–338). Beijing: Zhong Hua Book Company.

Ma, Y., & Han, S. (2009). Self-face advantage is modulated by social threat – Boss effect on self-face recognition. *Journal of Experimental Social Psychology, 45*, 1048–1051.

Ma, Y., & Han, S. (2010). Why respond faster to the self than others? An implicit positive association theory of self advantage during implicit face recognition. *Journal of Experimental Psychology: Human Perception and Performance, 36*, 619–633.

Ma, Y., & Han, S. (2011). Neural representation of self-concept in sighted and congenitally blind adults. *Brain, 134*, 235–246.

Ma, Y., & Han, S. (in press). Functional dissociation of the left and right fusiform gyrus in self-face recognition. *Human Brain Mapping*.

Macrae, C. N., Moran, J. M., Heatherton, T. F., Banfield, J. F., & Kelley, W. M. (2004). Medial prefrontal activity predicts memory for self. *Cerebral Cortex, 14*, 647–654.

Markus, H. R., & Kitayama, S. (1991). Culture and the self: Implications for cognition, emotion, and motivation. *Psychological Review, 98*, 224–253.

Markus, H. R., & Kitayama, S. (2003). Culture, self, and the reality of the social. *Psychological Inquiry, 14*, 277–283.

Markus, H. R., & Kitayama, S. (2010). Cultures and selves: A cycle of mutual constitution. *Perspective on Psychological Science, 5*, 420–430.

Mitchell, J. P., Banaji, M. R., & Macrae, C. N. (2005). General and specific contributions of the medial prefrontal cortex to knowledge about mental states. *Neuroimage, 28*, 757–762.

Mitchell, J. P., Macrae, C. N., & Banaji, M. R. (2006). Dissociable medial prefrontal contributions to judgments of similar and dissimilar others. *Neuron, 50*, 655–663.

Moran, J. M., Macrae, C. N., Heatherton, T. F., Wyland, C. L., & Kelley, W. M. (2006). Neuroanatomical evidence for distinct cognitive and affective components of self. *Journal of Cognitive Neuroscience, 18*, 1586–1594.

Ng, S. H., Han, S., Mao, L., & Lai, J. C. L. (2010). Dynamic bicultural brains: A fMRI study of their flexible neural representation of self and significant others in response to culture priming. *Asian Journal Social Psychology, 13*, 83–91.

Nisbett, R. E. (2003). *The geography of thought: How Asians and Westerners think differently, and why.* New York: Free Press.

Northoff, G., Heinzel, A., de Greck, M. D., Bermpohl, F., Dobrowolny, H., & Panksepp, J. (2006). Self-referential processing in our brain. A meta-analysis of imaging studies on the self. *NeuroImage, 31*, 440–457.

Platek, S. M., Keenan, J. P., Gallup, G. G., & Mohamed, F.B. (2004). Where am I? The neurological correlates of self and other. *Brain Research, Cognitive Brain Research, 19*, 114–122.

Platek, S. M., Loughead, J. W., Gur, R. C., Busch, S., Ruparel, K., & Phend, N. (2006). Neural substrates for functionally discriminating self-face from personally familiar faces. *Human Brain Mapping, 27*, 91–98.

Rego, S. A. (2009). *Culture and anxiety disorder.* In S. Eshun & R. A. R. Gurung (Eds.), *Culture and mental health* (pp. 197–220). Malden, MA: John Wiley & Son Ltd.

Rogers, T. B., Kuiper, N. A., & Kirker, W. S. (1977). Self-reference and the encoding of personal information. *Journal of Personality and Social Psychology, 35*, 677–688.

Sproul, R. C. (Ed.) (1995). *New Geneva Study Bible*. Nashville, TN: Thomas Nelson Publishers.

Singelis, T. M. (1994). The measurement of independent and interdependent self-construals. *Personality and Social Psychology Bulletin, 20*, 580–591.

Sugiura, M., Kawashima, R., Nakamura, K., Okada, K., Kato, T., Nakamura, A., . . . Fukuda, H. (2000). Passive and active recognition of one's own face. *NeuroImage, 11*, 36–48.

Sugiura, M., Watanabe, J., Maeda, Y., Matsue, Y., Fukuda, H., & Kawashima, R. (2005). Cortical mechanisms of visual self-recognition. *Neuroimage, 24*, 143–149.

Sui, J., & Han, S. (2007). Self-construal priming modulates neural substrates of self-awareness. *Psychological Science, 18*, 861–866.

Sui, J., Liu, C. H., & Han, S. (2009). Cultural difference in neural mechanisms of self-recognition. *Social Neuroscience, 4*, 402–411.

Sui, J., Zhu, Y., & Han, S. (2006). Self-face recognition in attended and unattended conditions: An ERP study. *NeuroReport, 17*, 423–427.

Tong, F., & Nakayama, K. (1999). Robust representations for faces: Evidence from visual search. *Journal of Experiment Psychology: Human Perception and Performance, 25*, 1016–1035.

Trafimow, D., Triandis, H. C., & Goto, S. G. (1991). Some tests of the distinction between the private self and the collective self. *Journal of Personality and Social Psychology, 60*, 649–655.

Uddin, L. Q., Kaplan, J. T., Molnar-Szakaca, I., Zaidel, E., & Iacoboni, M. (2005). Self-face recognition activates a frontoparietal "mirror" network in the right hemisphere: An event-related fMRI study. *Neuroimage, 25*, 926–935.

Wang, G., Mao, L., Ma, Y., Yang, X., Cao, J., Liu, X., . . . Han, S. (2012). Neural representations of close others in collectivistic brains. *Social Cognitive and Affective Neuroscience, 7*, 222–229.

Zhu, Y., & Han, S. (2008). Cultural differences in the self: From philosophy to psychology and neuroscience. *Social and Personality Psychology Compass, 2*, 1799–1811.

Zhu, Y., Zhang, L., Fan, J., & Han, S. (2007). Neural basis of cultural influence on self-representation. *NeuroImage, 34*, 1310–1316.

Shihui Han
Department of Psychology
Peking University
5 Yiheyuan Road
Beijing 100871
China
E-mail: shan@pku.edu.cn

Chapter 3

The Self and Its Emotional Brain

Georg Northoff*[1] and Jaak Panksepp*[2]

[1]University of Ottawa Institute of Mental Health Research, University of Hangzhou, China
[2]Washington State University, Pullman, WA, USA

Abstract

The concept of the self and how it relates to emotion remains largely unclear. While various neuronal correlates of self and emotion have been investigated recently, their interaction and dependence is not clear. We here propose the characterization of the self by self-related processing, which means that every stimulus is processed in relation to the organism and, more specifically, his brain and its intrinsic activity. By linking the stimuli to the organism, the stimulus is assigned a degree of self-relatedness. High degrees of self-relatedness go along with strong emotions, which, depending on the value assigned, will be positive or negative. We assume self-related processing to be associated with activity in predominantly the subcortical-cortical midline system. Since this system is an ancient system in evolutionary terms and thus present in many species, we assume the self and self-related processing to be present in various animals in different degrees.

Keywords: self, cortical, subcortical, midline structures, self-related processing, emotions, animals

Introduction

Consciousness, as one of the most crucial features of human existence, is increasingly becoming a topic of neuroscientific inquiry. This forces us to reconsider what it means for humans to possess a "self." Likewise, evolutionary perspectives coax us to entertain such issues in other organisms, for they too may possess such attributes of mentality. If we have core selves, perhaps they do also. This is rather likely since a basic level of self-representation would surely allow organisms to better relate to their environments,

* Both authors contributed equally to this chapter.

giving them a felt "ownership" of experiences. The most basic form of self is thus at its core relational, in the sense that it constitutes the selective and adaptive relation of the organism to its inner feelings and how they relate to the environment. Such relational self, which later we will call proto-self, provides the basis for subjective experience and phenomenal consciousness of existence as characterized by primary process consciousness – the ability to perceive the world and to experience various affective states (Merker, 2007; Panksepp, 1998a, 2005a). In contrast to Merker (2007), who focused largely on perceptual experiences, we focus more heavily on the affective-emotional aspects of core consciousness. Although our views overlap, they have emerged independently from rather distinct intellectual traditions. Thus, the aim of this chapter is to discuss the possible existence of an affective, nomothetic core-self in all mammals that may be the foundation for the diversity of selves and the many idiographic forms of selfhood that can emerge during human development.

Just like most brain/mind processes, self-representation is reiterated at many levels of the brain, requiring different concepts at different neuro-evolutionary levels. At minimum, these are: (1) primary-processes, namely the intrinsic unconditional tools for living (these we call the *nomothetic,* or universal, aspects of consciousness); (2) secondary-processes, namely the basic mechanisms of learning and memory; and (3) tertiary-processes, the higher brain mechanisms that elaborate reflecting on past experiences, thinking, and planning (which become highly *ideographic,* or individualized, depending on each person's temperament, storehouse of memories, and capacity to reflect on past events and future possibilities).

The clearest data for the primary-process neural nature of experiential brain/mind processes is available from the study of basic emotional processes in animals, where one can identify brain systems for specific emotions using localized electrical stimulation of the brain (ESB). Such artificially evoked instinctual arousals yield not only distinct emotional displays, but also clear indications that animals like or dislike such brain states. These effects are obtained in homologous brain regions in all mammals studied (Panksepp, 1998a; Panksepp & Bivin, 2011), and suggest that affect is a neurodynamic property of subcortical instinctual emotional arousal. The fact that humans, who can provide verbal self-reports, have comparable affective feelings during such evoked states, with full felt ownership of the evoked experiences, validates the cross-species nature of such primal emotional processes (Heath, 1996; Panksepp, 1982).

The fact that all basic emotional operating systems converge on primitive brain regions such as the periaqueductal gray (PAG) suggests how the affective foundation for a core-self may be constructed within the most ancient medial strata of all mammalian nervous systems (Panksepp, 1998a, 1998b). The massive interconnectivities of these medial brainstem regions to medial frontal cortical regions (Holstege & Saper, 2005), brain regions long implicated in self-related processing of information in human brain imaging work (Northoff et al., 2006), provide a coherent vision of how nomothetic core-self processes, homologous in all mammals, are related to higher mental functions that are unique in the human species. The primary-processes are easier to study in animals and the higher processes in humans, but for both we need to consider epigenetic-developmental issues in the experimental refinement of all levels of the brain/mind.

It is difficult to study experiential states of animals in cognitive domains (i.e., experiences derived directly from exteroceptive information processing), but the complex behavioral strategies exhibited by many vertebrate species strongly suggest they do have cognitive experiences (e.g., Clayton, Bussey, & Dickinson, 2003; Foote & Crystal, 2007; Smith, Shields, & Washburn, 2003). In contrast, the neural nature of primal emotional feelings is much easier to study in animals (Panksepp, 1998a, 2005a). Thus, bringing both human and animal data to bear on the issue of what it means to have a self and consciousness may allow more progress to envision how rich emotional experiences are a birthright of subneocortical limbic circuits, as first discussed by the late Paul MacLean (1990).

The proto-self may be assumed to be constituted empirically by what we called above, self-related processing (SRP). At its core, SRP describes the integration of interoceptive and exteroceptive stimuli from body and environment in relation to the intrinsic organismic functions – the basic emotion and motivation systems of the brain that generate a purely affective form of consciousness (Panksepp, 2007a) – and hence elaboration of animals' various goal-orientated survival activities (see below and Alcaro, Huber, & Panksepp, 2007; Northoff et al., 2006; Panksepp, 1998a for details). As such, the higher reaches of self-related processing, in medial frontal cortical regions, may be crucial in constituting what might be the first glimmers of the high cognitive self – that is, not only having the feeling tone of being a living creature as most animals and humans share, but awareness of being a certain type of creature within a specific environment that may be specific for higher-order animals, including humans. If coupled with higher-order cognitive functions in neocortically well-endowed animals, especially humans, SRP may also go beyond mere self-relating (see below for further explanation) by providing the basis for higher forms of self-awareness, self-consciousness, self-image, self-enhancement, self-regulation, self-cognition, and the great variety of coalesced idiographic selves that constitute a fully-developed personality. While the foundational SELF, characterized by raw affective feelings that mediate one's own bodily needs and emotional urges, as well as primary-process perceptual relatedness to social and physical environments, provides the very basis for the organism's orientation within and adaptation to the world. The more cognitive higher-order forms of self may allow for more refined, selective, and manipulative relation to the environment, often conceptualized as free will, and one's emerging interests and desires. We assume that the lower-order more basic form of an affective "core-SELF" that generates raw emotional and motivational feelings (Panksepp, 2007a) is shared homologously across different species, whereas the higher-order cognitive forms of core self may be more diverse across species, depending more on differences in sensory-perceptual abilities and cortical architectures.

Neurobiologically, such evolutionarily provided coherent affective-cognitive integration with these core-SELF/core-self processes may permit the emergence of coherently operating neural networks across different species that integrate incoming stimuli from the environment with internal needs, drives, and basic affects (Alcaro et al., 2007; Northoff & Bermpohl, 2004; Panksepp, 1998a, 1998b). We summarize evidence that a coherently operating subcortical-cortical midline system (SCMS) is the critical central neural processing network that mediates SRP across different species. At its lowest levels, it is largely instinctual, affective, but deeply embedded within life-supportive environments. At its higher levels it becomes immersed and molded by individual learning and cognitive functions as well as ecological and cultural issues.

In so doing, we begin to articulate a common *psychobiological* basis for constituting diverse emergent expressions of self across species – a trans-species, neurobiologically based, multilayered concept of an nomothetic self that is foundational for the emergence of diverse idiographic forms of selfhood. Thus, we would again reemphasize that this multi-tiered process is more homologous at its lower levels (e.g., PAG and medial diencephalons) and ecologically and experientially diversified in its higher medial frontal regions, which are richly connected to the rest of the higher cerebral apparatus. However, more detailed cross-species investigation is necessary since homology of structures like subcortical regions does not imply homology of function across animals and humans.

Definition of Self-Related Processing (SRP)

In keeping with, but in substantial contrast to the recent analysis by Bekoff and Sherman (2004), we emphasize that SRP is not just limited to cognition, but is a fundamental process allowing the organism to experience a variety of affective states. SRP strongly relates externally derived sensory stimuli, cognitive perspectives to basic organismic needs, and affective feelings according to their relevance for survival, as indexed by various positive and negative affects. The term "relevance" is assumed to reflect intrinsic biological values that are coded as affective feelings (Panksepp, 2005a, 2005b) that help create relational values within the brain/mind that are related to the organisms' growing knowledge of their environment. "Self-related" refers to the processes of coherently associating intero- and exteroceptive stimuli within an organism by means of which the organism becomes integrated with its environment. These potentialities are actualized within specific sensory, motor, attentional, emotional, motivational, morphological, and psychoethological conformation of each species. However, anchored in genetically provided and ancient, subcortical neurosymbolic representations of organisms as coherent creatures, we believe them to be laid out in ancient viscero-somatic coordinates, where intrinsic affective-instinctual processes provide a center of gravity for organismic actions (Panksepp, 2000a, 2000b, 2000c, 2002, 2007b).

This coherent brain function must be ancient and should not require a great deal of cortical encephalization. In this view, it is noteworthy that total neodecortication of all young mammals appears not to compromise the autonomic and sensory-motor manifestations of organismic coherence, nor their ability to experience the world affectively and thus to have a basic sense of self (Kolb & Tees, 2000; Merker, 2007; Panksepp,

Normansell, Cox, & Siviy, 1994; Panksepp, 2005a, 2005b; Shewmon, Holmse & Byrne, 1999). We postulate that this ancient brain function allows SRP to occur in homologous ways across all mammalian species and perhaps other vertebrates. Most importantly, we assume that the primordial coherence of this kind of core-self allows for epigenetic processing of external sensory-perceptual and cultural information within the extended, more cognitively oriented self in a self-referential manner, which in turn enables organisms to selectively adapt to their respective environmental contexts in "self-projective" ways (Buckner & Caroll, 2007).

Conceptualized in this way, higher SRP can be characterized by intrinsic integration of the following four features: (1) relation and colonization, (2) appropriateness and belongingness, (3) increasingly subtle affectivity and emotions, and (4) the phenomenal dimension of *mineness* in experience as organisms relate to their environment. To elaborate on these themes: (1) external stimuli may be related to and "colonized" by the organism (become established in a new mental ecosystem) primarily through the learning of new sensory-perceptual and motor function. (2) Appropriateness and belongingness implicate the process of valuing, i.e., whether the stimulus is relevant for the organism in biological terms, as for survival or reproduction within its actual goal-orientation. (3) Affectivity and emotions signal the linkage between evolutionarily ingrained values and those that are assigned epigenetically to the actual stimuli by SRP (see below for details). (4) Finally, phenomenal experience and mineness signal the relational and affective character of SRP and thus the emergence of self-perspectival organization that will be explained in further detail in the next section.

Only if all four criteria are met may one speak of a core-self. Though many organisms meet all four criteria, plants, for instance, do not. Even if we do not know whether plants may have some kind of proto-phenomenal experience of "mineness," they at least lack the first and third criteria, sensorimotor and affective involvement. Therefore, we would not speak of a self in the case of plants, since they lack what we call self-perspectival organization.

SRP and Self-Perspectival Organization

Once there exists a primordial neural representation of the body that can generate raw affective experiences (Panksepp, 1998a, 1998b), the guiding developmental concept, elaborated by higher medial frontal brain regions, becomes, as already noted, what we call Self Related Processing. SRP is the process that transforms stimuli from simple signals to a meaningful (i.e., valuative) part of the organism's functioning. Stimuli are "colonized" by an organism's intrinsic neural organization, through their appropriation and self-related belongingness, which in turn generates complex meaningful experiences. By such a relationship, sensory stimuli become linked to intrinsic affective values (via conditioning and other forms of learning), yielding the addition of the evaluative "for me" by means of which that particular stimulus becomes "mine," resulting in "mineness" (Metzinger, 2003; Lambie & Marcel, 2002). By becoming "mine," *stimuli make "something informational or neurophysiological into something phenomenological" (Lambie & Marcel, 2002).*

Conceptualized in this way, SRP intrinsically integrates affectivity, appropriateness, and belongingness, and the phenomenal dimension of mineness into the ownership of experience. By being deeply affective and motivational, the ancient universal core-self allows the external world to be related to the organism and consequently to be imbued with vast diversities and varieties of "meanings." By means of SRP the large variety of universal affective experiences (sensory affects, bodily-homeostatic affects, and emotional affects), the genetically provided tools of the core-SELF (as outlined in Panksepp, 1998b) are transformed into organisms' more cognitive phenomenal experiences, and in the most well-cerebrated species, into the development of awareness of themselves (perhaps reflecting the learned emergence of mirror-neurons in higher regions of the brain), their environments with specific spatial/temporal and conceptual organization of their ecological surrounds (see van Gulick, 2004).

There are a variety of basic affects, including various sensory feelings (from pleasant sweetness to disgust) and bodily imbalances (hunger, thirst, etc). The types of experiences that have been most studied in animals are the basic emotions, where a dual-aspect monism strategy (e.g., that raw emotional experiences arise from the same brain networks that generate complex instinctual behaviors, Panksepp, 2005a, 2005b), allows us to envision at least seven basic emotional feelings in all mammals. The appetitive desire is characterized by activation of (1) the SEEKING system; (2) a state of irritable anger when the RAGE system is aroused; (3) feelings of scared-trembling trepidation when the FEAR system is activated; (4) strong erotic feelings when somewhat distinct male and female LUST systems are activated; (5) nurturing, caring feelings when maternal CARE systems are engaged; (6) a form of psychic pain when arousal of the separation-distress PANIC system is triggered; and (7) social joy and laughing playful feelings when PLAY networks are engaged (Panksepp, 1998a, 2005a; Panksepp & Biven, 2011). Many of these feelings are initially "objectless" with object-relations being learned through real-world interactions. As learning and higher cognitive systems come into play, these primary-process affects can serve as fundamental substrates for many secondary- and tertiary-process feelings that are much harder to study in animals since the behavioral indicators become more subtle (Mendl, Burman, & Paul, 2010). The massive colonization of these feelings within complex human cognitive structures, guided by environmental events, have enormous implications for the varieties of subjective selves that can emerge in the human mind.

The ability to organize such external "stimulus colonizations" of higher cognitive regions of the brain into an extended self by the very existence of a basic core-self, which is almost completely affective and relational, is a neuroscience project that has barely begun. However, the particularities of such developmental-epigenetic progressions are surely differentiated not only according to each species' morphology, physiology, and ecological/cultural embeddedness, but also between individuals in a species depending on their affective temperamental differences. These idiographic varieties of subjective selves, which are extremely diverse across human beings and cultures by being linked to the objective self-processes we focus on in this chapter, may sustain many of the attributes of the nomothetic core-selves. In any event, through SRP a phenomenal sense of "mineness" emerges, and each organism's structure of phenomenal experience takes on a character that is philosophically described as self-perspectival organization (van Gulick, 2004).[1]

Self-perspectival organization describes experiences reflecting a certain point of view from which one experiences one's self, one's body, and one's environment singly in relation to others. According to Zahavi (2003, p. 72), self-perspectival organization and "mineness" arise from a primitive form of selfhood, what Damasio (1999) and Panksepp (1998a, 1998b) describe as core-self and the SELF, respectively. Drawing on the phenomenological tradition (Zahavi, 2003), we assume that at this basic lower-order level, self-perspectival organization and "mineness" constitute a conjoint phenomenal experience of both the environment and oneself. One may consequently speak of co-occurrence within phenomenal consciousness, as distinguished from reflective consciousness, and pre-reflective self-instantiation, as distinguished from reflective self-awareness.

Two features need to be emphasized here. First, the level described is what the phenomenologists call pre-reflective, precognitive, and prelinguistic, which must be distinguished from a reflective, cognitive, and linguistic level – this distinction might correspond (more or less, which needs more in-depth discussion than can be pursued here) with the one advanced by Ned Block between phenomenal and access consciousness. Second, most importantly, at this pre-reflective, precognitive, and prelinguistic level, phenomenal consciousness and pre-reflective self-instantiation are inseparably linked to each other. This implies that the occurrence of some kind of basic self in the sense described here is linked to the occurrence of the most basic forms of phenomenal consciousness, which may be deeply affective on the one hand (Panksepp, 2005a, 2005b; Northoff et al. 2009) and sensory-perceptual affected on the other (it is possible that in brain evolution, the latter was built upon the former).

Following and extending this distinction, we would like to distinguish three different levels of the self. (1) First, the relational self/proto-self, which is characterized as prephenomenal and preconsciousness since it is not accessible to subjective experience at this level. (2) Second, the affective self/core-self, which can be described as prelinguistic, preconceptual, and pre-reflective and may be characterized by phenomenal consciousness. (3) Finally, the reflective or cognitive self that allows one to thoughtfully reflect upon the organism's own relation to the environment, which may be associated with access or reflective consciousness (for the sake of simplicity we do not distinguish here).

The relational self/proto-self may be characterized by some kind of "sense of relatedness" between organism and environment, as a primordial attachment of the organ-

---

1 A rather broad meaning of the term phenomenal is assumed here to include various features like qualia, intentionality, unity and homogeneity, transparency, etc., which, due to reasons of space, cannot be discussed in further detail here.

ism to and integration within its respective environment. We assume that this "sense of relatedness" describing the co-occurrence between self and consciousness at this basic level is shared across species. However, this may no longer be true for higher forms of consciousness and self. At higher, more cognitive levels, both self and consciousness may dissociate from each other; for instance, higher-order cognition may allow introspection of one's self, thereby allowing an organism to distinguish and demarcate itself clearly from the environment. This demarcation may be experienced as a "sense of distinction" between self and environment. Due to different cognitive equipment, this "sense of distinction" and thus higher-order more cognitive forms of self (like "extended self," narrative self," dialogical self," "autobiographical self," etc.; see Damasio, 1999, Northoff et al., 2006, Bekoff & Sherman, 2004) may no longer be shared across species.

Of course the various levels of self surely interact with each other. The basic sense of self may be considered the foundation upon which higher-order forms of self may be implemented; the former may thus be considered the "core" around which, similar to an onion, different layers are constituted. There may consequently be a two-way interaction among the various layers of the self. The proto- and core-self may drive and determine the higher-forms of self; if the former is deficient (e.g., too much separation distress and insecurity during development), the latter may be rather fragile and volatile, as is the case in psychiatric problems like borderline personality disorder, where patients no longer experience some stable "sense of relatedness" and "core-self." However, the reverse direction may also be possible; that is, the higher-order cognitive forms of self modulating the basic "core-self," for instance, overriding the "sense of relatedness" and the associated emotions with a stronger "sense of distinction" and the respective cognitions.

One critical empirical question is, are neural substrates and mechanisms involved in such self-related processes, and thus is the core-self common among species? From an evolutionary perspective, the lower aspects are by necessity closely related (homologous). We here assume an SCMS, running from midbrain with greatest concentrations in the periaqueductal grey, which is well connected to higher midline cortical regions, constituting a core set of interrelated structures involved in creation of a basic sense of self – the "sense of relatedness" across different species. The lowest aspects of this network are genetically provided, and they appear sufficient to sustain raw perceptual and affective levels of phenomenal consciousness co-occurring with a "sense of relatedness" (Merker, 2007; Panksepp, 1998a; Shewmon et al., 1999). The higher aspects of the system allow the rest of the brain to become molded to fit cultural and ecological environments. It has been much easier to clarify the lower substrates scientifically through animal brain research, where very similar basic emotional processes are elaborated across all mammalian species that have been studied (Panksepp, 1982, 1998a, 1998b) and to empirically study the higher substrates through human neuropsychological and brain imaging approaches (Northoff et al., 2006). The conjunction of findings has fostered the present integration of perspectives to yield a more complete picture of the core-self.

SRP and the Subcortical-Cortical Midline System (SCMS)

Recent imaging studies in humans show various cortical regions, predominantly the so-called cortical midline structures (CMS), to be involved in SRP (see Northoff & Bermpohl, 2004; Northoff et al., 2006; Uddin, Iacobini, Lange, & Keenan, 2007) that are integrated with subcortical SELF processes to yield an integrated subcortical-cortical midline system (SCMS). Although some authors, like Gillihan and Farah (2005), do not yet see supporting evidence for localizing the epicenters of selfhood in particular brain regions, that may be because the concept covers so much territory and needs to be parsed at minimum into nomothetic and idiographic variants as we do here. In our estimation, as supported by a mass of empirical evidence (Northoff et al., 2006), there are specific brain regions most critically important for constituting the higher reaches of a core-nomothetic self-referential network. The question arises whether the very same higher medial frontal brain regions are present and also implicated in self-relatedness in animals. The stream of evidence runs thinner here than with respect to the deeper, subcortical midline SELF systems (Holstege & Saper, 2005; Panksepp, 1998a, 1998b). Thus, even if the higher midline regions are structurally homologous across species, this does not yet confirm that there is functional homology (e.g., they mediate SRP in animals as well as humans). How, then, does one develop translational models of SRP across species?

Trans-species investigations could employ various strategies to establish trans-species models of the self. One might investigate the same brain regions in human and animal resting states with the same imaging methodology as fMRI or PET and then directly compare regional neural activity and its intrinsic connectivity. Indeed, some recent work of this type has revealed that the aforementioned cortical midline structures do show a similar pattern of neural activity and connectivity (see below for details as well as Vincent et al. 2007; Rilling et al. 2007). Such trans-species anatomical models might be extended by employing the same task, with the same behavioral parameters, in both animals and humans during imaging. One such example is Gallup's self-face recognition, which is a mirror test in monkeys (Gallup, 1998) and other animals (Plotnik, de Waal, & Reiss, 2007, Reiss & Marinao 2001) that has already been applied in human imaging (Keenan, Freund, Hamilton, Ganis, & Pascual-Leone, 2000). Or one could stimulate pets (dogs, cats) and humans with the same empathy task (Vitulli, 2006) during brain imaging, thus establishing what might be called a trans-species anatomical-functional model of the self. Finally, even the relationship between self-relatedness and consciousness may be studied across species. A recent study by Northoff et al. (2009) distinguished between subjective experience of emotions and self-relatedness and found both dissociation and overlap in their respective neural correlates, for example, in different subcortical and cortical midline regions. Such investigations could also be done in animals, though in a slightly modified way with, for instance, food preference stimuli and stimuli inducing anger. These various strategies might allow one to investigate not only structural, but also functional homologies across species.

These higher regions of the brain provide abundant regulatory control over subcortical brain regions (Liotti & Panksepp, 2004), permitting robust top-down modulation of instinctual urges. However, as already noted, from a fully integrated system perspective, there should also be abundant bottom-up modulation in the form of nested-hierarchies that permit not only bottom-up intrinsic linkages, but top-down controls to emerge (Northoff, Quin, & Feinberg, 2011). Indeed, there is likely to remain substantial primacy of the primordial levels, for damage to the lower substrates of this midline system impairs consciousness more than damage to higher brain regions (see Panksepp, 1998b; Watt & Pincus, 2004), and stimulation of the subcortical regions in humans and other animals powerfully control affective-cognitive processing (Heath, 1996; Northoff et al., 2011). In short, we envision the bottom-up control to prevail during early development, when organismic behaviors are controlled more by instinctual urges reflecting powerful (unconditional) emotional and motivational states, and the top-down to prevail in mature animals, especially in everyday decision making when affective states are more diverse and cognitively modulated.

The lowest regions of this distributed SCMS network include the Periaqueductal grey (PAG), the superior colliculi (SC), and the adjacent mesencephalic locomotor region (MLR) as well as preoptic areas, the hypothalamus, and dorsomedial thalamus (DMT) (Holstege, Bandler, & Saper, 1996; Panksepp, 1998a, 1998b). For example, the colliculi and the PAG are among the most richly connected areas of the brain (Strehler, 1991); both receive afferents from several exteroceptive sensory regions (occipital, auditory, somatosensory, gustatory, and olfactory cortex) and while receiving afferents from other interoceptive subcortical regions (Holstege et al., 1996; for an overview of this area, see Watt, 2000). In addition, the PAG and the colliculi are connected with the cortical midline structures (CMS) (Dujardin & Jürgens, 2005; Holstege & Saper, 2005). Since the same is true for the other subcortical midline regions mentioned, it is important to conceptualize the self-integrative lower brain systems to have intimate relationships with the higher CMS structures, which is anatomically the case (see Strehler, 1991, for overview); thus yielding a highly integrated SCMS in normal organisms and providing a complex infrastructure for self-referential processing of external information. Functionally, higher cortical regions might represent the functions that are primarily represented subcortically in a more detailed, specific, and reined way. This is, for example, clearly realized in the case of sensory and motor functions. Though both sensory and motor functions are already represented in subcortical regions like the PAG, basal ganglia, mesencephalic locomotor system, they are again represented in cortical regions, for example, somatosensory and motor cortices. This may allow these functions to be elaborated in more detail, complexly and specifically resolved, than is possible on the subcortical level.

Such an analysis is consistent with various lines of research showing that core self-related functioning involves both cortical and subcortical regions (Panksepp, 1998a; Northoff et al., 2009; Phan et al., 2004). Many imaging studies in humans have focused on cortical regions, in part because of the involvement of strong cognitive components such as evaluative judgments in the respective tasks (see Northoff et al., 2006). A recent human imaging study on SRP pursuing a less cognitive approach (i.e., without an evaluative judgment in the task) observed involvement of various subcortical regions like the hypothalamus, the DMT, the PAG, and the superior colliculi in addition to the higher cortical midline structures during evaluative SRP (Northoff, 2004; Northoff et al., 2009; Heinzel et al., 2005). Interestingly, these subcortical regions are enriched in the preeminent anatomies of basic emotional systems in all mammals (MacLean, 1990; Panksepp, 1998a). This provides empirical support for the trans-species involvement of an SCMS in SRP in humans as well as other vertebrates. In further support, Mobbs et al. (2007) recently imaged the cascade of brain arousal in these regions from the higher cognitive structures (even to the amygdala) when threat was far away to the most basic animal instinctual-emotional integrative systems (e.g., PAG) when it was nearby, using a predatory imminence task during human brain imaging.

The assumption of the SCMS as common across species implies that it should be independent of particular sensory modalities and other domains. This has indeed been demonstrated in a recent meta-analysis that compared all imaging studies on SRP conducted in different sensory modalities (e.g., auditory, visual, olfactory) and different domains such as verbal/vocal, emotional, social, facial, spatial, and memory (Northoff et al., 2006). These results support the idea of SRP domain-independence, reflecting a common process whose coordinated functioning comprises the basic sense of self. Since the SCMS is ubiquitous in all mammals, we propose a coherent cross species self-referential network for core consciousness that has more evolutionary homologies (universality) among the lower neural substrates and more diversity in the upper ones.

SRP and Emotions

SRP is not just a process of ownership identification. Each stimulus is either implicitly (e.g., affectively and autonomically) or explicitly (e.g., cognitively) evaluated according to its possible value for the organism. Value is expressed in action as well as affect (Panksepp, 1998a, 1998b, 2005a, 2005b). When objects and events are viewed *through the "eyes" of the organism*, stimuli are presumably no longer simply objective aspects of the world, but as in most humans, they become subjective and thereby emotionally colored with various positive or negative associations. For example, the Implicit Association Task (IAT) used in humans and based upon reaction time measures, assesses the degree of association between the self and positive versus negative concepts. Greenwald and Farnham (2000) observed that participants were much faster to respond when self-related items (e.g., their birth month) were paired with pleasant words than when self-related items were paired with unpleasant words. Hermans (1999) introduced a so-called valuation theory, a phenomenological theory of the self, where the self is conceived of as an organized process of valuation. This has also been a prominent theme in psychoanalysis (Green, 1999) and in neuroscience (Panksepp, 1998a, 2005a).

A valuation is considered any unit of meaning as having positive (pleasant) or negative (unpleasant) value by the individual – each valuation has an affective connotation, a feeling, which results in what William James (1892) described as "self-feeling" or "self-qualia" (Kircher & David, 2003). The process of valuation is therefore closely tied to what we describe as SRP. Subsequently, SRP may be understood more broadly as the characterization of stimuli as self-related through their association with specific affective or emotional qualities. Although experimental social psychology commonly only accepts two primordial affects, negative and positive (e.g., Barrett, 2006), in fact the evidence suggests the brain is genetically provided with the capacity to experience many distinct affects, and an epistemology has been outlined for how we can causally link them to neuroscientific understanding (Panksepp, 2005b, 2007a, 2007b, 2007c, 2007d), and recent meta-analysis of human brain imaging corroborate the segregation of various affective processes (Vytal & Hamann, 2010) with perhaps less variability in the memory encoding aspects of emotions (Murty, Ritchey, Adcock, & Labar, 2010). At the primary process (i.e., unconditioned) level, we conceive these to be the basic tools of the core-self, which allowed at least one major form of mentality – experienced affective states of the nervous system – to emerge in brain evolution. It remains possible that this was the primordial neural scaffolding for all forms of consciousness, especially since damage to the primary convergence zone of emotional systems in the core-SELF, the PAG, have devastating effects on consciousness (Bailey & Davis, 1942, 1943).

The close psychological linkage between self and emotions makes it rather difficult to dissociate both SRP and emotional processing in neural terms. Several studies investigating emotions observed activation in anterior CMS including the vmPFC (e.g., ventromedial prefrontal cortex), the ACC, and the dmPFC (e.g., dorsomedial prefrontal cortex; see Phan, Wager, Taylor, & Liberzon, 2002 for an overview). Does this involvement of anterior CMS during emotions indicate self-related processing? (Phan et al., 2002; Phan et al., 2004) investigated the degrees of self-relatedness during emotional processing. Subjects had to appraise the extent of personal association of emotionally salient pictures during fMRI. The fMRI results were correlated with subjective ratings (conducted after imaging) appraising the degree of self-relatedness of the picture content in a visual analogue scale. Regions associated with self-relatedness were located in the CMS including vmPFC, pACC (e.g., perigenual anterior cingulate cortex), and dmPFC, the latter two appearing only with increasing degrees of self-relatedness (other regions activated in relation to self-relatedness concerned the insula and the nucleus accumbens). The more self-related the picture content was appraised, the more activation was observed in these regions.

Other studies directly compared ratings of self-relatedness and emotional intensity/valence and observed neural activity in the dmPFC to be directly linked to SRP (Moran, Macrae, Heatherton, Wyland, & Kelley, 2006; Macrae, Moran, Heatherton, Banfield, & Kelley, 2004; see also Northoff et al., 2009; Heinzel et al., 2005). Subcortically, the nucleus accumbens was also found to be parametrically modulated by the degree of self-relatedness (Northoff et al., 2009), which suggests that self-related processing, as suggested by studies of reward seeking, somehow involves the anticipation of events and associated feelings of aliveness and eager anticipation rather than mere consummatory pleasure (Alcaro et al., 2007; Ikemoto & Panksepp, 1999; Panksepp, 1998a). Interestingly, the right amygdala, generally deemed to be *the* key integrator of negative emotions (in fact, many other brain regions are as important), has also been implicated in SRP (see Northoff et al., 2009; Phan et al., 2004; Phan et al., 2002; Murphy, Nimmo-Smith, & Lawrence, 2003) and emotional memories (Murty et al., 2010) reflecting already secondary-processing of emotionality. The apparent participation of these subcortical regions in self-relatedness is thus strongly indicative of the involvement of valuation and affective processes in self-related processing. We tentatively consider the amygdala and the nucleus accumbens as major convergence zones for self-related and emotional processing where the self-related relationships between core affects and valuation of external stimuli are solidified.

However, there is such a large number of basic affective processes that apply to primal *emotional* affects (e.g., anger, fear, etc.) and do not as clearly apply to *homeostatic* (e.g., hunger, thirst, etc.) and *sensory* affects (e.g., tastes, touches, and other stimuli on the body surface). For instance, it is clear that the insula has a primal affective mapping system that appears to integrate various bodily-homeostatic conditions to sensory environments (Craig, 2002, 2003). Thus, these more laterally situated limbic regions of the brain, long implicated in affective issues (MacLean, 1990), should be envisioned as places in the brain where meta-representations of sensory affects different from the basic emotional concerns of the self are organized. Providing the integration between intero- and exteroceptive stimuli, these regions may be crucial in intrinsically linking the organism to the environment in an implicit and automatic way and it is here where the basic sense of self, the trans-species core-SELF, may become reconstituted in an embedded and contextualized way.

SRP Is Implicit and Automatic

We assume that self-related information processing does not typically occur on an explicit and consciously *aware* level even though it may be rich in affective consciousness (Panksepp, 2000a, 2007c). Thus, we assume much of SRP to be either *cognitively* preconscious or unconscious and thus implicit, but accompanied by experienced shifts in affective feeling states that are prepropositional and hence hard to put into words. Koole, Dijksterhuis, and Knippenberg (2001) demonstrated that the so-called "name letter effect" or initial preference, people preferring letters that are contained in their own names especially at the beginning of their first name, occurs without conscious awareness. People judged words and letters associated with their own name as more beautiful than nonassociated ones while not reporting to have any thoughts about this. Another test tapping implicit self-esteem is the IAT as described above. Therefore, Lieberman, Jarcho, and Satpute (2004; see also Satpute and Lieberman, 2006) speaks of an X-system – an intuition-based implicit and automatic self-knowledge that is largely responsible for the social, intuition-based, context-dependent, affective, and automatic processes that guide our habits and impulses in daily life. The X-system is contrasted with a C-system, an evidence-based self-knowledge that involves cognitive and controlled (i.e., nonautomatic and conscious) processes of reflection that guide our cognitions when conflicts arise. Broadly speaking, the X-system may imply an implicit nomothetic self and thus what we called SRP, whereas the C-system may refer to an explicit or cognitive self that is more variable across individuals and hence idiographic (see below). Interestingly, Lieberman et al. (2004) investigated the neural correlates of these two systems of self-knowledge. They observed activation in the vmPFC, the nucleus accumbens, and amygdala during intuition-based self-knowledge whereas evidence-based self-knowledge induced activation in the lateral prefrontal cortex, hippocampus, and posterior parietal cortex.

Automatic processing can be defined in terms of various characteristics such as lack of conscious awareness, effortlessness, lack of intentionality, and an inability to control the process (see Anderson, Reznik, & Glassman, 2005; Koole et al., 2001). For example, SRP cannot be activated and deactivated at will. An individual may be able to influence and modulate the degree of self-relatedness a stimulus is attributed but we remain unable to escape the process of SRP as such altogether. The term "automatic processing" thus implies at least partial if not complete independence of SRP from cognitively conscious modulation as would be achieved through directed attention and explicit evaluation. Correspondingly, the concept of an automatic self (Koole et al., 2001) has been suggested and characterized by operating automatically at an implicit, cognitively nonreflective level, yielding automaticity in self-evaluation without deliberative thought, often in situations with decreased cognitive control, and commonly associated with positive emotions. This highlights a key dilemma in consciousness studies – namely, what may be cognitively subconscious may be affectively experienced, and what is affectively experienced may often be hard to specify cognitively.

Automatic and implicit processing of the self may be relevant in both linguistic and nonlinguistic species. Automatic and implicit SRP may account for a basic relation between organism and environment, the "sense of relatedness," which in turn may enable the organism to communicate nonverbally, independent of any linguistic abilities. Much of this could be expressed in emotional sounds, which directly reflect internal affective states. Conceptually, William James' assumption of rapid emotional processing occurring before cognitive awareness and Damasio's concept of background feelings may reflect some automatic processing in nonlinguistic species, which provides the basis for subjective experience and primary (e.g., affective) consciousness to occur. There is indeed evidence for such assumptions. For instance, even rats make positive affective sounds that fulfill many of the characteristics of social laughter (Panksepp, 2007c); the circuitry of this response lies along the SCMS and mediates rewarding feelings (Burgdorf, Wood, Kroes, Moskal, & Panksepp, 2007). A more complex example of such nonverbal communication is empathy, whereby an organism can relate to another one emotionally, which is present in both animals and humans. It is increasingly realized that animals do exhibit empathic behavioral processes, from mice (Chen, Panksepp, & Lahvis, 2009; Langford et al., 2006) to primates (Preston & de Waal, 2002), and that such abilities are dependent very much on social emotional systems (Watt, 2007), which may constitute the very foundation of higher forms of social communication, even human language (Panksepp, 2008, 2009/2010; Shanahan, 2007). Accordingly, the automatic and implicit processing of self-relatedness may provide us with a basic nonverbal means of communication with others, which as such remains independent of the presence or absence of linguistic abilities, but that may have been a key communicative substrate upon which linguistic abilities were built (Zinken, Knoll, & Panksepp, 2008) (see Figures 3.1 and 3.2).

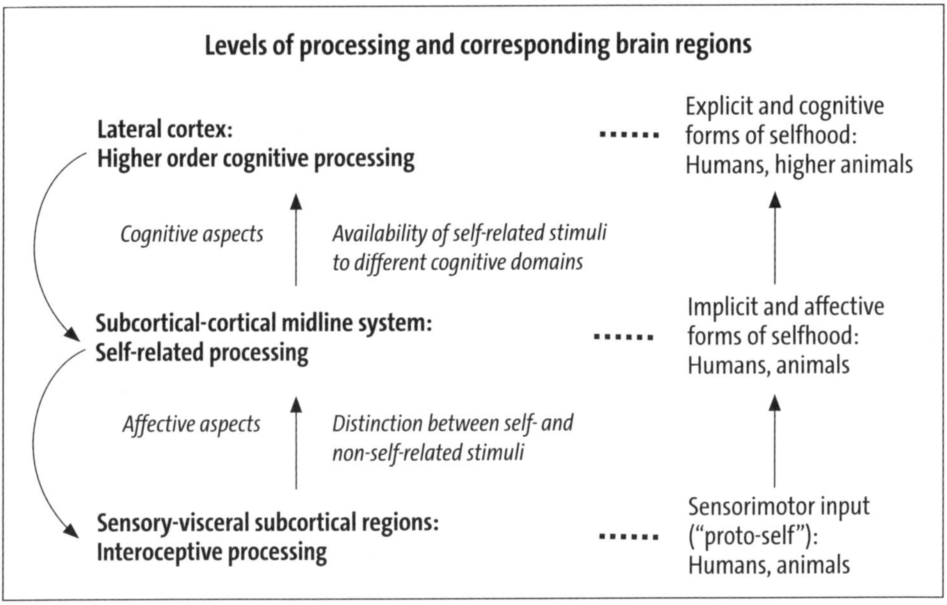

Figure 3.1. The figure presents the different characteristic features of the self that may be shared between humans and animals. This amounts to a trans-species representation of a basic sense of self.

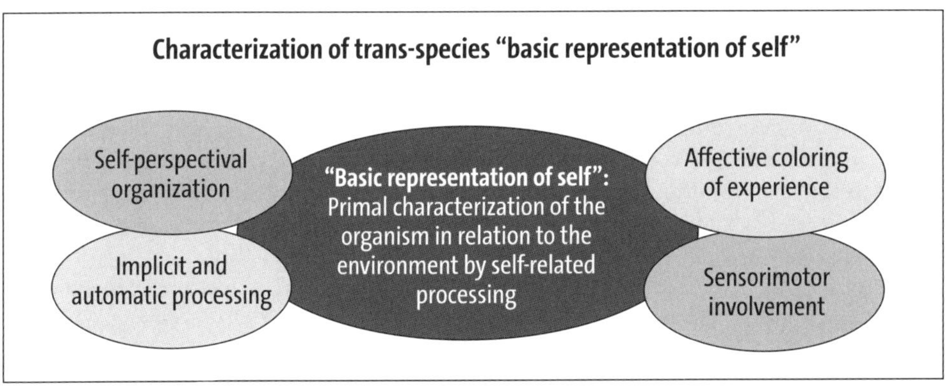

Figure 3.2. The figure shows the different levels of processing of the self in association with possible neural and psychological substrates in relation to different concepts of self given by a different author. Also pointed out is the level that may be shared between animals and humans.

Conclusion: Self and Emotions

Taken together, these results suggest that the linkage between self and emotions occur implicitly and therefore remains pre- or unconscious. SRP may consequently be characterized as affective and automatic and must therefore be distinguished from self-conscious awareness that is rather cognitive and explicit. How are the "implicit and affective forms of selfhood" (we assume these are the nomothetic aspects of the self) and the various "explicit and cognitive forms of selfhood" (the idiographic aspects) related to each other in neurobiological terms? Some studies reported activation (and increased functional connectivity) in anterior and posterior CMS during self-related tasks with low cognitive load (Kjaer, Nowak, & Lou, 2002; Greicius, Krasnow, Reiss, & Menon, 2003; Wicker et al., 2003; Lou et al., 2004). Conversely, deactivation (and low functional connectivity) in CMS has been observed in tasks with high cognitive load and low degrees of self-relatedness (Gusnard, Akbudak, Shulman, & Raichle, 2001; Gusnard & Raichle, 2001; Raichle et al., 2001; Simpson, Drevets, Snyder, Gusnard, & Raichle, 2001; Kelley et al., 2002; Greicius et al., 2003; Wicker et al., 2003; Vogeley et al., 2004).

These findings suggest reciprocal modulation between self-related and higher-order cognitive processing. Activation in CMS corresponds to SRP predominating, with higher-order processing remaining in the background. In contrast, deactivation in CMS reflects increased higher-order processing while SRP shifts into the background. The assumption of reciprocal modulation between self-related and higher-order deliberate cognitive processing is clearly compatible with the recent observation of reciprocal modulation between medial and lateral prefrontal cortex during emotional-cognitive interaction (Goel & Dolan, 2003; Northoff & Bermpohl, 2004; Northoff et al., 2004). At present, however, comparable reciprocal modulation between medial and lateral prefrontal cortex remains to be demonstrated for the interaction between self-related and higher-order information processing.

In addition to the apparently reciprocal modulation between medial and lateral prefrontal cortical regions, we assume convergence in the interaction between subcortical and cortical midline regions. Subcortical regions may determine the basic self-relatedness of the organism by coding the relation between different stimuli: interoceptive, motor, and exteroceptive. This relation is expressed in affective and valuative terms. The resulting "sense of relatedness" may then be further elaborated in cortical midline regions in cognitive and temporal terms. Higher-order cognitive abilities like attention, impulse control, working memory, executive functions, and so forth, may allow a representation of the "sense of relatedness" on a cognitive or mental level independent of any actual stimulus. This allows an organism to distinguish one's "sense of relatedness" from others' "sense of relatedness," and thus from the environment, resulting in what we earlier called a "sense of distinction." Depending on the cognitive equipment and the prefrontal cortical development, different species may or may not share the ability to explicitly distinguish themselves to varying degrees from others and from their environment. However, the data stream runs thin on such a conjecture. In fact, even laboratory rats and mice are quite adept at distinguishing individual others via their olfactory signatures, a test that has been effectively used as a measure of social memory (Dantzer, 1998).

Beside such cognitive elaborations, cortical midline regions may also regulate the subcortically established "sense of relatedness" temporally. Recent studies in humans indicate that the cortical midline structures are involved in both anticipating future events and recollecting past events (Schacter, Addis, & Buckner, 2007; Szpunar & McDermott, 2008; Buckner and Carroll, 2007; Addis, Wong & Schacter, 2007). Furthermore, a recent human imaging study demonstrated that self-relatedness induced delayed signal changes in cortical midline structures when compared to subcortical ones (Schneider et al., 2008). However, further confirmation of these findings, not only in humans, but also in animals, is needed. Taken together, this leads to a rather speculative assumption that cortical midline structures may be crucially involved in temporally extending the subcortically processed self-relatedness. By delaying or anticipating neural activity and dissociating it from the presence of actually impinging stimuli, cortical midline structures may put the already established self-relatedness into a wider temporal mental context when compared to subcortical regions where it seems to be tied to the actual presence of internal or external stimuli and state-control functions (e.g., basic homeostatic and emotional states).

The main difference between different species might then lie not so much in the presence or absence of self-relatedness but rather in the width of the temporal span (e.g., from the disappearance of the stimulus on) across which the stimulus' degree of self-relatedness can be processed and thus maintained. In other terms, cortical elaboration may extend the temporal window of self-relatedness (and consciousness) and may potentially make it more independent of the actual stimulus presence, which in turn allows for higher cognitive abilities like introspection (i.e., the so-called *mind's eye*) to interact with phenomenal consciousness and pre-reflective self-awareness, resulting in reflective consciousness and reflective self-awareness (see above). We must admit though, this neuro-temporal subcortical-cortical hypothesis remains hypothetical at this point since the underlying neurophysiological mechanisms for such psychic functions remain to be empirically clarified. Still, certain lines of thought would implicate ascending medially situated ascending dopamine systems, essential for SEEKING urges in all animals, which innervate higher brain more extensively in primates than rodents (Berger, Gaspar, & Verney, 1991), to expand and extend spatio-temporal processes in the brain (Previc, 1999). Further analysis of such subtle issues will require the development of much better empirical network analysis tools than we currently have.

References

Addis D. R., Wong A. T., & Schacter D. L. (2007). Remembering the past and imagining the future: Common and distinct neural substrates during event construction and elaboration. *Neuropsychologia, 45*, 1363–1377.

Alcaro, A., Huber, R., & Panksepp, J. (2007). Behavioral functions of the mesolimbic dopaminergic system: An affective neuroethological perspective. *Brain Research Reviews, 56*, 283–321.

Anderson, S., Reznik, I., & Glassman, N. (2005). The unconscious relational self. In B. Hassin, J. S. Uleman, & J. A. Bargh (Eds.), *The new unconscious* (pp. 421–485). Cambridge, MA: MIT Press.

Bailey, P., & Davis, E. W. (1942). Effects of lesions of the periaqueductal gray matter in the cat. *Proceedings of the Society for Experimental Biology and Medicine, 351*, 305–306.

Bailey, P., & Davis, E. W. (1943). Effects of lesions of the periaqueductal gray matter on the Macaca Mulatta. *Journal of Neuropathology and Experimental Neurology, 3*, 69–72.

Barrett, L. F. (2006). Solving the emotion paradox: Categorization and the experience of emotion. *Personality and social psychology review, 10*(1), 20–46.

Bekoff, M., & Sherman, P. W. (2004). Reflections on animal selves. *Trends in Ecology and Evolution, 19*, 176–180.

Berger, B., Gaspar, P., & Verney, C. (1991). Dopaminergic innervation of the cerebral cortex: Unexpected differences between rodents and primates. *Trends in Neurosciences, 14*, 21–27.

Buckner, R. L., & Carroll, D. C. (2007). Self-projection and the brain. *Trends in Cognitive Sciences, 11*, 49–57.

Burgdorf, J., Wood, P. L., Kroes, R. A., Moskal, J. R., & Panksepp, J. (2007). Neurobiology of 50–kHz ultrasonic vocalizations in rats: Electrode mapping, lesion, and pharmacology studies. *Behavioral Brain Research, 182*, 274–283.

Clayton, N. S., Bussey, J. T., & Dickinson, A. (2003). Can animals recall the past and plan the future? *Nature Reviews Neuroscience, 4*, 685–691.

Chen, Q., Panksepp, J. B., & Lahvis, G. P. (2009). Empathy is moderated by genetic background in mice. *PlosOne, 2*, e351.

Craig, A. D. (2002). How do you feel? Interoception: The sense of the physiological condition of the body. *Nature Reviews Neuroscience, 3*(8), 655–666.

Craig, A. D. (2003). Interoception: The sense of the physiological condition of the body. *Current Opinion in Neurobiology, 13*, 500–505.

Damasio, A. R. (1999). *The feeling of what happens: Body and emotion in the making of consciousness.* New York: Harcourt Brace.

Dantzer, R. (1998). Vasopressin, gonadal steroids and social recognition. *Progress in Brain Research, 119*, 409–414.

Dujardin, E., & Jürgens, U. (2005). Afferents of vocalization-controlling periaqueductal regions in the squirrel monkey. *Brain Research, 1034*(1–2), 114–131.

Foote, A. L. & Crystal, J. D. (2007). Metacognition in the rat. *Current Biology, 17*, 551–555.

Gallup, G. G., Jr. (1998). Self-awareness and the evolution of social intelligence. *Behavioural Processes, 42*, 239–247.

Gillihan, S. J., & Farah, M. J. (2005). Is self special? A critical review of evidence from experimental psychology and cognitive neuroscience. *Psychological Bulletin, 131*(1), 76–97.

Goel, V., & Dolan, R. J. (2003). Reciprocal neural response within lateral and ventral medial prefrontal cortex during hot and cold reasoning. *Neuroimage, 20*, 2314–2321.

Green, A. (1999) *The fabric of affect in the psychoanalytic discourse*. London: Routledge.

Greenwald, A., & Farnham, S. (2000). Using the implicit association test to measure self-esteem and self-concept. *Journal of Personality and Social Psychology, 79*, 1022–38.

Greicius, M. D., Krasnow, B., Reiss, A. L., & Menon, V. (2003). Functional connectivity in the resting brain: A network analysis of the default mode hypothesis. *Proceedings of the National Academy of Sciences, USA, 100*, 253–258.

Gusnard, D. A., Akbudak, E., Shulman, G. L., & Raichle, M. E. (2001). Medial prefrontal cortex and self-referential mental activity: Relation to a default mode of brain function. *Proceedings of the National Academy of Sciences, USA, 98*, 4259–4264.

Gusnard, D. A., & Raichle, M. E. (2001). Searching for a baseline: Functional imaging and the resting human brain. *Nature Reviews Neuroscience, 2*, 685–694.

Heath, R. (1996). *Exploring the mind-body relationship.* Baton Rouge, LA: Moran Printing.

Heinzel, A., Bermpohl, F., Niese, R., Pfennig, A., Pascual-Leone, A., Schlaug, G., & Northoff, G. (2005). How do we modulate our emotions? Parametric fMRI reveals cortical midline structures as regions specifically involved in the processing of emotional valences. *Brain Research Cognitive Brain Research, 25*, 348–358.

Hermans, H. J. (1999). Self-narrative as meaning construction: The dynamics of self-investigation. *Journal of Clinical Psychology, 55*(10), 1193–1211.

Holstege, G. R., Bandler, R., & Saper, C. B. (1996). The emotional motor system. In G. Holstege, R. Bandler, & C. B. Saper (Eds.), *Progress in brain research: Vol 170. The emotional motor system* (pp. 3–6). Amsterdam: Elsevier.

Holstege, G. R., & Saper, C. B. (2005). Special Issue: The anatomy of the soul. *Journal of Comparative Neurology, 493*, 1–176.

Ikemoto, S., & Panksepp, J. (1999). The role of nucleus accumbens dopamine in motivated behavior: A unifying interpretation with special reference to reward-seeking. *Brain Research Reviews, 31*, 6–41.

James, W. (1892). *Psychology*. New York: Henry Holt and Company.

Keenan, J. P., Freund, S., Hamilton, R. H., Ganis, G., & Pascual-Leone, A. (2000). Hand response differences in a self-face identification task. *Neuropsychologia, 38*, 1047–1053.

Kelley, W. M., Macrae, C. N., Wyland, C. L., Caglar, S., Inati, S., & Heatherton, T. F. (2002). Finding the self? An event-related fMRI study. *Journal of Cognitive Neuroscience, 14*, 785–794.

Kircher, T., & David, A. (2003). *The self in neuroscience and psychiatry*. Oxford/New York: Oxford University Press.

Kjaer, T. W., Nowak, M., & Lou, H. C. (2002). Reflective self-awareness and conscious states: PET evidence for a common midline parietofrontal core. *Neuroimage, 17*, 1080–1086.

Kolb, B., & Tees, C. (Eds.). (2000). *The cerebral cortex of the rat.* Cambridge, MA: MIT Press.

Koole, S., Dijksterhuis, A., & Knippenberg, A. (2001). What's in a name: Implicit self-esteem and the automatic self. *Journal of Personality and Social Psychology, 80*, 669–685.

Lambie, J. A., & Marcel, A. J. (2002). Consciousness and the varieties of emotion experience: A theoretical framework. *Psychological Review, 109*(2), 219–259.

Langford, D. J., Crager, S. E., Shehzad, Z., Smith, S. B., Sotocinal, S. G., Levenstadt, J. S., . . . Mogil, J. S. (2006). Social modulation of pain as evidence for empathy in mice. *Science, 312*, 1967–1970.

Lieberman, M. D., Jarcho, J. M., & Satpute, A. B. (2004). Evidence-based and intuition-based self-knowledge: An FMRI study. *Journal of Personality and Social Psychology, 87*, 421–435.

Liotti, M., & Panksepp, J. (2004). Imaging human emotions and affective feelings: Implications for biological psychiatry. In J. Panksepp (Ed.), *Textbook of Biological Psychiatry* (pp. 33–74). Hoboken, NJ: Wiley.

Lou, H. C., Luber, B., Crupain, M., Keenan, J. P., Nowak, M., Kjaer, T. W., ... Lisanby, S. H. (2004). Parietal cortex and representation of the mental Self. *Proceedings of the National Academy of Sciences, USA, 101*(17), 6827–6832.

MacLean, P. D. (1990). *The Triune Brain in Evolution: Role in Paleocerebral Functions*. New York: Plenum.

Macrae, C. N., Moran, J. M., Heatherton, T. F., Banfield, J. F., & Kelley, W. M. (2004). Medial prefrontal activity predicts memory for self. *Cerebral Cortex, 14*, 647–654.

Mendl, M., Burman, O. H. P., & Paul, E. S. (2010). An integrative and functional framework for the study of animal emotion and mood. *Proceedings of Royal Society. Biological Sciences, 277*, 2895–2904.

Merker, B. (2007). Consciousness without a cerebral cortex: A challenge for neuroscience and medicine. *Behavioral and Brain Sciences, 30*(1), 63–81.

Metzinger, T. (2003). *Being no one: The self-model theory of subjectivity*. Cambridge, MA: MIT Press.

Mobbs, D., Petrovic, P., Marchant, J. , Hassabis, D., Seymour, B., Weiskopf, N., … Frith, C. D. (2007). When fear is near: Threat imminence elicits prefrontal-periaqueductal gray shifts in humans. *Science, 317*, 1079–1083.

Moran, J. M., Macrae, C. N., Heatherton, T. F., Wyland, C. L., & Kelley, W. M. (2006). Neuroanatomical evidence for distinct cognitive and affective components of self. *Journal of Cognitive Neuroscience, 18*, 1586–1594.

Murphy, F. C., Nimmo-Smith, I., & Lawrence, A. D. (2003). Functional neuroanatomy of emotions: A meta-analysis. *Cognitive, Affective, & Behavioral Neuroscience, 3*, 207–233.

Murty, V. P., Ritchey, M., Adcock, R. A., & Labar, K. S. (2010). Reprint of: fMRI studies of successful emotional memory encoding: A quantitative meta-analysis. *Neuropsychologia, 49*(4), 695–705.

Northoff, G. (2004). *Philosophy of the brain. The brain problem*. Amsterdam: John Benjamins.

Northoff, G., & Bermpohl, F. (2004). Cortical midline structures and the self. *Trends in Cognitive Sciences, 8*, 102–107.

Northoff, G., Heinzel, A., Bermpohl, F., Niese, R., Pfennig, A., Pascual-Leone, A., & Schlaug, G. (2004). Reciprocal modulation and attenuation in the prefrontal cortex: An fMRI study on emotional-cognitive interaction. *Human Brain Mapping, 21*, 202–212.

Northoff, G., Heinzel, A., de Greck, M., Bermpohl, F., Dobrowolny, H., & Panksepp, J. (2006). Self-referential processing in our brain – a meta-analysis of imaging studies on the self. *Neuroimage, 31*, 440–457.

Northoff, G., Schneider, F., Walter, M., Bermpohl, F., Heinzel, A., Tempelmann, C., . . . Panksepp, J. (2009). Differential parametric modulation of self-relatedness and emotions in different brain regions. *Human Brain Mapping, 30*(2), 369–382.

Northoff, G., Quin, P., & Feinberg, T. E. (2011). Brain imaging of the self – conceptual, anatomical and methodological issues. *Consciousness and Cognition, 20*, 52–63.

Panksepp, J. (1982). Toward a general psychobiological theory of emotions. *The Behavioral and Brain Sciences*, *5*, 407–467.

Panksepp, J. (1998a). *Affective neuroscience: The foundations of human and animal emotions.* New York: Oxford University Press.

Panksepp, J. (1998b). The periconscious substrates of consciousness: Affective states and the evolutionary origins of the SELF. *Journal of Consciousness Studies, 5,* 566–582.

Panksepp, J. (2000a). Affective consciousness and the instinctual motor system: The neural sources of sadness and joy. In R. Ellis & N. Newton (Eds.), *The caldron of consciousness: Motivation, affect and self-organization, advances in consciousness research* (pp. 27–54). Amsterdam: John Benjamins.

Panksepp, J. (2000b). The cradle of consciousness: A periconscious emotional homunclus? *Neuro-Psychoanalysis, 2,* 24–32.

Panksepp, J. (2000c). A home for the soul: The neuroanatomy of the primal self. (Review of Damasio's "The feeling of what happens: Body and emotion in the making of consciousness"). *Neuro-Psychoanalysis, 2,* 81–88.

Panksepp, J. (2002). The self and "its" vicissitudes: Critique of the commentaries. *Neuropsychoanalysis, 4*, 44–61.

Panksepp, J. (2005a). Affective consciousness: Core emotional feelings in animals and humans. *Consciousness and Cognition, 14*(1), 30–80.

Panksepp, J. (2005b). On the embodied neural nature of the core emotional affects. *Journal of Consciousness Studies, 5,* 158–184.

Panksepp J. (2007a). Affective Consciousness. In M. Velmans, & S. Schneider (Eds.) *The Blackwell Companion to Consciousness.* (pp. 114–129). Malden, MA: Blackwell Publishing, Ltd.

Panksepp, J. (2007b). Emotional feelings originate below the neocortex: Toward a neurobiology of the soul. Behavioral and Brain Sciences, 30, 101–103.

Panksepp, J. (2007c). The neuroevolutionary and neuroaffective psychobiology of the prosocial brain. In R. I. M. Dunbar & L. Barrett (Eds.), *The Oxford handbook of evolutionary psychology* (pp. 145–162). Oxford: Oxford University Press.

Panksepp, J. (2007d). Neuroevolutionary sources of laughter and social joy: Modeling primal human laughter in laboratory rats. *Behavioral Brain Research, 182*, 231–244.

Panksepp, J. (2008). The power of the word may reside in the power of affect. Integrative Physiological and Behavioral Science, 42, 47–55.

Panksepp, J. (2009/2010). The emotional antecedents to the evolution of music and language. Special Issue of *Musicae Scientiae,* devoted to "Music and Evolution," 229–259.

Panksepp, J., & Biven, L. (2011). *The archaeology of mind: Neuroevolutionary origins of human emotions.* New York: Norton.

Panksepp, J., Normansell, L. A., Cox, J. K. F., & Siviy, S. (1994). Effects of neonatal decortication on the social play of juvenile rats. *Physiology & Behavior, 56*, 429–443.

Phan, K. L., Taylor, S. F., Welsh, R. C., Ho, S. H., Britton, J. C., & Liberzon, I. (2004). Neural correlates of individual ratings of emotional salience: A trial-related fMRI study. *Neuroimage, 21*, 768–780.

Phan, K. L., Wager, T., Taylor, S. F., & Liberzon, I. (2002). Functional neuroanatomy of emotion: A meta-analysis of emotion activation studies in PET and fMRI. *Neuroimage, 16*, 331–348.

Plotnik, J. M., de Waal, F. B. M., & Reiss, D. (2007). Self-recognition in an Asian elephant. *Proceedings of the National Academy of Sciences of the United States of America, 103*, 17053–17057.

Preston, S. D., & de Waal, B. M. (2002). Empathy: Its ultimate and proximate bases. *Behavioral and Brain Sciences, 25*, 1–72.

Previc, F. H. (1999). Dopamine and the origins of human intelligence. *Brain and Cognition, 41*, 299–350.

Raichle, M. E., MacLeod, A. M., Snyder, A. Z., Powers, W. J., Gusnard, D. A., & Shulman, G. L. (2001). A default mode of brain function. *Proceedings of the National Academy of Sciences, USA, 98*(2), 676–682.

Reiss, D., & Marinao, L. (2001). Mirror self-recognition in the bottlenose dolphin: A case of cognitive convergence. *Proceedings of the National Acadamey of Sciences of the United States of America, 98*(10), 5937–5942.

Rilling, J. K., Glenn, A. L., Jairam, M. R., Pagnoni, G., Goldsmith, D. R., Elfenbein, H. A., & Lilienfeld, S. O. (2007). Neural correlates of social cooperation and non-cooperation as a function of psychopathy. *Biological Psychiatry, 61*, 1260–1271.

Satpute, A. B., & Lieberman, M. D. (2006). Integrating automatic and controlled processes into neurocognitive models of social cognition. *Brain Research, 1079*, 86–97.

Schacter, D. L., Addis, D. R., & Buckner, R. L. (2007). Remembering the past to imagine the future: The prospective brain. *Nature Reviews Neuroscience, 8*, 657–667.

Schneider, F., Bermpohl, F., Heinzel, A., Rotte, M., Walter, M., Tempelmann, C., ... Northoff, G. (2008). The resting brain and our self: Self-relatedness modulates resting state neural activity in cortical midline structures. *Neuroscience, 157*(1), 120–131.

Shanahan, D. (2007). *Language, feeling, and the brain.* New Brunswick, NJ: Transaction Publishers.

Shewmon, D. A., Holmse, D. A., & Byrne, P. A. (1999). Consciousness in congenitally decorticate children: Developmental vegetative state as self-fulfilling prophecy. *Developmental Medicine and Child Neurology, 41*, 364–374.

Simpson, J. R., Jr., Drevets, W. C., Snyder, A. Z., Gusnard, D. A., & Raichle, M E. (2001). Emotion-induced changes in human medial prefrontal cortex: II. During anticipatory anxiety. *Proceedings of the National Academy of Sciences, USA, 98*, 688–693.

Smith, J. D., Shields, W. E., & Washburn, D. A. (2003). The comparative psychology of uncertainty monitoring and metacognition. *Behavioural Brain Sciences, 26*, 317–373.

Strehler, B. L. (1991). Where is the self? A neuroanatomical theory of consciousness. *Synapse, 7*, 44–91.

Szpunar, K. K., & McDermott, K. B. (2008). Episodic future thought: Remembering the past to imagine the future. In K. Markmam, J. A. Suhr, & W. M. P. Klein (Eds.), *The handbook of imagination and mental simulation* (pp. 119–129). New York: Psychology Press.

Uddin, L. Q., Iacoboni, M., Lange, C., & Keenan, J. P. (2007). The self and social cognition: The role of cortical midline structures and mirror neurons. *Trends in Cognitive Sciences, 11*, 153–157.

Van Gulick, R. (2004). Consciousness. *Stanford Encyclopedia of Philosophy*. Retrieved from http://plato.stanford.edu/entries/consciousness/

Vincent, J. L., Patel, G. H., Fox, M. D., Snyder, A. Z., Baker, J. T., Van Essen, D. C., . . . Raichle, M. E. (2007). Intrinsic functional architecture in the anaesthetized monkey brain. *Nature, 447*, 83–86.

Vitulli, W. F. (2006). Attitudes toward empathy in domestic dogs and cats. *Psychological Reports, 99*(3), 981–991.

Vogeley, K., May, M., Ritzl, A., Falkai, P., Zilles, K., & Fink, G. R. (2004). Neural correlates of first-person perspective as one constituent of human self-consciousness. *Journal of Cognitive Neuroscience, 16*, 817–827.

Vytal, K., & Hamann, S. (2010). Neuroimaging Support for Discrete Neural Correlates of Basic Emotions: A Voxel-Based Meta-Analysis. *Journal of Cognitive Neuroscience, 22*, 1–22.

Watt, D. F. (2000). The centrencephalon and thalamocortical integration. Neglected contributions of periaqueductal gray. *Consciousness & Emotion, 1*, 91–114.

Watt, D. F. (2007). Towards a neuroscience of empathy: Integrating affective and cognitive perspectives. *Neuro-Psychoanalysis, 9*, 119–140.

Watt, D. F., & Pincus, D. I. (2004). Neural substrates of consciousness: Implications for clinical psychiatry. In J. Panksepp (Ed.), *Textbook of Biological Psychiatry* (pp. 627–660). Hoboken, NJ: Wiley.

Wicker, B., Keysers, C., Plailly, J., Royet, J. P., Gallese, V., & Rizzolatti, G. (2003). Both of us disgusted in my insula: The common neural basis of seeing and feeling disgust. *Neuron, 40*(3), 655–664.

Zahavi, D. (2003). Phenomenology of the self. In T. Kircher & A. S. David (Eds.), *The self in neuroscience and psychiatry* (pp. 56–75). Cambridge, UK: Cambridge University Press.

Zinken, J., Knoll, M., & Panksepp, J. (2008). Universality and diversity in the vocaliztion of emotions. In K. Izdebski (Ed.), *Emotions in the human voice, Vol. 1. Foundations* (pp. 185–202). San Diego, CA: Plural Publishing Inc.

Georg Northoff
Institute of Mental Health Research
University of Ottawa
1145 Carling Avenue
Ottawa, ON K1Z 7K4
Canada
E-mail: georg.northoff@theroyal.ca

III. The Interplay Between Culture and Emotion Regulation

Implications for Mental Health

Chapter 4

Socialization of Emotions and Emotion Regulation in Cultural Context

Gisela Trommsdorff and Tobias Heikamp

University of Konstanz, Germany

Abstract

In this chapter, universal and culture-specific aspects of socialization of emotion regulation are discussed. Emotions and emotion regulation are socialized and develop in cultural contexts. Cultural views on self-other relations are the basis for the child's agentic self and emotion regulation affecting the socio-emotional adjustment in the respective culture. Cultural models of self-other relations are transmitted through socialization processes such as parenting beliefs and practices, which can differ in their specific cultural meaning and therefore affect emotion regulation differently. This chapter discusses cross-cultural studies on the function of parental support, control, and sensitivity for emotional development and regulation. Cultural differences shed light on the importance of taking the cultural context into account when studying emotion regulation and socio-emotional competence. Possible consequences for planning intervention programs are discussed.

Keywords: culture, socialization, development, emotions, emotion regulation, self

Children grow up in a developmental niche as part of the broader culture. The socialization goals for emotion regulation aim to foster the development of culturally adequate regulation in accordance with the respective cultural values. The resulting cultural fit can be understood as cultural emotional competence (Friedlmeier & Trommsdorff, 2002; Trommsdorff, 2007a). However, research on emotion regulation and related concepts is usually based on Western studies, usually of adult (student) samples from WEIRD (Western, Educated, Industrialized, Rich, and Democratic) societies (Henrich, Heine, & Norenzayan, 2010).

So far, only a few culture-informed studies on the development and socialization of emotion regulation are available (for reviews see Cole, Dennis, Martin, & Hall, 2008;

Cole & Tan, 2006; Friedlmeier, Corapci, & Cole, 2011; Heikamp, Trommsdorff, & Fäsche, in press; Mesquita & Albert, 2007; Rothbaum & Rusk, 2011; Trommsdorff, 2006, 2012; Trommsdorff & Cole, 2011; Trommsdorff & Rothbaum, 2008). Empirical findings have shown cultural and individual differences in the preference of open versus restricted emotional expression or socially disengaging (anger) versus engaging (shame) emotions (Kitayama, 2001; Markus & Kitayama, 1991). These findings can be interpreted as indicating different cultural values and models of agency that affect development of emotion regulation. It will be questioned whether claims for a generalization of such species-specific samples is justified. Before we review some research findings, which call this generalization into further question, we need to clarify the meaning of the term *emotion regulation*.

Emotion regulation is defined here as a skill and as a motivated goal-directed behavior based on agency, a major factor in the general development of self-regulation. Emotion regulation generally refers to the regulation of emotion-related physiological responses, motivational states, experience, and associated behaviors "in the service of accomplishing affect-related biological or social adaptation or achieving individual goals" (Eisenberg & Spinrad, 2004, p. 338). From a developmental perspective, maturational and experience-based changes in effortful inhibitory control (e.g., voluntary behavior inhibition, attention processes) are associated with the development of emotion regulation and related responses (e.g., coping with stress) (Blair, 2010).

Taking a functionalist approach to emotion Saarni, Campos, Camras, and Witherington (2006) emphasize that emotions result from cognitive appraisals of events and influence evaluations of capacities to act: "Emotion is thus the person's attempt or readiness to establish, maintain, or change the relation between the person and his or her changing circumstances on matters of significance to that person" (p. 227). According to this view emotions are subject to regulation and have the capacity to influence other psychological processes (e.g., attention, motivation, cognition; Gross & Thompson, 2007). In line with this view on emotion, agentic regulation is assumed to be an activity that is motivated by the goal to fulfill one's needs in accordance with one's self-construal and self–other relations. "To be an agent is to intentionally influence one's functioning and life-circumstances" (Bandura, 2006, p. 164). Bandura (2006) describes the major properties of subjective (perceived) agency as intentionality, forethought, self-regulation, and self-reflectiveness. Agency is the dynamic force in regulatory goal-directed behavior underlying individual development in context (Trommsdorff, 2007a).

The ability for emotion regulation is complemented by the motivation and intention to self-regulate in order to achieve self-focused (e.g., improving one's individual status) or other-focused (e.g., improving the outcomes of the group) goals (Trommsdorff, 2009, 2012; Trommsdorff & Cole, 2011). Emotion regulation therefore is seen here as an intended or as an agentic, goal-directed act that develops in different stages. These stages range from infants' early understanding of physical and social agency influencing objects and people through behavior to children's more mature understanding of the self and of others as mental agents (see Gergely, 2002; Meltzoff, 1995; Tomasello, 1999, 2009; Wellman, 2009).

Early in development, caretakers play an important role as socialization agents for the development of emotion regulation within the family context (Morris, Silk, Steinberg, Myers, & Robinson, 2007). Socialization conditions are influenced by the broader sociocultural context and mediate between culture and individual development (Rothbaum, Pott, Azuma, Miyake, & Weisz, 2000; Rothbaum & Trommsdorff, 2007; Super & Harkness, 1997; Trommsdorff, 2007a). Taking culture into account suggests that socialization should be studied in relation to caretakers' intuitive beliefs about emotion socialization and parenting practices. These beliefs are seen as part of the developmental niche of the child, which is anchored in a cultural context based on a culture-specific meaning system for constructing the self, others, and social relations. The cultural context affects socialization conditions and thereby the development of emotion regulation. According to this theoretical framework the child is seen as agentic, contributing to his or her own development, both being influenced by proximate settings (e.g., family, school) and the wider sociocultural context (e.g., culture), and influencing the respective sociocultural context.

To summarize, emotion regulation is influenced by motivation, cognitive abilities, and subjective beliefs in self-other relations. Moreover, emotions influence the cognitive evaluation of capacities to act and the selection, initiation, and execution of actions. In the next sections we discuss relations of emotion regulation to cultural models of agency and control beliefs (and related views on the self and the world) and how these affect specific forms of regulatory behavior. In the first section, we examine some universal and some culture-specific aspects of emotion regulation (and aspects of coping). In the second section, we present a culture-informed perspective on the development of emotion regulation and discuss the role of parenting beliefs and practices for emotional development and development of emotion regulation. The summary underlines the importance of culture-informed studies for a better understanding of emotional development and emotion regulation.

Individualistic and Social-Oriented Approaches to Emotion Regulation: A Cultural View

Cultural Models of Agency and Their Relation to Emotion Regulation

Cultures are not homogenous entities, and socialization and developmental outcomes can comprise individualistic and relational facets depending on situational conditions (Greenfield, 2010; Raeff, 2010). Therefore, a simple dichotomy (e.g., individualism versus collectivism) may have a heuristic value but cannot account for the inter- and intra-cultural variance (see meta-analysis by Oyserman, Coon, & Kemmelmeier, 2002). The authors describe core elements of individualism as the value of independence and uniqueness, whereas core elements of collectivism are described as duty to in-group and maintaining harmony. These world views differ in the issues and values they make salient (Kağitçibaşi, 1997). There is no perfect solution to solve the problem of simplification by grouping cultural phenomena into types (such as individualism, collectivism; or "Gemeinschaft" and "Gesellschaft"). Both types, a purely descriptive approach illustrating a variety of phenomena and an "address" approach only naming the societies, lack a theoretical perspective on the psychological variables. To unpack culture (e.g., "Asian" societies), theoretically-based descriptions are needed (Bond & van de Vijver, 2011; Trommsdorff, 2012).

Trommsdorff (2009) suggested in line with others (Rothbaum & Trommsdorff, 2007) that development of emotion regulation is related to cultural models of agency and self-regulation. Cultural differences in models of agency have been described along the lines of independence and interdependence, individualism and collectivism, or disjoint and conjoint agency (see Markus & Kitayama, 1991, 1994, 2004; Markus, Uchida, Omoregie, Townsend, & Kitayama, 2006; Morris, Menon, & Ames, 2001). A basic difference between these models is the concern with individual autonomy and self-related goals versus the concern with social goals and harmony control. A major assumption of an individual-centered approach is that people strive for independence, self-fulfillment, and authentic expression of emotions based on autonomy. In contrast, for the majority of many non-Western (e.g., Asian) societies, a social-oriented approach is more appropriate because people there strive for interdependence and relatedness, regarding the self as embedded in social relationships (Kitayama, 2000; Markus & Kitayama, 1991; Triandis, 1989; see chapter 14). The related culture-specific development of emotions has been characterized as fostering socially disengaging (e.g., anger, pride) versus engaging (e.g., empathy) emotions (Kitayama, Mesquita, & Karasawa, 2006).

Most research on emotion regulation has taken an individual-centered approach, which is based on Western values emphasizing clear boundaries between one's self and others (Sampson, 1988; Spence, 1985). Accordingly, most psychological research on emotion regulation has focused on the individual person and the inner self. However, recent research on intergroup phenomena (Vohs, Lasaleta, & Fennis, 2009) as well as on cultural phenomena (Cohen & Hoshino-Browne, 2005; Rothbaum & Wang, 2010; Trommsdorff, 2009) has taken a social-oriented perspective into consideration, suggesting that emotion regulation can be motivated by the goal to act in accordance with relevant others' expectations. This perspective is in line with the notion of the interdependent self (Markus & Kitayama, 1991), and a broader view on the "cultural self" (different from the "conceptual" self) (Shweder et al., 1998), assuming a multifaceted, permeable, and context-dependent self. According to an individual-centered approach, self- and emotion regulation are agentic processes aimed at fostering independence and promoting self-focused emotions (e.g., pride). In contrast, according to a social-oriented approach of a cultural self, self- and emotion regulation are agentic processes aimed at fostering interdependence and promoting other-focused emotions (e.g., empathy).

The two types of emotion regulation are assumed to be related to different views of the self in relation to the world. Therefore, culture-informed studies on control beliefs and attributions and their relation to emotion regulation will be addressed next.

Control Beliefs and Attributions: Social-Cognitive Factors in Emotion Regulation

Important but infrequently considered factors involved in emotion regulation are attributions and beliefs about the self and world (Rothbaum & Wang, 2010). The belief in an entity self (fixed traits) and a malleable world gives rise to a tendency to pursue high intensity happiness and to change the world. On the contrary, a belief in a malleable self and an entity view on the world gives rise to a tendency to pursue calmness and to change the self to fit the world. Although coping and emotion regulation are discussed as different concepts, there is conceptual overlap and the study of emotion regulation has implications for understanding the development of coping and vice versa (Eisenberg, Valiente, & Sulik, 2009).

For instance, referring to the distinction of primary and secondary control, agentic regulation can either aim to change the environment (fixed self and a malleable world) or to adapt the self to environment (malleable self and fixed world) in order to satisfy one's needs depending on salient self-construals (Rothbaum, Weisz, & Snyder, 1982; Weisz, Rothbaum, & Blackburn, 1984). The direct personal control attempting to change the environment is typical for Western cultures where autonomy is highly valued. Cultural differences in primary and secondary control have been demonstrated in cross-cultural studies on coping (Essau & Trommsdorff, 1996; See & Essau, 2010). The prevalence of secondary control in societies that value harmony (Essau & Trommsdorff, 1996; Weisz et al., 1984) can be seen in the aforementioned value of effort and self-improvement in East Asian cultures (e.g., Heine, Lehman, Markus, & Kitayama, 1999; Li, 2002, 2005). Morling and Fiske's (1999) concept of harmony control as separate from primary and secondary control suggests the importance of social-oriented regulation. According to the cultural model of interdependence, agency serves the motivation for relatedness and is directed to fitting in socially by adjusting one's own goals and behavior to the goals and expectations of others (fit-focused secondary control; Morling & Evered, 2006). In contrast, in the cultural model of independence, primary control serves to maintain individual autonomy.

Emotion regulation also operates through such culture-specific ways of self- and world views. These are indicated in attributions and everyday explanations (Miller, 1984). For example, successful emotion regulation can be enhanced by the belief in external or internal causes of one's own behavioral outcomes, indicating a belief in entity (fixed traits) or malleability of the self (Dweck, 1999). The belief in malleability (variable factor) allows for further effort and striving even after failure because one's ability (stable factor) is not seen as primarily influencing achievement outcomes. Through the practice of training and related effortful regulation, East Asian children tend to internalize the model of the malleable self and engage in emotion regulation fostering effort and exercise, thereby accommodating to parental expectations (Trommsdorff, 2012).

Further, the belief in external causes of another person's behavior allows for discounting negative behavioral outcomes (aggression); this reduces one's own frustration and disappointment. For example, another person's aggression is interpreted by Balinese and Japanese adolescents as a non-intended act resulting from bad luck or even from one's own (the victim's) misbehavior (Kornadt, 2011). This interpretation reduces anger and the tendency for revenge (see chapter 10). Accordingly, emotion regulation and coping differ depending on the individual's control beliefs and attributions, which are socialized in the respective culture (Trommsdorff, 2007b).

In Confucian societies, striving for virtue by learning and exercise are the preferred control strategies for achieving mastery and contributing to society (Li, 2002, 2005; Rothbaum & Rusk, 2011; Trommsdorff, 2012). Striving for self-improvement (Heine et al., 1999) and self-cultivation are part of self-regulation (Hwang & Chang, 2009), whereas self-enhancement is not (see Sedikides & Gregg, 2008, for different kinds of self-enhancement). Thus, depending on the cultural preference of causal attributions (e.g., malleability beliefs), different modes of emotion regulation are preferred. These modes are in line with the cultural model of self and agency and respective self-other relations.

Therefore, this chapter on the socialization of emotions and emotion regulation goes beyond an individual-oriented approach and attempts to reduce possible biased theorizing by extending the discussion to a social-oriented approach. The development of emotion regulation is related to control beliefs (causal attributions and fit-focused control) in line with the respective cultural models of self-orientations (independent vs. interdependent). These different orientations develop as part of the attachment relationship between caretaker and child and result from a culturally different focus on autonomy and relatedness and its relations (Morelli & Rothbaum, 2007; Rothbaum et al., 2000; Rothbaum & Trommsdorff, 2007). Useful methods for achieving this goal are cross-cultural comparisons of socialization conditions and developmental outcomes of emotion regulation. Therefore, we will discuss cultural difference in development of emotion regulation in the next sections.

Cultural Differences in the Development of Emotion Regulation and Emotion Socialization

Development of Intra- and Interpersonal Emotion Regulation

Emotion regulation has often been described to develop through the experience of regulation provided by the actions of caretakers. In early development the caretaker responds to a child's needs, and supports the child's attempts to regulate emotions on his or her own as part of interpersonal regulation. Most studies on the development of emotion regulation have postulated a shift from interpersonal regulation (organized by the caretaker) to intrapersonal regulation organized by the child in more or less autonomous ways (see Holodynski & Friedlmeier, 2006; Thompson, 1994). These two modes of regulation are based on different models of agency: social interaction in the case of the infant's interpersonal (asymmetric) regulation, and activation of internalized models of regulation in the case of the child's intrapersonal regulation.

This raises the question whether these two modes indicate a developmental process that is based on an individualistic orientation. The concept of intrapersonal emotion regulation conceives of the self as independent with emotion regulation serving to maintain autonomy. However, emotion regulation may also be a means to achieve other-oriented (more or less far-reaching) social goals such as acting in accordance with group values, promoting group interests, or solving/avoiding social conflicts (e.g., Mulder, 1992; Vohs et al., 2009). Sameroff (2009) assumes an integration of individual and social factors when defining "behavioral self-regulation as an emergent of social regulation" (p. 2). This implies a broader view of the "cultural" self (Shweder et al., 1998).

Here we assume that individuals may differ in their preference for intrapersonal or interpersonal regulation, and that those preferences may be related to self- versus other-focused emotional development. Either preference depends on the self- or other-focused self-construal, the motivation to act in accordance with personal desire or norms and situational demands, and the prevalent cultural model of independence or interdependence. Self- and emotion regulation require agency for both the development and for the activation of either regulatory skills. The activation of self- or other-focused emotions and intra- or interpersonal regulation is based on the internalization of culture-bound values and goals. Both modes exist within as well as between cultures, although cultures differ in the prevalence of situations evoking each mode (Trommsdorff, 2012).

Since the individual-centered approach of intrapersonal regulation does not suffice to explain the development of an extended interpersonal regulation, we are suggesting here to distinguish two types, the interpersonal intimate and the interpersonal extended regulation, taking into account basic needs, individual goals and values, and attributional and motivational preferences (see Table 4.1). In early development, a precondition for self-regulation is the intimate interpersonal regulation with the primary caretaker. In later development, the social and cultural context may require an extended

Table 4.1. Development of emotion regulation as influenced by the cultural model of agency

	Development of emotion regulation		
	Interpersonal intimate	**Intrapersonal**	**Interpersonal extended**
Context	Parent-child interaction	Self-other differentiation	Self-other bonds
Universal needs	Attachment	Autonomy	Relatedness
Regulating agent	Caretaker	Self	Internalized social expectations
Self-regulation	Dependent	Independent	Shared (related)
Self-construal	Dependent	Independent	Interdependent
Agency		Disjoint agency	Conjoint agency

relational quality of interpersonal regulation. For example, the commitment to social roles and the social group motivate people to exert self-control and engage in interpersonally engaging regulatory processes. Especially in a cultural and situational context where the cultural model of interdependence and relatedness prevails, interpersonal extended emotion regulation is given priority (see Table 4.1).

Both forms of regulation, intrapersonal (independent) and interpersonal extended regulation, are seen as agentic modes of emotion regulation. We define here interpersonal-extended regulation as a form of shared regulation based on empathic relatedness with others, assuming cultural and individual differences in both forms of regulation. We will address this issue in more detail when we discuss cultural differences in parent-child relationships and development of emotion regulation.

Cultural Differences in the Development of Emotion Regulation

As mentioned earlier, the cultural model of interdependence facilitates adjustment to other people and interpersonal emotion regulation. These individuals tend to prefer the outsider mode, in which one looks at the self through the eyes of others and regulates one's emotions in order to maintain social harmony and tight social norms (Cohen & Hoshino-Browne, 2005). For European-American populations, relatively loose social norms are related to the insider mode of looking at the self through one's own eyes. Here, the belief in authentic expression of emotions influences the socialization of emotion regulation. For example, emotion regulation in the Confucian tradition follows the goal of fostering a relational self. This requires the person to maintain "face" and social harmony by taking into consideration other's expectations and by fulfilling one's role obligations in relationships, particularly to family members (see Miller, 1997). A goal for emotion regulation in many Confucian-influenced communities is self-cultivation and self-perfection (Hwang & Chang, 2009).

In a cultural context of relatedness and social harmony, two of the most valued developmental tasks are empathy and perspective taking. Emotions are regulated in a way that fosters harmony. Accordingly, the expression of socially disengaging emotions such as anger, disappointment, and distress is rather discouraged in cultures that favor the interdependent model of agency (Kitayama, 2001; see chapter 5). This is also the case in cultures that, though not following the Confucian tradition, favor value systems in line with Hindu or Buddhist beliefs. For example, in Japan, Nepal, Java, and in many Indian communities, children are socialized to know that expressing anger when frustrated is socially undesirable and considered as immature behavior (see Cole, Tamang, & Shrestha, 2006; Cole & Tan, 2007; Kornadt, 2011; Trommsdorff, 2012).

In Asian cultures, caretakers refrain from supporting children's expression of negative emotions based on the belief that this may endanger the child's socio-emotional competence. This is in contrast to European American parents who show relative support and encouragement of children's expression of negative emotions based on the belief that suppression may harm the child's socio-emotional competence (Tromms-

Table 4.2. Cultural model of socializing emotion regulation

	Independence	Interdependence
Child's emotional reaction	• socially disengaging • authentic self • anger, pride	• socially engaging • empathic, other-focused • shame, sadness
Parent's socialization of emotion regulation by	• promotion focus – expressive encouragement – reactive sensitivity	• prevention focus – minimization – proactive sensitivity
Agentic emotion regulation	• disjoint	• conjoint

dorff, Cole, & Heikamp, 2012). Here, one can see the importance of taking into account the cultural meaning of both supportive parenting and socio-emotional competence.

In Asian cultures, regulating socially disengaging emotions serves the goals of social belonging, relatedness, and maintaining social harmony and thereby contributes to socio-emotional competence. For example, Japanese or Chinese caretakers socialize children to become aware of other person's feelings (e.g., Hayashi, Karasawa, & Tobin, 2009; Lebra, 1994; Wang, 2003). The development of interpersonally based other-focused (in contrast to self-focused) emotion regulation such as empathy and shame in the service of harmonious interpersonal relations ("relational emotional competence") has been reported in several culture-informed studies for Japanese, Korean, Chinese, Javanese, Nepalese, or Indian children (for an overview see Friedlmeier et al., 2011; Trommsdorff, 2006, 2012; Trommsdorff & Cole, 2011; see Table 4.2 and Figure 4.1).

However, besides the different quality of negative emotions (e.g., anger versus sadness versus shame) the process and outcome of emotion regulation has to be taken into account in order to illustrate emotional competence. Since most studies are based on self-reports, the process of emotion regulation remains unclear. In our own observational

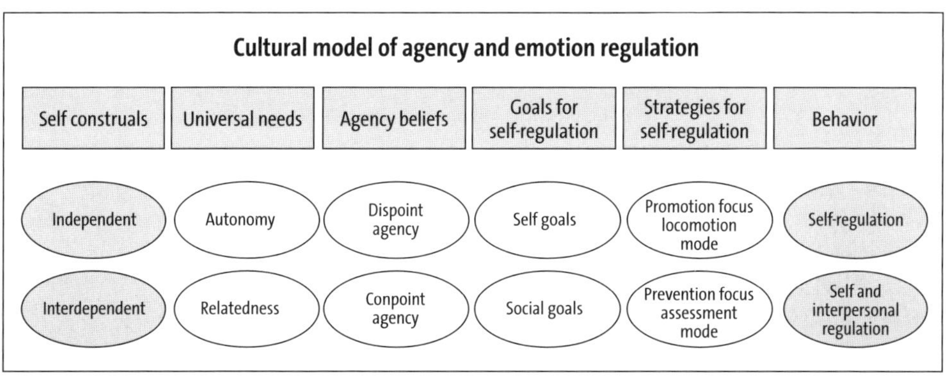

Figure 4.1. Cultural model of agency and emotion regulation (adapted from Trommsdorff (2009), p. 69)

studies, significant differences between Japanese and German children with respect to the regulation of negative emotions (Friedlmeier & Trommsdorff, 1999) and the process of regulation (related to different negative emotions) occurred (Trommsdorff & Friedlmeier, 2010). In the latter study, the experimental conditions differed with respect to self-focused negative emotions (disappointment, failure) and other-focused negative emotions (e.g., empathic distress for another person's misfortune) of preschoolers. In the self-focused condition, children were asked to draw a picture within a limited time. Japanese, as compared to German girls, showed less distress when they realized before the time elapsed that they were not able to complete the task successfully. German and Japanese children showed an increased distress reaction after the given time elapsed and the experimenter took the incomplete picture away for evaluation (stress induction).

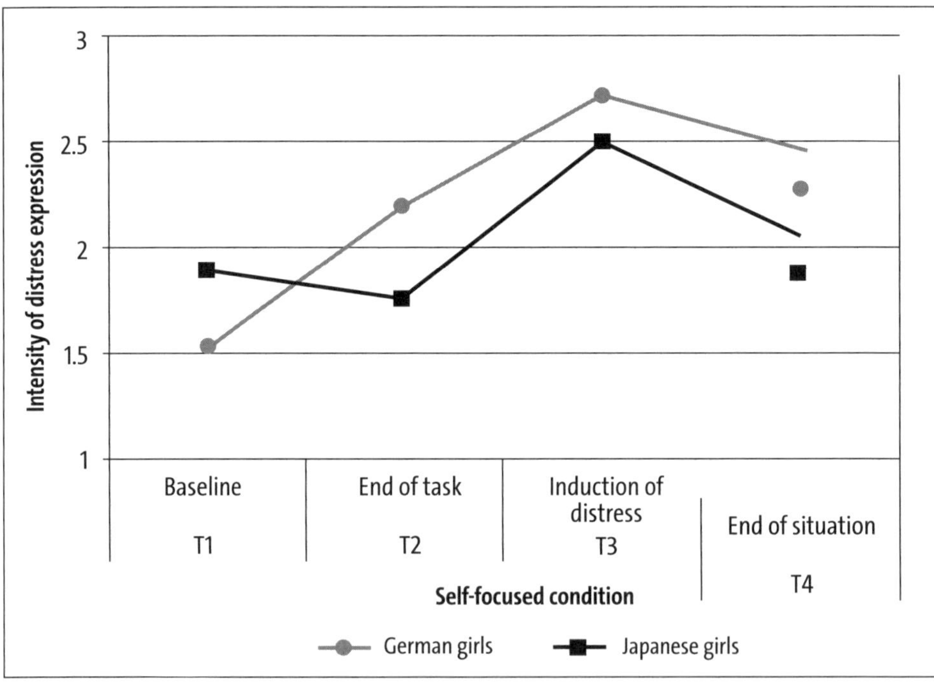

Figure 4.2. Emotion regulation in self-focused condition: Experiencing own failure. German girls showed a significant increase of distress expression during the task (from T1 to T2), whereas Japanese girls did not. Both groups showed a significant increase from the end of the task (T2) to the distress induction (T3). Distress expression decreased significantly (T4 compared to T3) for Japanese girls but not for German ones. German girls showed a significantly higher intensity of distress expression than Japanese girls at the end of the task (T2) and at the end of the situation (T4). (From: Trommsdorff, G., & Friedlmeier, W. (2010). Preschool girls' distress and mothers' sensitivity in Japan and Germany. *European Journal of Developmental Psychology, 7*, 350–370. Reprinted by permission of Taylor & Francis Ltd, http://www.tandf.co.uk/journals)

However, Japanese girls were less distressed at the end of the situation after some minutes than German girls (see Figure 4.2); they seemingly had regulated their distress and showed again a relaxed mood. In the other-focused situation, Japanese girls (as compared to German ones) became increasingly more distressed witnessing the misfortune of another person. As compared to German girls, the Japanese, could regulate their self-focused negative emotions more successfully and their other-focused negative emotions less so (see Figure 4.3). Moreover, in line with other studies (e.g., Trommsdorff, Friedlmeier, & Mayer, 2007), these findings also suggest that at a rather early age children interpret the same situations differently across cultures, leading to different emotional reactions. The self- and other-focused emotions may indicate emotional costs for valuing independence or interdependence, respectively (Trommsdorff & Friedlmeier, 2010).

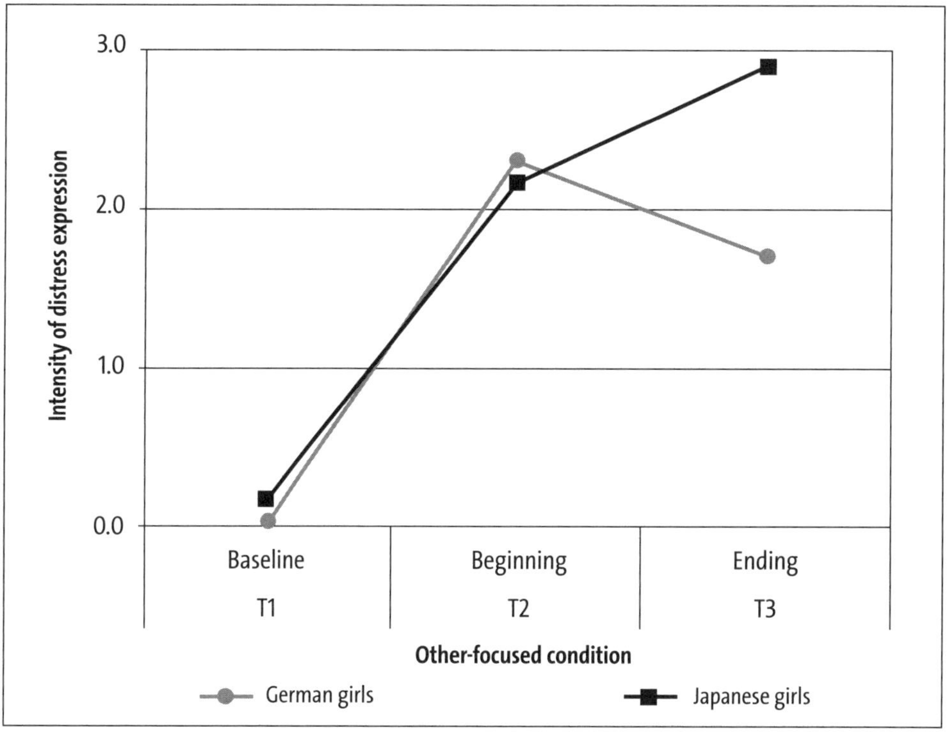

Figure 4.3. Emotion regulation in other-focused condition: Experiencing another person's misfortune. German girls showed a significant decrease of distress expression from the beginning (T2) to the end of the situation (T3), whereas Japanese girls showed a significant increase. Intensity of distress expression at the end of the situation was significantly higher for Japanese girls than for German girls. (From: Trommsdorff, G., & Friedlmeier, W. (2010). Preschool girls' distress and mothers' sensitivity in Japan and Germany. *European Journal of Developmental Psychology, 7,* 350–370. Reprinted by permission of Taylor & Francis Ltd, http://www.tandf.co.uk/journals)

Cultural Differences in Socialization of Emotion Regulation

Parents' socialization goals and practices are usually influenced by predominant cultural values and related agency beliefs (i.e., disjoint, conjoint models of agency). Socialization can be based on direct parenting (e.g., supportive, nonsupportive) or indirect parenting (e.g., modeling; Morris et al., 2007). Further, intuitive parenting beliefs ("naïve theories") and goals are part of the socialization processes and help to better understand the cultural meaning of specific parenting practices (e.g., parental control) (Trommsdorff et al., 2012).

Self-reported direct parental reactions to children's negative emotions have often been found to influence children's development of emotional competence. Usually, "supportive" (e.g., encouragement of emotion expression, giving instrumental or emotional support) and "nonsupportive" (e.g., dismissing, minimizing, ignoring) parental responses to children's negative emotions have been assessed by the Coping with Children's Negative Emotions Scale (CCNES) consisting of hypothetical scenarios (Fabes, Poulin, Eisenberg, & Madden-Derdich, 2002). Most studies including European American samples show that "supportive" parenting fosters successful emotion regulation (e.g., Davidov & Grusec, 2006) and social adaptation (e.g., internalization of rules of conduct; Suchodoletz, Trommsdorff, & Heikamp, 2011). However, is the meaning of "supportive" parenting in Asian cultures the same as in the European American context?

Cross-cultural studies showed significant differences in mothers' reactions. For example, more minimizing reactions and less expressive encouragement were reported by Indian and Nepalese as compared to German and European American mothers of 6- to 7-year-old children. Further, Asian mothers reported more distress as a reaction to the child's expression of negative emotions (Fäsche et al., 2011; Trommsdorff et al., 2012). In another study, German mothers of preschoolers, compared to Indian mothers, reported less distress and more encouragement of negative emotional expression of their preschool children (Heikamp, Mishra, Suchodoletz, & Trommsdorff, 2008). This is in line with results from the study by Raval and Martini (2009) on Indian mothers' high endorsement of minimization and low value for expressive encouragement of negative emotions. The authors also showed that traditional in comparison to urbanized Indian mothers were more likely to perceive the child's expression of negative emotions as socially undesirable.

These results are consistent with the literature on socialization of emotions in Asian countries. For example, Japanese (Lebra, 1992; Trommsdorff & Kornadt, 2003), and Chinese parents (Chan, Bowes, & Wyver, 2009) discourage the expression of negative, socially disengaging emotions. Chinese parents value the relational compared to individualistic emotional competence of their children higher. Therefore, Asian parents rather prefer "conjoint" (i.e., proactive sensitivity) as compared to "disjoint" (i.e., reactive sensitivity) agency in emotion regulation (see Table 4.2 and Figure 4.1). Emotion regulation as part of socio-emotional competence has a different meaning in Asian as compared to European American cultures. An important goal in Asian cultures is that children learn to maintain social harmony and not to disappoint social expectations (i.e., prevention focus). In contrast, in European American cultures, autonomy, self-confidence, and authentic expression of emotions, are relatively more highly valued parental goals (i.e., promotion focus; see Table 4.2).

Cross-cultural studies have shown that two modes of caretaker's sensitivity have to be distinguished: proactive (i.e., caretaker anticipates child's emotion experience) and reactive (i.e., caretaker reacts to child's emotion expression) sensitivity. Proactive sensitivity is based on an empathic understanding of the child's feelings, and the mother's anticipation of the child's needs. This results from a very close mother-child bonding, her felt responsibility to fulfill the child's needs, the goal to save her child from negative emotions (prevention focus), and her conceptualization of the child as a child (see Trommsdorff & Kornadt, 2003; Trommsdorff & Rothbaum, 2008). These studies suggest that an important cultural difference in socialization conditions is related to the value of autonomy and relatedness and its culture-specific meaning (Rothbaum & Trommsdorff, 2007; Trommsdorff & Rothbaum, 2008). Both pro- and reactive sensitivity have different effects on the child's emotion and self-regulation (Rothbaum, Nagaoka, & Ponte, 2006; Trommsdorff & Friedlmeier, 2010; Trommsdorff & Rothbaum, 2008; see Table 4.2).

Preliminary results from an ongoing cross-cultural study on self-reported parental cultural beliefs in Nepal, India, Korea, Germany, and the US (about $N = 100$ in each country) illustrate cultural differences in mothers' reactions when their 6- to 7-year-old child experiences a disturbing or frustrating situation (Fäsche et al., 2011; Trommsdorff et al., 2012). Caretakers from contexts valuing interdependence (i.e., Nepal, India) preferred proactive (in contrast to reactive) sensitivity in comparison to caretakers from independence-oriented socialization contexts (i.e., Germany, the US).

Typical examples of Asian mothers who take the initiative in regulating the child's needs before the child regulates their own needs include: "By guessing in advance we can fulfill the needs of the child in time." "Being a mother I would know her needs before she tells me." "The child is still small and does not know what he has to do." "We have to teach the child what behavior to learn. This depends on the mothers." "Children do not know so much what they need and when." Typical examples of Western mothers who reject such interventions and who instead demonstrate the belief that the child is a separate entity from the mother who can regulate his or her own needs include: "Because with anticipating the child's personal opinion leads to forcing the parent's will/preferences on the child." "I can only act on what I think, and the child can think completely differently." "The child should have experiences of her own." "The child should cope with the situation herself." "If I interfere, I disturb her development."

The data consistently showed a higher preference of proactive than of reactive sensitivity for Nepalese and Indian as compared to German and US mothers. However, the response patterns of the Korean mothers were less consistent. Also, Asian compared to Western mothers showed more proactive sensitivity and also reacted to their child's distress with more concern (distress), less expressive encouragement, and more minimization (playing down the distressing event and the child's negative emotions). Further analyses of our interview data on mothers' beliefs about sensitivity based on the method by Rothbaum et al. (2006) showed that most Indian and Nepalese mothers clearly preferred to immediately comfort the child, whereas half of the Korean mothers, and the majority of German and US mothers, expected the child to clearly express his or her needs. The results also showed cultural differences in the associations between mothers' implicit theories regarding reactive and proactive sensitivity and their reactions to the child's distress. Only for Indian and Nepalese mothers did a substantial association between proactive sensitivity and lower level of expressive encouragement and higher level of minimization occur. This indicates the aforementioned culture-specific meaning of parental support, which is in contrast to European American studies on supportive parenting.

While these self-report studies focus on specific parental reactions to children's distress, observational studies provide more insight into the interaction process between caretaker and child. The observational methods further clarify the culture-specific meaning of certain caretaker's behavior such as sensitivity (Rothbaum et al., 2006; Trommsdorff & Friedlmeier, 2010). Observational studies of German and Japanese mothers who witnessed distress of their child are in line with these results. Mothers of 2-year-old toddlers regulated their child's negative emotions by engaging in interpersonal regulation, not leaving the child regulating alone. Intrapersonal regulation did not occur in this age group, even in the German sample. Mothers' strategies differed in line with the respective cultural model: German mothers used verbal strategies while Japanese mothers preferred nonverbal behavior, using physical closeness and avoiding eye contact (Trommsdorff & Friedlmeier, 1993). These different strategies of emotion regulation indicate a different prevalence of independent and interdependent regulation in both cultures. The child is considered a separate entity in the German context where verbal communication between independent persons is prevalent and necessary, while it is in unity with the mother in the Japanese context where physical contact fosters intimate interdependence between mother and child.

Other cross-cultural studies on behavioral observations of Asian and Western mothers who are witnessing distress of their child confirm the assumption of culturally different emotion regulation processes (see Table 4.2 and Figure 4.1). For example, German and Indian mothers used different strategies to regulate their preschool child's negative emotions (disappointment for not receiving an expected gift; Heikamp et al., 2008). German mothers openly expressed (verbally and nonverbally) their emotions (disappointment, surprise, dissatisfaction, anger). They also focused verbally on their child's disappointment, thereby increasing the child's distress. In contrast, Indian mothers remained calm; they continued smiling and showed no negative emotions. In line with our hypothesis that Indian mothers display higher proactive sensitivity, they took the initiative by reversing the unpacking of the empty box. They also invited their child to do the same by acting on an object in line with social norms and behavioral rules, ignoring their child's disappointment. Therefore the child does not become fully aware of his or her distress, making it likely that emerging distress is alleviated without much need for suppression. This striking example of effective interpersonal norm-oriented regulation in Indian mother-child interactions can be seen as a special form of sensitive behavior: Ignoring the child's disappointment indicates a form of minimization that would not be regarded as supportive parenting from a Western perspective. However, this seemingly "nonsupportive" parenting helps the child to regulate negative emotions effectively.

Role of Emotions for Parent-Child Relationships

The above reported results suggest that "supporting" socialization practices can have a different function in different cultures, depending on the cultural meaning. For example, European American parents' negative reactions to children's negative emotions were related to harsh parenting and children's poor adjustment (Eisenberg, Fabes, Carlo, & Karbon, 1992; Fabes, Leonard, Kupanoff, & Martin, 2001). Also, European American's parents' dismissing in contrast to accepting and encouraging expression of children's negative emotions has been shown to impede children's socio-emotional competence (Friedlmeier et al., 2011). It is unlikely that the meaning of "nonsupportive" parenting is the same in Asian cultures.

Culture-informed studies have indeed shown that parenting styles and practices can have a different function for children's development in Asian cultures. For example, Tao, Zhou, and Wang (2010) have reported for samples from Hong Kong and mainland China that authoritarian (e.g., directiveness, verbal hostility) and authoritative parenting styles (e.g., warmth, reasoning) are more predictive for the child's outcomes as compared to parents' reactions to children's negative emotions. One reason may be that the cultural validity of measures of the parental responses to children's negative emotions has not yet been tested, and certain items are related to different cultural beliefs. For example, Indian mothers who report to feel distressed when their child expresses negative emotions, for instance anger (measured by the CCNES; self-report), explain in a subsequent structured interview that they feel empathy with their child. They report that their child's feels sad and reacts angrily. The mothers believe that it is their responsibility to calm down their child.[1] This finding supports the notion that parents' distress reactions to their child's negative emotion indicate culture-specific beliefs about child development and the role of the parent.

Cross-cultural studies have shown that seemingly the same kind of parenting can function differently depending on the respective cultural model of agency. For example, parental support or parental practices like warmth, parental sensitivity, or parental control as aspects of socialization can be experienced by the child in different ways. This not only depends on the child's developmental age, gender, socialization situation, and parent-child relationship, but moreover, on the cultural context.

It should be noted that the meaning of specific caretaking behavior may vary according to the parents' goals and parents' general parenting style. For example, "parental control" may be related to guidance, or monitoring, or the expression of affect and

[1] R. C. Mishra (personal communication, 2011)

involvement (Grolnick & Pomerantz, 2009). All self-report measures of parenting suffer from the problem that objective and subjective measures imply different constructs. When the child's experience of parenting is of theoretical interest since the child's development is largely based on the child's internal model of the self and the world, parents' self-reports are only partially informative. Empirical studies show that the function of parental behavior (e.g., control) for socializing their children differs depending on the respective meaning of such behavior for the children (Grusec & Goodnow, 1994); this can be moderated by culture and also by the specific domain in the socialization context. For example, sensitivity (i.e., responsiveness to child's needs) and warmth (i.e., positive expressivity) have for a long time been seen as aspects of "positive parenting" that foster social adaptation in the same way. However, both aspects have a domain-specific function (Grusec & Davidov, 2007, 2010). Whereas responsiveness to children's distress is positively related to regulation of negative emotions and empathy, warmth is associated with regulation of positive emotions and peer acceptance (e.g., Davidov & Grusec, 2006).

For our discussion, the ways in which the cultural context influences children's experience of their parents' behavior are of interest. Cross-cultural studies have shown that Japanese and Korean adolescents, but not German and American adolescents, felt neglected by their parents when they experienced low control (Rohner & Pettengill, 1985; Trommsdorff, 1985). In cultural contexts where independence and autonomy are highly valued, parental control may be less accepted by adolescents; this differs from cultures in which interdependence is highly valued (Rudy & Grusec, 2001). Chinese children experience their parents' "control" as related to the value of training, and as guidance, warmth, and support (Chao, 1994, 2001; Chao & Tseng, 2002). However, children from individual-oriented cultures experience parental "control" as nonsupportive – a threat to their autonomy and a constraint of their agency (Rothbaum & Trommsdorff, 2007; Trommsdorff, 1985). Accordingly, the cultural context may moderate the relation between perceived parenting and children's outcomes (Cheah & Rubin, 2004; Kakihara & Tilton-Weaver, 2009).

A similar moderating effect of culture can be seen in studies on "psychological control," which has been reported to have negative effects on European American children's developmental outcomes (Barber, 1996, 2002). However, results for European American samples differ from other cultural groups. Rothbaum and Wang (2010) have discussed in detail why psychological control (e.g., inducing shame) has adverse effects in the United States but not in East Asia, referring to cultural differences in self-construal and related cultural values. These studies on caretaking and its effects on development therefore raise the question of an ethnocentric bias in generalizing from results on Western samples.

Taking culture into account suggests again that parenting behavior should be studied in relation to parenting beliefs and goals as part of the developmental niche of the child (Trommsdorff et al., 2012). Depending on the cultural meaning, the same kind of parenting goal can manifest itself in different behavior and vice versa (Kornadt & Trommsdorff, 1984; Trommsdorff & Kornadt, 2003). Further, the relations between general parenting style, specific practices, and parenting goals give a specific functional meaning to aspects of parenting.

Studies on parental style and emotion socialization in Hong Kong (Chan et al., 2009) and in mainland China (Tao et al., 2010) showed that authoritarian parenting style was related to less supportive strategies, and authoritative parenting style was related to more supportive strategies for emotion socialization. Interestingly, authoritative parenting was related to both individualistic and social-relational goals for emotion competence, whereas authoritarian parenting was related only to social-relational goals. Furthermore, authoritarian parents' relational goals for emotion competence were related to dismissing and coaching practices; this was motivated to maintain authority. In contrast, authoritative parents' relational goals were associated to encouragement of emotion expression while the underlying goal was to foster interpersonal sensitivity.

Different regulation strategies are embedded in a cultural system of socialization promoting cultural values of independence and interdependence and the different cultural meanings of autonomy and relatedness (see Figure 4.1). In line with the cultural model of interdependence, the Indian and the Japanese child's agentic regulation is embedded, channeled, and fueled by the regulatory behavior of the mother with culture-specific variations in interdependence. This is in contrast to German mothers' regulation strategies, which are in line with the cultural model of independence. Whereas the German mothers used verbal strategies focusing on the child's distress, Indian mothers used strategies referring to social norms and obligations; Japanese mothers preferred anticipatory sensitivity and an emotion-based close unity with the child (amae) (Lebra, 1994; Rothbaum & Trommsdorff, 2007). While amae, a feeling of oneness and dependence, can be seen as a basis for emotion regulation in Japan, active disengagement from goals is a strategy for emotion regulation in India. In Confucian societies, a functionally equivalent regulatory strategy is the effortful striving for self-cultivation and perfection. However, even though there is a culturally different basis for emotion regulation in Asian societies, they all serve the goal to maintain social harmony. In contrast, fostering self-esteem and autonomy is of main importance for emotion regulation in European American societies (Trommsdorff, 2012). Accordingly, socio-emotional competence has a very different meaning in these cultural contexts. Therefore, the socialization conditions (e.g., the meaning of support and control) for fostering emotion regulation and socio-emotional competence differ in line with the respective cultural model of agency (Figure 4.1).

Summary, Conclusions, and Outlook

Different cultural models give a different meaning to socialization conditions of emotion regulation. Accordingly, the development of emotion regulation should be studied in the cultural context, thus combining the lens of culture with the lens of development. The studies discussed above can be organized according to the model of agency and self-regulation (see Figure 4.1).

The reported studies show that different kinds (e.g., conjoint and disjoint) of emotion regulation, as an aspect of self-regulation, are related to different cultural models of agency (Markus & Kitayama, 2004; Markus et al., 2006) that can be traced back to early development of self- and emotion regulation in the cultural context. Caretakers prefer culture-specific beliefs and parenting strategies for successfully socializing their child's emotion regulation. These beliefs and strategies are based on different views on the self and the world. Culture-specific self- and world views structure how caretakers interact with their children, how they perceive their role as parents, and related responsibilities.

German mothers, for instance, would rather promote their child's independent emotion regulation (intrapersonal regulation) in line with the belief in authentic expression of emotions. In comparison, Asian mothers would rather believe that their children are not yet independent, need to find their place within a social group, and need to establish a bond with their significant others. Therefore, they view their own responsibility in anticipating and fulfilling the child's needs (proactive sensitivity) and to guide their child's interpersonal harmony-oriented regulation (Trommsdorff & Rothbaum, 2008). However, Asian mothers also differ in their parenting strategies, indicating that the cultural model of interdependence embraces various patterns of parenting beliefs and practices that influence the child's socialization (Trommsdorff, 2012).

This chapter illustrates the limited empirical validity and restricted theoretical range of traditional theories on the development of emotion regulation based mostly on European American samples. Cross-cultural studies show that the assumption of a developmental shift from inter- to intrapersonal regulation should be modified by taking into account a shift to an extended interpersonal regulation. Further, aspects of "supportive" parenting and of related successful development of emotion competence can only be described on the basis of the respective cultural meaning. Culture-informed studies show how specific models of agency influence socialization conditions and developmental outcomes of socio-emotional competence in terms of achieving a fit between cultural values, personal goals, and emotion regulation.

Clinical Implications

Taking into account the cultural context and related values for emotion regulation is therefore unavoidable in many applied areas, for example, acculturation, intercultural adjustment, development in a multicultural context, development of psychopathology, or intervention programs on emotion regulation. However, most studies on emotion regulation have dealt with European American populations (for example, see the *Handbook of Emotion Regulation* edited by Gross, 2007). We cannot continue to avoid including populations from other cultures into psychological research. It is necessary to extend our studies on questions of how people from other cultures are coping with stress (Wong & Wong, 2006), and how children's emotion regulation develops in other cultural contexts. Studying the development of emotion regulation can be particularly informative for the understanding of coping (Eisenberg et al., 2009) and psychosocial functioning (e.g., depression; Caprara, Gerbino, Paciello, Di Giunta, & Pastorelli, 2010). Cross-cultural research needs to address both cultural differences and similarities regarding the psychological processes underlying well-being and psychosocial adjustment.

There is an increasing need for multicultural perspectives of psychopathology and for culture-informed intervention programs. Further research is needed to investigate, for instance, whether the same psychological processes (e.g., emotion regulation strategies) are conducive to well-being in different cultural contexts. Based on culture-informed studies it is doubtful that suppression of negative emotions necessarily is generally harmful and that open expression is the more adaptive strategy. An example is the famous Morita therapy in Japan (Chen, 2010). The main task is that the person engages in his or her unhappy feelings, such as anxiety or shame, by focusing on just these feelings and related episodes for a longer period of isolation. The goal of this therapy is to have the person engage in harmonious relations after having successfully accepted his or her anxiety. This therapy would presumably not be successful in an individualistic cultural context where accepting negative emotions and the goal to maintain social harmony is less valued. The Morita therapy can be seen as based on the belief in the malleability of the self and the fixed state of the world – a belief that is in sharp contrast to the belief in the malleable world and a fixed self (Rothbaum & Wang, 2010; Trommsdorff, 2012).

Future Perspectives

Further culture-informed studies on emotion and self-regulation may address the question to what extent goals of independence or interdependence are activated in different situations and vary in their relative importance during development, and how a balance between individual and relationship goals is achieved (Chan et al., 2009; Miller, 2003; Rothbaum & Trommsdorff, 2007; Trommsdorff, 2007a, 2007b; Trommsdorff & Cole, 2011). Probably future research will indicate that in times of social change previously prevalent forms of interdependent self-regulation will become less adaptive and forms of independent self-regulation will become more dominant. Therefore, empirical studies are needed in order to better understand the links between individual development and socio-cultural change (Chen, 2010; Chen & French, 2008). Especially in times of socioeconomic and political change, cultural tasks and models of agency undergo changes that may affect socialization conditions and children's emotion regulation and moreover, values underlying socio-emotional competence in specific cultural domains (Trommsdorff, 2000; Trommsdorff & Kornadt, 1995; Trommsdorff, Kornadt, & Hessel-Scherf, 1998).

In case of transitions and socioeconomic change, successful development of emotion regulation follows the path of cultural fit. Taking into account the subjective self and world views may allow for a better understanding of culture-specific developmental paths to socio-emotional competence, and may also serve for successful culture-informed intervention programs.

Acknowledgments

This research was supported by a grant from the German Research Foundation (DFG GZ, TR 169/1 4–2) as part of the project "Developmental Conditions of Intentionality and Its Limits," and as part of the Interdisciplinary Research Center "Limits of Intentionality" at the University of Konstanz. We are grateful to the late Fred Rothbaum for his most valuable comments. Special thanks to Holly Bunje for assistance in editing the manuscript.

References

Bandura, A. (2006). Toward a psychology of human agency. *Perspectives on Psychological Science, 1*, 164–180.

Barber, B. K. (1996). Parental psychological control: Revisiting a neglected construct. *Child Development, 67*, 3296–3319.

Barber, B. K. (Ed.) (2002). *Intrusive parenting: How psychological control affects children and adolescents.* Washington, DC: American Psychological Association.

Blair, C. (2010). Stress and the development of self-regulation in context. *Child Development Perspectives, 4*, 1–188.

Bond, M. H., & van de Vijver, F. J. R. (2011). Making scientific sense of cultural differences in psychological outcomes: Unpackaging the Magnum Mysterium. In D. Matsumoto & F. J. R. van de Vijver (Eds.), *Cross-cultural research methods in psychology* (pp. 75–100). New York: Cambridge University Press.

Caprara, G. V., Gerbino, M., Paciello, M., Di Giunta, L., & Pastorelli, C. (2010). Counteracting depression and delinquency in late adolescence: The role of regulatory emotional and interpersonal self-efficacy beliefs. *European Psychologist, 15*, 4–48.

Chan, S. M., Bowes, J., & Wyver, S. (2009). Parenting style as a context for emotion socialization. *Early Education and Development, 20*, 631–656.

Chao, R. K. (1994). Beyond parental control and authoritarian parenting style: Understanding Chinese parenting through the cultural notion of training. *Child Development, 65*, 1111–1119.

Chao, R. K. (2001). Extending research on the consequences of parenting style for Chinese Americans and European Americans. *Child Development, 72*, 1832–1843.

Chao, R., & Tseng, V. (2002). Parenting of Asians. In M. H. Bornstein (Ed.), *Handbook of parenting: Vol. 4. Social conditions and applied parenting* (2nd ed., pp. 59–93). Mahwah, NJ: Erlbaum.

Cheah, C. S. L., & Rubin, K. H. (2004). European American and Mainland Chinese mother's responses to aggression and social withdrawal in preschoolers. *International Journal of Behavioral Development, 28*, 83–94.

Chen, X. (2010). Socio-emotional development in Chinese children. In M. H. Bond (Ed.), *The Oxford handbook of Chinese psychology* (pp. 37–52). New York: Oxford University Press.

Chen, X., & French, D. C. (2008). Children's social competence in cultural context. *Annual Review of Psychology, 59*, 591–616.

Cohen, D., & Hoshino-Browne, E. (2005). Insider and outsider perspectives on the self and social world. In R. M. Sorrentino, D. Cohen, J. M. Olson, & M. P. Zanna (Eds.), *Cultural and social behavior: The Ontario Symposium.* (Vol. 10, pp. 49–76). Mahwah, NJ: Erlbaum.

Cole, P. M., Dennis, T. A., Martin, S. E., & Hall, S. E. (2008). Emotion regulation and the early development of psychopathology. In M. Vandekerckhove, C. von Scheve, S. Ismer, S. Jung, & S. Kronast (Eds.), *Regulating emotions: Culture, social necessity and biological inheritance* (pp. 171–188). Malden, MA: Blackwell.

Cole, P. M., Tamang, B. L., & Shrestha, S. (2006). Cultural variations in the socialization of young children's anger and shame. *Child Development, 77*, 1237–1251.

Cole, P. M., & Tan, P. Z. (2006). Capturing the culture in the cultural socialization of emotion. *ISSBD Newsletter, 49*, 5–7.

Cole, P. M., & Tan, P. Z. (2007). Emotion socialization from a cultural perspective. In J. E. Grusec & P. Hastings (Eds.), *Handbook of socialization: Theory and research* (pp. 516–542). New York: Guilford.

Davidov, M., & Grusec, J. E. (2006). Untangling the links of parental responsiveness to distress and warmth to child outcomes. *Child Development, 77*, 4–58.

Dweck, C. S. (1999). *Self-theories: Their role in motivation, personality, and development.* Philadelphia, PA: Psychology Press.

Eisenberg, N., Fabes, R. A., Carlo, G., & Karbon, M. (1992). Emotional responsivity to others: Behavioral correlates and socialization antecedents. In N. Eisenberg & R. A. Fabes (Eds.), *New directions in child development: Emotion and its regulation in early development* (pp. 57–73). San Francisco, CA: Jossey-Bass.

Eisenberg, N., & Spinrad, T. L. (2004). Emotion-related regulation: Sharpening the definition. *Child Development, 75*, 334–339.

Eisenberg, N., Valiente, C., & Sulik, M. J. (2009). How the study of regulation can inform the study of coping. In E. A. Skinner & M. J. Zimmer-Gembeck (Eds.), *Coping and development of regulation. New directions for child and adolescent development* (Vol. 124, pp. 75–86). San Francisco, CA: Jossey-Bass.

Essau, C. A., & Trommsdorff, G. (1996). Coping with university-related problems: A cross-cultural comparison. *Journal of Cross-Cultural Psychology, 27*, 315–328.

Fabes, R. A., Leonard, S. A., Kupanoff, K., & Martin, C. L. (2001). Parental coping with children's negative emotions: Relations with children's emotional and social responding. *Child Development, 72*, 907–920.

Fabes, R. A., Poulin, R. E., Eisenberg, N., & Madden-Derdich, D. A. (2002). The Coping with Children's Negative Emotions Scale (CCNES): Psychometric properties and relations with children's emotional competence. *Marriage & Family Review, 34*, 285–310.

Fäsche, A., Trommsdorff, G., Heikamp, T., Cole, P. M., Mishra, R. C., Niraula, S., & Park, S.-Y. (2011). Cultural differences in mothers' beliefs about sensitivity and maternal reactions to children's distress. In E. M. Leerkes & J. A. Nelson (Chairs), *Racial and cultural differences in parents' emotion socialization beliefs.* Symposium conducted at the SRCD Biennial Meeting, Montreal, Canada.

Friedlmeier, W., Corapci, F., & Cole, P. M. (2011). Emotion socialization in cross-cultural perspective. *Social and Personality Psychology Compass, 5*, 410–427.

Friedlmeier, W., & Trommsdorff, G. (1999). Emotion regulation in early childhood: A cross-cultural comparison between German and Japanese toddlers. *Journal of Cross-Cultural Psychology, 30*, 684–711.

Friedlmeier, W., & Trommsdorff, G. (2002). Emotionale Kompetenz im Kulturvergleich [Emotional competence in cross-cultural comparison]. In M. von Salisch (Ed.), *Emotionale Kompetenz entwickeln: Grundlagen in Kindheit und Jugend* (pp. 229–262). Stuttgart, Germany: Kohlhammer.

Gergely, G. (2002). The development of understanding self and agency. In U. Goswami (Ed.), *Blackwell handbook of childhood cognitive development* (pp. 26–46). Malden, MA: Blackwell.

Greenfield, P. M. (2010). Particular forms of independence and interdependence are adapted to particular kinds of sociodemographic environment: Commentary on "Independence and interdependence in children's developmental experiences." *Child Development Perspectives, 4*, 37–39.

Grolnick, W. S., & Pomerantz, E. M. (2009). Issues and challenges in studying parental control: Toward a new conceptualization. *Child Development Perspectives, 3*, 165–170.

Gross, J. J. (Ed.). (2007). *Handbook of emotion regulation.* New York: Guilford.
Gross, J. J., & Thompson, R. A. (2007). Emotion regulation: Conceptual foundations. In J. J. Gross (Ed.), *Handbook of emotion regulation* (pp. 3–24). New York: Guilford.
Grusec, J. E., & Davidov, M. (2007). Socialization in the family: The roles of parents. In J. E. Grusec & P. Hastings (Eds.), *Handbook of socialization: Theory and research* (pp. 284–308). New York: Guilford.
Grusec, J. E., & Davidov, M. (2010). Integrating different perspectives on socialization theory and research: A domain-specific approach. *Child Development, 81*, 687–709.
Grusec, J. E., & Goodnow, J. J. (1994). Impact of parental discipline methods on the child's internalization of values: A reconceptualization of current points of view. *Developmental Psychology, 30*, 4–19.
Hayashi, A., Karasawa, M., & Tobin, J. (2009). The Japanese preschool's pedagogy of feeling: Cultural strategies for supporting young children's emotional development. *Ethos, 37*, 32–49.
Heikamp, T., Mishra, R. C., Suchodoletz, A. v., & Trommsdorff, G. (2008). Cultural aspects of the development of regulatory behaviour: Maternal reactions to children's frustration in Germany and India. In X. Chen (Chair), *Children and adolescents' social competence in cultural context.* Invited Symposium conducted at 19th International Congress of Psychology (ICP), Berlin, Germany.
Heikamp, T., Trommsdorff, G., & Fäsche A. (in press). Development of self-regulation in context. In P. M. Gollwitzer, M. Schmitz, & G. Seebaß (Eds.), *Acting intentionally and its limits: Individuals, groups, institutions.* Berlin: De Gruyter.
Heine, S. J., Lehman, D. R., Markus, H. R., & Kitayama, S. (1999). Is there a universal need for positive self-regard? *Psychological Review, 106*, 766–794.
Henrich, J., Heine, S. J., & Norenzayan, A. (2010). The weirdest people in the world? *Behavioral and Brain Science, 33*, 61–83.
Holodynski, M., & Friedlmeier, W. (2006). *Development of emotions and emotion regulation.* New York: Springer.
Hwang, K.-K., & Chang, J. (2009). Self-cultivation. *The Counselling Psychologist, 37*, 1010–1032.
Kağitçibaşi, C. (1997). Individualism and collectivism. In J. W. Berry, M. H. Segall, & C. Kağitçibaşi (Eds.), *Handbook of cross-cultural psychology* (pp. 1–50). Needham Heights, MA: Allyn & Bacon.
Kakihara, F., & Tilton-Weaver, L. C. (2009). Adolescents interpretations of parental control: Differentiated by domain and types of control. *Child Development, 80*, 1722–1738.
Kitayama, S. (2000). Collective construction of the self and social relationships: A rejoinder and some extensions. *Child Development, 71*, 1143–1146.
Kitayama, S. (2001). Culture and emotion. In N. J. Smelser & P. B. Baltes (Eds.), *International encyclopedia of the social and behavioral sciences* (pp. 3134–3139). Oxford: Elsevier.
Kitayama, S., Mesquita, B., & Karasawa, M. (2006). Cultural affordances and emotional experience: Socially engaging and disengaging emotions in Japan and the United States. *Journal of Personality and Social Psychology, 91*, 890–903.
Kornadt, H.-J. (2011). *Aggression: Die Rolle der Erziehung in Europa und Ostasien* [Aggression: The role of education in Europe and East Asia]. Wiesbaden, Germany: VS Verlag.
Kornadt, H.-J., & Trommsdorff, G. (1984). Erziehungsziele im Kulturvergleich [Parenting goals in cross–cultural comparison]. In G. Trommsdorff (Ed.), *Jahrbuch für Empirische Erziehungswissenschaft 1984: Erziehungsziele* (pp. 191–212). Düsseldorf, Germany: Pädagogischer Verlag Schwann.
Lebra, T. S. (1992). Self in Japanese culture. In N. R. Rosenberger (Ed.), *Japanese sense of self: Publications of the Society for Psychological Anthropology* (pp. 105–120). New York: Cambridge University Press.
Lebra, T. S. (1994). Mother and child in Japanese socialization: A Japan-U.S. comparison. In P. M. Greenfield & R. R. Cocking (Eds.), *Cross-cultural roots of minority child development* (pp. 259–274). Hillsdale, NJ: Erlbaum.

Li, J. (2002). A cultural model of learning: Chinese "heart and mind for wanting to learn." *Journal of Cross-Cultural Psychology, 33*, 248–269.

Li, J. (2005). Mind or virtue: Western and Chinese beliefs about learning. *Current Directions in Psychological Science, 14*, 190–194.

Markus, H. R., & Kitayama, S. (1991). Culture and the self: Implications for cognition, emotion, and motivation. *Psychological Review, 98*, 224–253.

Markus, H. R., & Kitayama, S. (1994). The cultural construction of self and emotion: Implications for social behavior. In S. Kitayama & H. R. Markus (Eds.), *Emotion and culture: Empirical studies of mutual influence* (pp. 89–130). Washington, DC: American Psychological Association.

Markus, H. R., & Kitayama, S. (2004). Models of agency: Sociocultural diversity in the construction of action. In G. Berman & J. Berman (Eds.), *Nebraska Symposium on Motivation: Cross-cultural differences in the perspectives on the self* (Vol. 49, pp. 1–57). Lincoln, NE: University of Nebraska Press.

Markus, H. R., Uchida, Y., Omoregie, H., Townsend, S. S. M., & Kitayama, S. (2006). Going for the gold: Models of agency in Japanese and American contexts. *Psychological Science, 17*, 103–112.

Meltzoff, A. N. (1995). Understanding the intentions of others: Re-enactment of intended acts by 18-month-old children. *Developmental Psychology, 31*, 838–850.

Mesquita, B., & Albert, D. (2007). The cultural regulation of emotions. In J. J. Gross (Ed.), *Handbook of emotion regulation* (pp. 486–503). New York: Guilford.

Miller, J. G. (1984). Culture and the development of everyday social explanations. *Journal of Personality and Social Psychology, 46*, 961–978.

Miller, J. G. (1997). Cultural conceptions of duty: Implications for motivation and morality. In D. Munro, J. F. Schumaker, & S. C. Carr (Eds.), *Motivation and culture* (pp. 178–192). New York: Routledge.

Miller, J. G. (2003). Culture and agency: Implications for psychological theories of motivation and social development. In V. Murphy-Berman & J. Berman (Eds.), *Nebraska Symposium on Motivation: Cross-cultural difference in perspectives on the self* (Vol. 49, pp. 59–99). Lincoln, NE: University of Nebraska Press.

Morelli, G. A., & Rothbaum, F. (2007). Situating the child in context: Attachment relationships and self–regulation in different cultures. In S. Kitayama & D. Cohen (Eds.), *Handbook of cultural psychology* (pp. 500–527). New York: Guilford.

Morling, B., & Evered, S. (2006). Secondary control reviewed and defined. *Psychological Bulletin, 132*, 269–296.

Morling, B., & Fiske, S. T. (1999). Defining and measuring harmony control. *Journal of Research in Personality, 33*, 379–414.

Morris, M. W., Menon, T., & Ames, D. (2001). Culturally conferred conceptions of agency: A key to social perception of persons, groups, and other actors. *Personality and Social Psychology Review, 5*, 169–182.

Morris, A. S., Silk, J. S., Steinberg, L., Myers, S. S., & Robinson, L. R. (2007). The role of the family context in the development of emotion regulation. *Social Development, 16*, 1–388.

Mulder, N. (1992). *Individual and society in Java: A cultural analysis* (2nd ed.). Yogyakarta, Indonesia: Gadjah Mada University Press.

Oyserman, D., Coon, H. M., & Kemmelmeier, M. (2002). Rethinking individualism and collectivism: Evaluation of theoretical assumptions and meta-analyses. *Psychological Bulletin, 128*, 3–72.

Raeff, C. (2010). Independence and interdependence in children's developmental experiences. *Child Development Perspectives, 4*, 31–36.

Raval, V. V., & Martini, T. S. (2009). Maternal socialization of children's anger, sadness, and physical pain in two communities in Gujarat, India. *International Journal of Behavioral Development, 33*, 215–229.

Rohner, R. P., & Pettengill, S. M. (1985). Perceived parental acceptance–rejection and parental control among Korean adolescents. *Child Development, 56*, 524–528.
Rothbaum, F., Nagaoka, R., & Ponte, I. C. (2006). Caregiver sensitivity in cultural context: Japanese and U.S. teachers' beliefs about anticipating and responding to children's needs. *Journal of Research in Childhood Education, 21*, 23–39.
Rothbaum, F., Pott, M., Azuma, H., Miyake, K., & Weisz, J. (2000). The development of close relationships in Japan and the United States: Paths of symbiotic harmony and generative tension. *Child Development, 71*, 1121–1142.
Rothbaum, F., & Rusk, N. (2011). Pathways to emotion regulation: Cultural differences in internalization. In K. H. Rubin & X. Chen (Eds.), *Socioemotional development in cultural context* (pp. 99–130). New York: Guilford.
Rothbaum, F., & Trommsdorff, G. (2007). Do roots and wings oppose or complement one another? The socialization of autonomy and relatedness in cultural context. In J. E. Grusec & P. Hastings (Eds.), *The handbook of socialization* (pp. 461–489). New York: Guilford.
Rothbaum, F., & Wang, Y. Z. (2010). Fostering the children's malleable views of the self and the world: Caregiving practices in East Asian and European American communities. In B. Mayer & H.-J. Kornadt (Eds.), *Soziokultureller Kontext und menschliche Entwicklung* (pp. 101–120). Wiesbaden, Germany: VS Verlag.
Rothbaum, F., Weisz, J. R., & Snyder, S. S. (1982). Changing the world and changing the self: A two-process model of perceived control. *Journal of Personality and Social Psychology, 42*, 5–37.
Rudy, D., & Grusec, J. E. (2001). Correlates of authoritarian parenting in individualist and collectivist cultures and implications for understanding the transmission of values. *Journal of Cross–Cultural Psychology, 32*, 202–212.
Saarni, C., Campos, J. J., Camras, L. J., & Witherington, D. (2006). Emotional development: Action, communication, and understanding. In W. Damon & N. Eisenberg (Eds.), *Handbook of child psychology: Vol. 3. Social, emotional, and personality development* (6th ed., pp. 226–299). New York: Wiley.
Sameroff, A. J. (2009). Conceptual issues in studying the development of self-regulation. In S. L. Olson & A. J. Sameroff (Eds.), *Biopsychosocial regulatory processes in the development of childhood behavioral problems* (pp. 1–18). Cambridge: Cambridge University Press.
Sampson, E. E. (1988). The debate on individualism: Indigenous psychologies of the individual and their role in personal and societal functioning. *American Psychologist, 43*, 15–22.
Sedikides, C., & Gregg, A. P. (2008). Self-enhancement: Food for thought. *Perspectives on Psychological Science, 3*, 102–116.
See, C. M., & Essau, C. (2010). Coping strategies in cross-cultural comparison. In B. Mayer & H.–J. Kornadt (Eds.), *Psychologie – Kultur – Gesellschaft* (pp. 161–174). Wiesbaden, Germany: VS Verlag.
Shweder, R. A., Goodnow, J., Hatano, G., LeVine, R. A., Markus, H. R., & Miller, P. (1998). The cultural psychology of development: One mind, many mentalities. In W. Damon & R. M. Lerner (Eds.), *Handbook of child psychology: Theorectical models of human development* (5th ed., Vol. 1, pp. 865–937). Hoboken, NJ: Wiley.
Spence, J. T. (1985). Achievement American style: The rewards and costs of individualism. *American Psychologist, 40*, 1285–1295.
Suchodoletz, A. v., Trommsdorff, G., & Heikamp, T. (2011). Linking maternal warmth and responsiveness to children's self-regulation. *Social Development, 20*, 486–503.
Super, C. M., & Harkness, S. (1997). The cultural structuring of child development. In J. W. Berry, P. R. Dasen, & T. S. Saraswathi (Eds.), *Handbook of cross-cultural psychology: Vol. 2. Basic processes and human development* (2nd ed., pp. 1–39). Boston, MA: Allyn & Bacon.
Tao, A., Zhou, Q., & Wang, Y. (2010). Parental reactions to children's negative emotions: Prospective relations to Chinese children's psychological adjustment. *Journal of Family Psychology, 24*, 135–144.

Thompson, R. A. (1994). Emotion regulation: A theme in search of definition. In N. A. Fox (Ed.), *The development of emotion regulation: Biological and behavioural considerations. Monographs of the Society for Research in Child Development* (Vol. 59, Issue 2-3, Series 240, pp. 25–52). Chicago, IL: University of Chicago Press.

Tomasello, M. (1999). Having intentions, understanding intentions, and understanding communicative intentions. In P. D. Zelazo, J. W. Astington, & D. R. Olson (Eds.), *Developing theories of intention: Social understanding and self-control* (pp. 63–75). Mahwah, NJ: Erlbaum.

Tomasello, M. (2009). *Why we cooperate.* Cambridge, MA: MIT Press.

Triandis, H. C. (1989). The self and social behavior in differing cultural contexts. *Psychological Review, 96*, 506–520.

Trommsdorff, G. (1985). Some comparative aspects of socialization in Japan and Germany. In I. Reyes Lagunes & Y. H. Poortinga (Eds.), *From a different perspective: Studies of behavior across cultures* (pp. 231–240). Amsterdam: Swets & Zeitlinger.

Trommsdorff, G. (2000). Effects of social change on individual development: The role of social and personal factors and the timing of events. In L. Crocket & R. K. Silbereisen (Eds.), *Negotiating adolescence in times of social change* (pp. 58–68). Cambridge: Cambridge University Press.

Trommsdorff, G. (2006). Development of emotions as organized by culture. *ISSBD Newsletter, 49*, 1–4.

Trommsdorff, G. (2007a). Entwicklung im kulturellen Kontext [Development in cultural context]. In G. Trommsdorff & H.-J. Kornadt (Eds.), *Enzyklopädie der Psychologie: Themenbereich C Theorie und Forschung, Serie VII Kulturvergleichende Psychologie. Band 2: Kulturelle Determinanten des Erlebens und Verhaltens* (pp. 435–519). Göttingen, Germany: Hogrefe.

Trommsdorff, G. (2007b). Intentionality of action in cultural context. In J. Wassmann & K. Stockhaus (Eds.), *Experiencing new worlds* (pp. 58–77). New York: Berghahn.

Trommsdorff, G. (2009). Culture and development of self-regulation. *Social and Personality Psychology Compass, 3*, 687–701.

Trommsdorff, G. (2012). Development of agentic regulation in cultural context: The role of self and world views. *Child Development Perspectives, 6*, 9–26.

Trommsdorff, G., & Cole, P. M. (2011). Emotion, self-regulation, and social behaviour in cultural contexts. In X. Chen & K. H. Rubin (Eds.), *Socioemotional development in cultural context* (pp. 131–163). New York: Guilford.

Trommsdorff, G., Cole, P. M., & Heikamp, T. (2012). Cultural variations in mothers' intuitive theories: A preliminary report on interviewing mothers of five nations about their socialization of children's emotions. *Global Studies of Childhood, 2*, 158–169.

Trommsdorff, G., & Friedlmeier, W. (1993). Control and responsiveness in Japanese and German mother–child interactions. *Early Development and Parenting, 2*, 65–78.

Trommsdorff, G., & Friedlmeier, W. (2010). Preschool girls' distress and mothers' sensitivity in Japan and Germany. *European Journal of Developmental Psychology, 7*, 350–370.

Trommsdorff, G., Friedlmeier, W., & Mayer, B. (2007). Sympathy, distress, and prosocial behavior of preschool children in four cultures. *International Journal of Behavioral Development, 31*, 284–293.

Trommsdorff, G., & Kornadt, H.-J. (1995). Prosocial and antisocial motivation of adolescents in East and West Germany. In J. Youniss (Ed.), *After the wall: Family adaptations in East and West Germany* (pp. 39–56). San Francisco, CA: Jossey-Bass.

Trommsdorff, G., & Kornadt, H.-J. (2003). Parent–child relations in cross-cultural perspective. In L. Kuczynski (Ed.), *Handbook of dynamics in parent–child relations* (pp. 271–306). Thousand Oaks, CA: Sage.

Trommsdorff, G., Kornadt, H.-J., & Hessel-Scherf, M. (1998). Soziale Motivation ost- und westdeutscher Kinder [Social motivation of East and West German children]. In H. Oswald (Ed.), *Sozialisation und Entwicklung in den neuen Bundesländern: Ergebnisse empirischer Längsschnittstudien* (pp. 121–136). Weinheim, Germany: Juventa.

Trommsdorff, G., & Rothbaum, F. (2008). Development of emotion regulation in cultural context. In S. Ismer, S. Jung, S. Kronast, C. V. Scheve, & M. Vandekerckhove (Eds.), *Regulating emotions: Social necessity and biological inheritance* (pp. 85–120). New York: Blackwell.

Vohs, K. D., Lasaleta, J. D., & Fennis, B. (2009). Self-regulation in the interpersonal sphere. In J. P. Forgas, R. F. Baumeister, & D. M. Tice (Eds.), *Psychology of self-regulation: Cognitive, affective, and motivational processes* (pp. 289–302). New York: Psychology Press.

Wang, Q. (2003). Emotion situation knowledge in American and Chinese preschool children and adults. *Cognition and Emotion, 17*, 725–746.

Wellman, H. M. (2009). Understanding the psychological world: Developing a theory of mind. In U. Goswami (Ed.), *Handbook of childhood cognitive development* (pp. 167–187). Oxford: Blackwell.

Weisz, J. R., Rothbaum, F. M., & Blackburn, T. C. (1984). Standing out and standing in: The psychology of control in America and Japan. *American Psychologist, 39*, 955–969.

Wong, P. T. P., & Wong, L. C. J. (Eds.). (2006). *Handbook of multicultural perspectives on stress and coping.* New York: Springer.

Gisela Trommsdorff
Department of Psychology
University of Konstanz
P.O. Box D 14
78457 Konstanz
Germany
E-mail: Gisela.Trommsdorff@uni-konstanz.de

Chapter 5

Emotion Regulation in Cultural Context

Implications for Wellness and Illness

Emily A. Butler

Norton School Family and Consumer Sciences, University of Arizona, Tucson, AZ, USA

Abstract

Emotion regulation can be conceptualized in at least three ways (Butler, 2011). First, emotions can be seen as one component of a general self-regulatory system that modifies our ongoing behavioral responses in order to achieve our goals. From this perspective emotions help to regulate much of our behavior. Second, emotions arise from internal feedback processes within the brain and between the brain and the body that help to keep our physical and psychological systems in balance and within an optimal range of functioning. In this context, it is the emotion system itself that is internally regulated. Third, emotions can become the target of self-regulatory efforts, such as when we try to hide what we are feeling. Each of these views emphasizes slightly different connections between emotion regulation and well-being. In addition, emotion regulation is not constrained to within a person; it is embedded in larger sociocultural contexts that influence most aspects of emotional responding (Markus & Kitayama, 1991, 1994; Mesquita, 2001; Oyserman, Coon, & Kemmelmeier, 2002; Scherer, 1997; Wierzbicka, 1994). This chapter considers the ways in which cultural contexts modulate emotion regulatory processes and the implications this has for well-being.

Keywords: emotion, regulation, culture, suppression, reappraisal, health, well-being

Introduction

Emotional states arise from a dynamic process involving interacting components such as feelings, cognitive appraisals, behaviors, and physiology (Barrett, Ochsner, & Gross, 2007; Cacioppo et al., 1992; Hoeksma, Oosterlaan, & Schipper, 2004; Lewis, 2005; Scherer, 1987, 2000; Thayer & Lane, 2000). These coordinated responses are grounded in an interconnected network of structures within the brain that integrates appraisals, attention, and biological responses to mount an organized behavioral response to environmental demands (Lewis, 2005; Ochsner & Gross, 2007; Thayer & Lane, 2000). Subjective states, such as feeling angry or happy, are assumed to reflect a person's summary perception of how successfully he or she is responding to personally relevant threats or opportunities (Thayer & Lane, 2000). Emotional states have a significant impact on self-regulation, for example, subjective feelings provide feedback to the other emotional components, especially cognition, allowing internal modulation of the total emotional response (Hoeksma et al., 2004). Furthermore, emotions guide behavioral responses to important events, tune decision making, enhance memory for important events, and facilitate social relationships (Campos, Mumme, Kermoian, & Campos, 1994; Cole, Martin, & Dennis, 2004; Gross, 1998, 1999; Witherington & Crichton, 2007).

Given this backdrop, emotions and emotion regulation have implications for wellness and illness because emotions involve coordinated responses across physical, experiential, and behavioral systems. Due to this, emotions can have direct physiological effects relevant to well-being (e.g., increased blood pressure), effects on behaviors relevant to well-being (e.g., drinking too much alcohol), and social effects relevant to well-being (e.g., increased hostility). In addition, well-regulated emotional responding is critical for our ability to respond flexibly to the environment and flexibility has emerged as a critical factor for healthy functioning (Hollenstein, Granic, Stoolmiller, & Snyder, 2004; Kashdan & Rottenberg, 2010). Our physical systems are in constant flux, responding in organized patterns to environmental demands (Friedman, 2007). Imbalance or rigidity in these systems is predictive of poor health and even death (Thayer & Brosschot, 2005; Thayer & Lane, 2007; Thayer & Sternberg, 2006). Similarly, cognitive and emotional flexibility are important for modulating our behavior to successfully meet the demands of life (Bonnano, Papa, O'Neill, Westphal, & Coifman, 2004; Thompson, 1994). In addition, a lack of interpersonal flexibility has been linked to psychological problems in families (Granic, O'Hara, Peplar, & Lewis, 2007; Hollenstein et al., 2004).

Despite the fact that emotions clearly have implications for well-being, the research reviewed in this chapter shows that understanding emotion regulation in cultural context is necessary if we are to fully appreciate how emotions contribute to wellness and illness. Before addressing these issues, however, we need to consider the term *emotion regulation* in greater detail.

The Concept of Emotion Regulation

The relationship between emotion and self-regulation can be conceptualized in at least three ways. First, emotions play an important role in overall self-regulation, which entails generating, inhibiting, exaggerating, or otherwise changing our own global response (Baumeister, Bratslavsky, Muraven, & Tice, 1998; Baumeister, Zell, & Tice, 2007; Muraven, Tice, & Baumeister, 1998). Emotions arise when a situation is seen as relevant to our goals and coordinate a full-body response that allows us to quickly change our overall behavioral reaction to optimize achieving those goals (Gross, 1999). Thus emotions help to motivate and guide much of our behavior. Second, the emotion system itself operates through internal feedback processes that modulate our emotional responding (Hoeksma, Oosterlaan, Schipper, & Koot, 2007; Lewis, 2005). For example, anxiety may arise through a positive feedback loop involving attention to danger cues, followed by increased fight-or-flight physiological responses (e.g., increased heart rate), which then increase attention to danger cues, which increase physiological activation, and so forth (Mathews, 1990). From this perspective, a well-functioning emotion system is a well-regulated one, meaning that the emotions that arise are optimal in kind, strength, and duration for promoting adaptive behaviors, with suboptimal emotional responses being inhibited (Rottenberg & Gross, 2003). Third, emotions can themselves become the target of self-regulatory efforts. For example, we may try to hide what we are feeling from other people, take a few deep breaths to calm down, or try to think about a situation differently so that we also feel differently. In this context emotion regulation is defined as any self-regulatory action that modulates any aspect of emotional processing, including which emotions we have, when we have them, and how we experience and express them (Gross & Thompson, 2007).

Implications of Emotion Regulation in Cultural Context for Wellness and Illness

How might cultural context impact individuals' emotion regulation and its implications for illness and wellness? First, different emotions, such as anger or happiness, support different forms of goal achievement (Tamir, Mitchell, & Gross, 2008). For example, anger may improve our performance in a confrontational situation, but happiness is more conducive to cooperation. In addition, cultural contexts vary in the priority given to different high-level goals, such as achieving individual success versus maximizing group outcomes (Markus & Kitayama, 1991). To achieve these divergent goals, different emotions would be optimal. Thus the role of emotion in self-regulation should vary across cultural contexts to the extent that higher-level goals vary. Second, internal regulation of the emotion system is sculpted by social learning from birth to promote well-regulated responding within a given cultural context (Camras, Chen, Bakeman, Norris, & Cain, 2006; Camras et al., 1998; Wang, 2001). Thus cultural contexts contribute to the types, strength, and range of emotions we spontaneously experience and express across the life span. Third, the ways in which we target our own emotions for self-regulation, and toward what ends, will vary as we attempt to achieve our goals within the constraints, affordances, and meaning systems of a particular cultural context (Kitayama, Karasawa, & Mesquita, 2004). The following sections first clarify the terms *cultural context*, *wellness*, and *illness* in greater detail and then consider research relevant to these issues from the perspectives of each of the three views of emotion regulation.

Cultural Context

Following Kroeber and Kluckholm (1952), I use the term cultural context to refer to the "[e]xplicit and implicit patterns of historically derived and selected ideas and their embodiment in institutions, practices, and artifacts" (p. 357). One important aspect of this definition is that it does not imply that all people from one cultural background are alike. Instead, similarities between people arising from cultural context depend upon the extent to which they share particular ideas, values, experience with practices, learned habits, and so on (Mauss, Butler, Roberts, & Chu, 2010). From this view, culture is not "in the head." It is out there in the world in the form of institutions, practices, and meaning systems (Kitayama, 2002). Each person's psychological processes, such as emotions, are organized through coordinating with the cultural system of practices and public meanings. Cultural values are important because they shape the system of institutions, daily practices, lay theories, and so forth, which in turn shape individuals' habits, beliefs, emotions, sense of self, and the like (Kitayama, Mesquita, & Karasawa, 2006). Shared experiences of adapting to these cultural affordances and constraints contribute to a sense of being at home in a particular group (Shweder, 2007). In other words, being a member of a cultural group arises through thinking and acting in a certain way, in the light of particular goals, values, and beliefs of the world (Berlin, 1976). Individuals and cultures are thus mutually constituted, emerging from each other in a continuously evolving discourse in which individual actions accumulate in cultural patterns and those patterns in turn constrain future individual acts (Adams & Markus, 2004; Kitayama, 2002; Ryder, Ban, & Dere, in press).

Wellness and Illness

For a long time research on health focused on its opposite, disease, and considered only biological factors. A shift has occurred over the last 40 years with the advent of the biopsychosocial model (Borrell-Carrio, Suchman, & Epstein, 2004; Engel, 1977; Gross, 1989; Lindau, Laumann, Levinson, & Waite, 2003). The basic tenet of this model is that health is influenced by interactions across levels of the human system including biological, psychological, and social influences. Given this premise, physical, psychological, and social well-being are tightly intertwined. In addition, increasing emphasis has been placed on well-being and thriving (Fava, Rafanelli, Cazzaro, Conti, & Grandi, 1998; Izquierdo, 2005). Health is now seen as not only the lack of disease, but the ability to flourish as well, including relating to others in mutually satisfying ways, working productively, and feeling comfortable when alone (Gross & Munoz, 1995). In contrast to wellness, disease has been defined as the malfunctioning of biological and/or psychological processes, while the term illness refers to the psychosocial experience and meaning of perceived disease (Kleinman, 1988). This suggests that health needs to be considered within a larger sociocultural context: Although people in most cultures desire a lack of physical disability, what constitutes well-being and thriving varies, with some groups placing greater value on biological indices and others placing more importance on things like the quality of one's social relationships and moral goodness (Izquierdo, 2005).

Emotions as Part of Overall Self-Regulation

Emotions provide motivation for behavior and influence our decision-making processes, thereby providing an important component of our overall self-regulatory system (Baumeister et al., 2007; Thayer & Lane, 2000). One way emotions guide our behavior is through affective forecasting, which occurs when we choose to do – or not do – something based on the expected emotional impact it will have on us (Cooper, Flanagan, Talley, & Micheas, 2006). Although affective forecasting may be a universal psychological process, different cultures prioritize different goals and have corresponding differences in ideals for emotional experience (Tsai, Knutson, & Fung, 2006). For example, European Americans tend to hold influence goals, such as wanting to change or improve their environment, and value high-arousal positive emotions that support achieving influence. In contrast, Asians are more likely to have goals compatible with adjusting to their environment and value low-arousal positive emotions that promote such accommodation (Tsai et al., 2006). Similarly, American culture emphasizes individual achievements and Americans report high levels of disengaging emotions, such as pride and anger, as well as hedonistic positive emotions such as enjoyment, all of which support individual goal striving. Asian culture, however, prioritizes collective achievements and Asians report greater engaging emotions, such as friendliness and guilt, as well as greater self-critical emotions such as shame, which all contribute to group cohesion and striving to meet social obligations (Falk, Dunn, & Norenzayan, 2010; Kitayama, Markus, & Kurokawa, 2000; Kitayama et al., 2006).

Given these cultural differences in goals and desired emotions, affective forecasting should promote different behaviors in different contexts for different cultures (Mesquita & Frijda, 1992). In support of this, in one study European Canadians tended to make choices that optimized enjoyment, while Asian Canadians were more likely to choose activities that were useful. In addition, the Asian Canadians placed less weight on expected enjoyment when making hypothetical choices, and bicultural Asian Canadians primed with interdependent self-construals placed less weight on enjoyment than if they were primed with independent construals (Falk et al., 2010). These results could have implications for illness and wellness because they suggest there may be cultural differences in the extent to which people pursue enjoyable but unhealthy behaviors, such as eating candy, versus more useful activities such as following prescribed health guidelines like getting enough exercise. The answer to whether this is true or not, however, awaits future research.

In addition to differences in which emotions are pursued, there may also be cultural differences in the weight given to future emotions as a guide to behavior. For example, cultures that emphasize individualism appear to value emotions more as a source of information and guide for behavior than cultures that emphasize collectivism. In contrast, more collectivistic cultures appear to value norms more as a guide to behavior. Evidence for this comes from a large cross-national study that showed that emotions and life satisfaction were strongly correlated in more individualistic countries, while emotions and norms were both correlated with satisfaction in more collectivistic countries (Suh, Diener, Oishi, & Triandis, 1998). Again, this could have implications for health, since people in more individualistic cultures may allow emotions to play a larger role in guiding their health behaviors, while those in more collectivistic cultures may pay more attention to established health guidelines. I am not aware of any research addressing this question, however, making it an important direction for future research.

In addition to expected future emotions guiding behavior, cultural differences also exist in how people respond to currently experienced emotions. In other words, the same emotion can guide self-regulation differently. One example of this is a study in which Dutch and Phillipino salespeople responded to shame differently. The Dutch became self-protective and their sales performance suffered, but the Phillipinos tried to mend their relationships and their performance did not suffer (Bagozzi, Verbeke, & Gavino, 2003). Similarly, in a study of interpersonal negotiations, expressing anger elicited higher concessions from European Americans, but smaller concessions from Asians and Asian Americans. Furthermore, these effects were shown to be due to cultural norms regarding the appropriateness of anger expression. Specifically, the cultural differences were eliminated if anger expressions were manipulated to be appropriate or not. In that case all participants gave larger concessions in response to appropriate anger expression and smaller ones to inappropriate expressions (Adam, Shirako, & Maddux, 2010).

Internal Regulation of Emotion System

Emotions are partly a physical phenomenon, but they are also partly cognitively constructed in the context of moral and ideological values (Gross, 1999; Ryder et al., in press). Culture can therefore have a direct impact on the internal regulation of the emotion system due to influencing cognitive and interpretative aspects of emotional processing (Mesquita & Frijda, 1992; Scherer, 1997). One example comes from research showing that cultural differences in appraisals of agency give rise to different emotional experiences (Imada & Ellsworth, 2011). Americans attributed recalled and imagined success to their own agency but attributed failure to external factors. Japanese participants did the opposite. In addition, the Americans experienced pride due to success and anger when failing, but the Japanese experienced feeling lucky due to success and shame due to failing. Importantly, these cultural differences in emotional experience were greatly reduced when similar agency appraisals were induced. Similarly, perceptual biases can produce cultural differences in emotional processing. European Americans appear biased toward perceiving their own emotion in other's faces, while East Asians appear to be biased toward seeing the complementary emotion (Cohen & Gunz,

2002). Self-conception is also linked differently to emotional experience in different cultural contexts. Attending to individual aspects of the self increases emotional reactivity in European Americans compared to Asian Americans, but attention to relational aspects of the self produces similar or greater emotional reactivity in Asian Americans compared to European Americans (Chentsova-Dutton & Tsai, 2010). Finally, Asian dialectical thinking, which emphasizes the intertwining of good and bad and the need to find a middle-way for addressing contradictions, is associated with more balanced experience of positive and negative emotions, as compared to the negative correlation found in nondialectical cultural contexts (Miyamoto & Ryff, 2011; Schimmack, Oishi, & Diener, 2002; Shiota, Campos, Gonzaga, Keltner, & Peng, 2010).

Culture can also impact the internal regulation of the emotion system by affording (making some actions/responses easier) and reinforcing (rewarding and punishing) different emotions, resulting in differences in spontaneous emotional responding (Kitayama, 2002; Kitayama et al., 2004). In this way cultural contexts produce a different range of emotions in terms of both type and intensity (Kitayama et al., 2000; Matsumoto, 1993; Soto, Levenson, & Ebling, 2005; Tsai & Levenson, 1997). To give just a few examples, East Asians and Asian Americans, as compared to European Americans, report less emotional intensity and more neutral affect (Eid & Diener, 2001; Mesquita & Karasawa, 2002), experience more pride in affiliated others' accomplishments and stronger guilt due to their social transgressions (Stipeck, 1998), experience less high arousal positive emotion and socially disengaging emotions such as pride and anger (Kitayama et al., 2006; Tsai et al., 2006), and are less emotionally expressive (Kim & Markus, 2002; Kim & Sherman, 2007). Furthermore, these expressive differences are evident early in life. East Asian children display less emotion than American children and spontaneously refer to fewer emotions (Camras et al., 2006; Camras et al., 1998). In addition, American mothers use an "emotion-explaining" style (focus on individual understanding of emotions), while Chinese mothers use an "emotion-criticizing" style (emotions in service of proper social behavior and emotion restraint). Furthermore, the children's comments about emotions parallel their mothers' (Wang, 2001). These findings suggest that parents in different cultures socialize their children to modulate their emotional responding beginning at birth and this becomes internalized and automatic (Friedlmeier & Trommsdorff, 1999; Keller & Otto, 2009; see chapter 4).

Internal regulation of the emotion system becomes most apparent when regulation fails. Most psychopathologies, such as depression or anxiety, involve emotional dysregulation (Berking et al., 2008; Gross & Munoz, 1995; Moses & Barlow, 2006; Rottenberg & Gross, 2003). Some fascinating recent research suggests, however, that emotional dysregulation can take different forms depending on cultural context. In a sequence of studies, depressed European Americans showed blunted responding to positive and negative emotional stimuli, including less smiling and crying, and reduced emotional experience. Depressed Asian Americans, however, showed increased emotional reactivity (Chentsova-Dutton et al., 2007; Chentsova-Dutton, Tsai, & Gotlib, 2010). These effects suggest that depression reduces attention and the ability to adhere to dominant sociocultural norms for emotional experience and expression. At the same time, a failure to comply with social norms may contribute to developing depression. Also in keeping with this idea, higher positive emotions are associated with lower depressive symptoms for European Americans, but this association is reduced in Asian Americans and eliminated in immigrant Asians (Leu, Want, & Koo, 2011).

Self-Regulation Directed at Emotional Responses

All cultures have implicit and explicit display and feeling rules that specify which emotions are appropriate in what contexts for which people (Matsumoto, 1990; Mesquita & Frijda, 1992). Children are socialized from an early age to develop a psychological system of self-regulation that is responsive to these cultural norms (Ryder et al., in press). Thus our emotional responses can become the target of self-regulation as we attempt to modulate our responding to match the constraints of the social environment and to optimize our emotional state for attaining our goals. Recent research on gene by culture interactions provides a dramatic example of just how powerful cultural shaping of self-regulation can be. In a sequence of studies Kim and her colleagues have shown that a particular genotype of the oxytocin receptor gene (GG; homozygous for the G allele of the OXTRrs53576), which prior research with European Americans has shown to be connected to socioemotional sensitivity, is associated with different emotion regulation strategies in Americans and Koreans (Kim et al., 2011; Kim et al., 2010). Seeking social support and expressing emotions are normative in American cultural contexts, but are more likely to be discouraged in Korean culture. Individuals higher in socioemotional sensitivity should be more responsive to social feedback reinforcing appropriate behaviors and inhibiting inappropriate ones. It was predicted, therefore, that although the GG genotype may be associated with socioemotional sensitivity, culture would affect how socially sensitive people should regulate their emotions. In support of this, for Americans the GG genotype was associated with less self-reported suppression, but the opposite was true for Koreans. In addition, for Americans experiencing high distress, the GG genotype was associated with higher support seeking, but this was not true for Asians.

Cultural Differences in Values Regarding Emotion Expression and Suppression

Cultural shaping of individuals' emotion regulatory strategies likely occurs through multiple mechanisms (Kitayama et al., 2004). In our work my colleagues and I have focused on the role that cultural values play in shaping our emotion-regulatory efforts and outcomes. We adopt the viewpoint that cultural values and practices are reciprocally constituting (Kitayama, 2002; Kitayama et al., 2004; Markus & Kitayama, 1991, 1994; Matsumoto, 1993; Miller, 2002; Wierzbicka, 1993). That is, cultural practices embody cultural values, but those values are simultaneously reinforced by daily practices. Thus, cultural values are expected to be linked to differences in the everyday functions, frequency, and outcomes associated with different emotion regulation attempts.

In several of our studies we focused on emotion suppression, defined as not expressing the emotions that one is experiencing (Butler et al., 2003; Butler, Lee, & Gross,

2007). We join many other authors in proposing that Western European values such as independence and self-assertion encourage open emotion expression in most situations, while constraining the use of emotion suppression to primarily self-protective acts of withdrawal in the face of social threats (Markus & Kitayama, 1991; Matsumoto, 1990; Oyserman et al., 2002; Tsai & Levenson, 1997; Wierzbicka, 1993, 1994). Suppression can also function in a prosocial manner, however. For example, one can hide glee when beating a peer at a competitive game (Friedman & Miller-Herringer, 1991), or suppress anger with a friend to preserve the relationship (Tavris, 1984). Again following previous authors, we suggest that Asian values such as interdependence and relationship harmony might encourage suppression equally often for these prosocial goals and during positive social interactions, rather than constraining it to relatively self-protective purposes. If Asian cultures encourage suppression in a broad range of situations, while Western European cultures constrain it to self-protective functions, then this should be reflected in cultural differences in its frequency of use. Also, if suppression is typically associated with self-protection for Western Europeans, then it would not be surprising if it were also associated with negative emotions such as fear and anger. In contrast, if suppression was more normative for Asians, and often used prosocially, then this association might not hold for them. These hypotheses were supported in a study of European American and bicultural Asian American young women. Women with predominantly European values reported lower levels of habitual suppression than did women with bicultural European Asian values. In addition, for the women with high European values, suppression was associated with more self-protective goals and higher levels of negative emotion, while these associations were, if anything, reversed for the women with bicultural values (Butler et al., 2007).

Most research on emotion suppression has been limited to European American cultural contexts and has found that suppression has generally negative social consequences, such as reduced responsiveness and rapport (Butler et al., 2003). We reasoned, however, that if individuals with more Asian values suppress more often and across more contexts then they may be more practiced and comfortable with suppressing emotions, which may allow them to remain responsive and connected during social interactions even if they do inhibit emotional expression (see chapter 6). To test this hypothesis we randomly assigned European American and bicultural Asian American young women to participate in pairs in a study of conversations about an upsetting documentary war film (Butler et al., 2007). Each pair was randomly assigned to either a suppression group or a control group. In the suppression group one woman in each pair was randomly chosen to secretly receive suppression instructions asking her to hide her emotions during the conversation. The control participants, and the partners of the suppressors, heard instructions asking them to discuss the film as they normally would. Physiological responses were collected throughout the experiment and the conversations were videotaped and rated for behavioral expressions of hostility and for responsiveness. Participants also reported after the conversation on how hostile and withdrawn they found their partners to be. As predicted and shown in Figure 5.1, suppressors with more bicultural Asian European values were seen less hostile and withdrawn than sup-

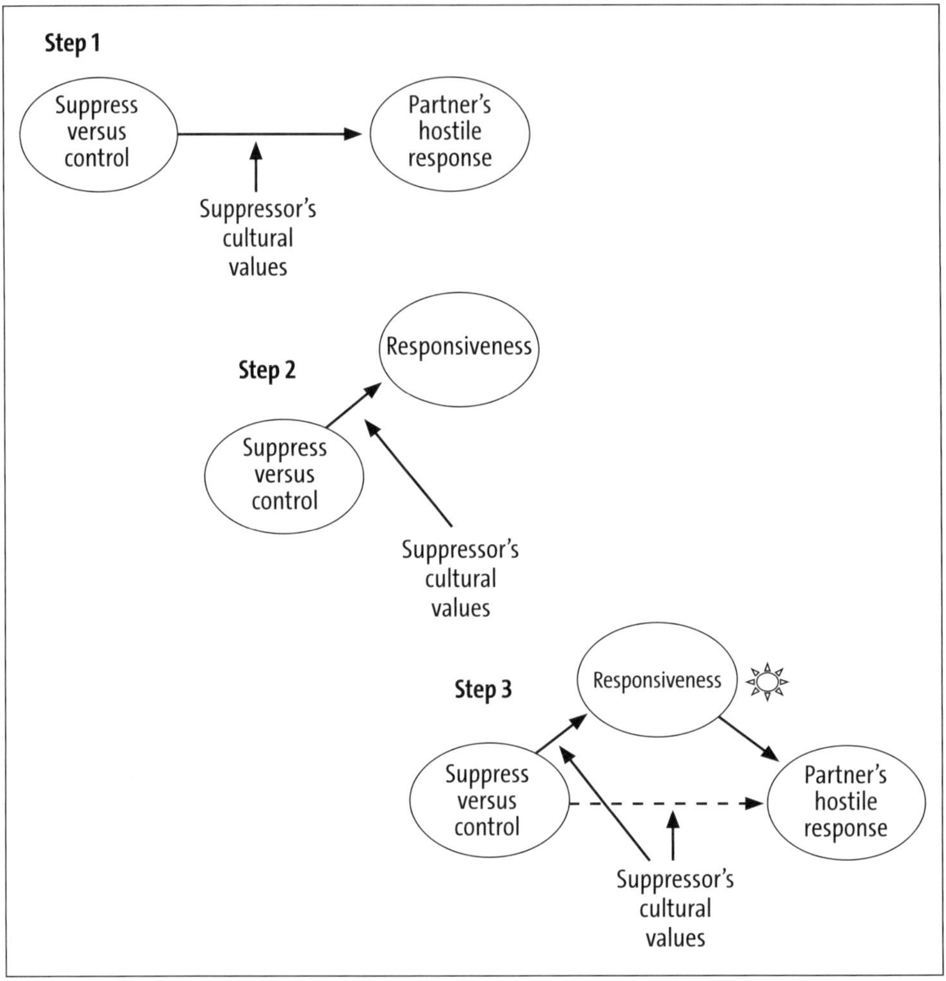

Figure 5.1. A mediated moderation model of the effects of emotion suppression on a social partner's hostile reactions, moderated by cultural values and mediated by responsiveness. Step 1: Suppressors with more European values elicited more hostile reactions from their partners than did suppressors with more bicultural values. Step 2: Suppressors with more European values became less responsive than suppressors with more bicultural values. Step 3: The effect of cultural values on the association between suppression and partner responses was accounted for by the effect of cultural values on the association between suppression and responsiveness.

pressors with predominantly European values. Their partners were also less hostile in their behavioral responses. In addition, these cultural differences in the outcomes of suppression were mediated by cultural differences in the suppressors' responsiveness.

Suppressors with bicultural values were more responsive than those with primarily European values, and this difference accounted for the reduction in negative outcomes.

In a separate analysis of the data from the previous study we reversed our focus and investigated uninhibited emotion expression, the converse of suppression (Butler, Lee, & Gross, 2009). We hypothesized that the social meaning of openly expressing emotion may differ across cultural contexts, with accompanying effects on the relationship between expression and physiological responding. European American culture values self-expression of most forms (Kim & Sherman, 2007). Children are encouraged to speak up and emotional expression is condoned both with in-group and out-group members (Matsumoto, 1990). High levels of expressiveness are seen as signs of competence and likeability and suppressing emotional behavior is associated with increased physiological responding and reduced affiliation (Butler et al., 2003; Gross & Levenson, 1993). In contrast, Asian Americans rate the expression of negative emotions and emotion expression with casual acquaintances as less appropriate than do European Americans (Matsumoto, 1993) and are less likely to seek social support due to concerns that self-expression may have negative relationship consequences (Kim, Sherman, Ko, & Taylor, 2006). Given these cultural differences we hypothesized that in interactions between European Americans, open expression would be normative and desirable, functioning as a marker of successful social interaction. As such, expressivity might be accompanied by physiological calming, such as occurs during socially sup-

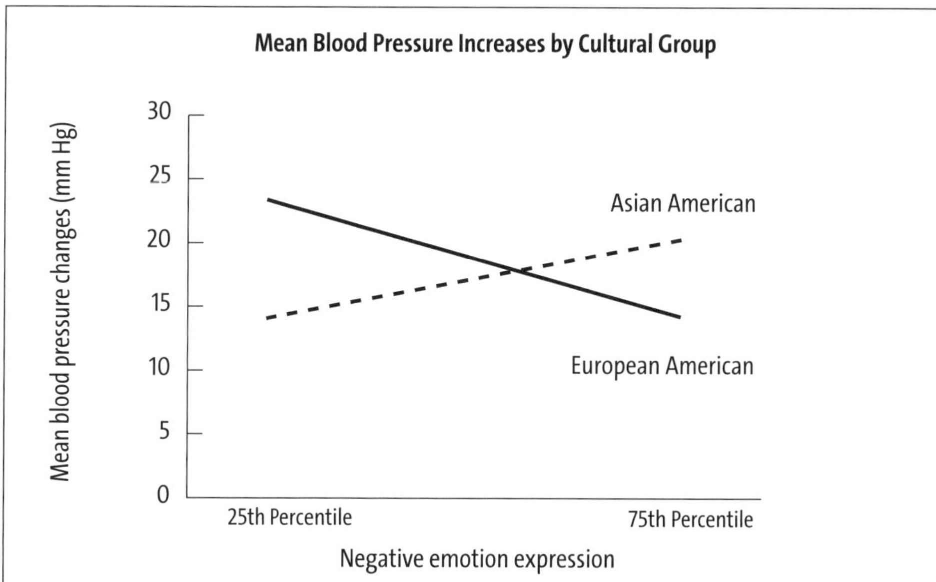

Figure 5.2. Mean blood pressure increases from baseline to conversation as a function of negative emotion expression in European American and Asian American dyads.

portive interactions (Lepore, Allen, & Evans, 1993). In contrast, in interactions between Asian Americans, cultural sanctions might make emotion-expressive behavior a potentially negative stimulus in its own right, requiring careful consideration before engaging in it and extensive evaluation afterward to establish its social impact. If this were the case, such ambivalence may exacerbate physiological responding. As shown in Figure 5.2, these hypotheses were supported. European American women who expressed their negative emotions about the upsetting film had smaller blood pressure increases than those who were less expressive. In contrast, negative expressivity and blood pressure were somewhat positively related for members of Asian American dyads.

Cultural Differences in Values Regarding Emotion Control

I turn now to a different line of research in which we focus on cultural differences in values specifically regarding emotion control. We reason that cultural differences in prescriptions of how emotions should be experienced and expressed may translate into differences in actual emotional responses and in turn have implications for individual well-being and interpersonal interactions. Many other researchers have also proposed that cultural differences in emotional responses are at least partly due to individuals' values about emotion (Eid & Diener, 2001; Markus & Kitayama, 1991, 1994; Matsumoto, Yoo, & Nakagawa, 2008), in addition to factors such as situational demands, genetic factors, or temperament. However, few studies have directly tested whether observed cultural differences can be accounted for by cultural values. To investigate this we compared European American and Asian American women's self-reported emotion control values (e.g., "People should not express their emotions openly," "People in general should control their emotions more," Mauss et al., 2010). We also compared their emotional responses (behavioral, experiential, and physiological) to a laboratory-based anger provocation and assessed whether emotion control values mediated any observed ethnic group differences in anger responding (Mauss et al., 2010). We found, as expected, that the Asian Americans endorsed higher emotion control values. Figure 5.3 shows that we also found that the Asian Americans reported less anger experience and showed less anger behavior when provoked. Furthermore, these group differences in emotional responding were mediated by group differences in values regarding emotion control. Notably we did not find any ethnic group differences in physiological aspects of emotional responding, perhaps because physiology is more difficult to self-regulate than experience or expression.

The previous findings show that cultural context affects people's values regarding emotions, as well as the levels of their experiential and behavioral, but not physiological, responses to emotional situations. We wondered, however, whether the associations between emotion control values and physiological responding might differ across cultural contexts, even if absolute levels of physiology did not. Specifically, depending on their cultural context, individuals' values about emotion control may have differing meanings, and as such, be associated with differing physiological responses in emotional situations, similar to our previous finding that emotion expression related differently to blood pressure for Asian Americans and European Americans. As reviewed

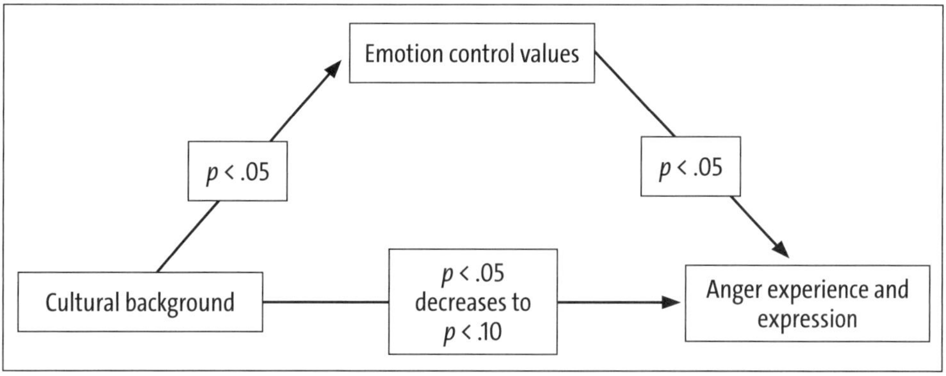

Figure 5.3. A mediation model of the effects of ethnic background (Asian American versus European American) on anger experience and expression, mediated by emotion control values. Asian Americans reported lower anger experience and showed less anger behavior in response to an anger provocation and these effects were mediated by the Asian Americans' higher emotion control values.

earlier, in Asian cultural contexts, emotion control is highly and relatively unambiguously valued. Accordingly, then, individuals in Asian American contexts who highly value emotion control should perceive high congruity with their cultural context and receive more frequent opportunity to "practice" and automatize emotion control. In turn, when they find themselves in a situation that requires emotion control, they should evaluate it as relatively unambiguous, requiring little effort, and perceive their emotion regulatory abilities to be high. This evaluative pattern has been referred to as a challenge response because it entails motivated responding and confidence in one's potential to cope with the demands of the situation (Mendes, Blascovich, Lickel, & Hunter, 2002; Tomaka, Blascovich, Kelsey, & Leitten, 1993). Challenge evaluations are associated with a specific cardiovascular response pattern involving high cardiac output, high left ventricular contractility, and low total peripheral resistance (Mendes et al., 2002; Mendes, Reis, Seery, & Blascovich, 2003; Tomaka et al., 1999). In contrast, in European American cultural contexts, emotion control is more ambiguous and on average less valued because it conflicts with individual self-expression and authenticity. In this context, then, individuals who highly value emotion control may perceive lower congruity with their cultural context and receive less frequent opportunity to practice it. In turn, when they find themselves in a situation that requires emotion control, they should evaluate the situation as more ambiguous, requiring greater effort, and evaluate their own regulatory abilities less confidently. This evaluative pattern has been referred to as a threat response and is associated with a cardiovascular pattern involving lower cardiac output, lower left ventricular contractility, and greater total peripheral resistance (Mendes et al., 2002; Mendes et al., 2003; Tomaka et al., 1999).

To assess whether emotion control values are associated differently with cardiovascular responding in different cultural contexts, we reanalyzed the data from the previ-

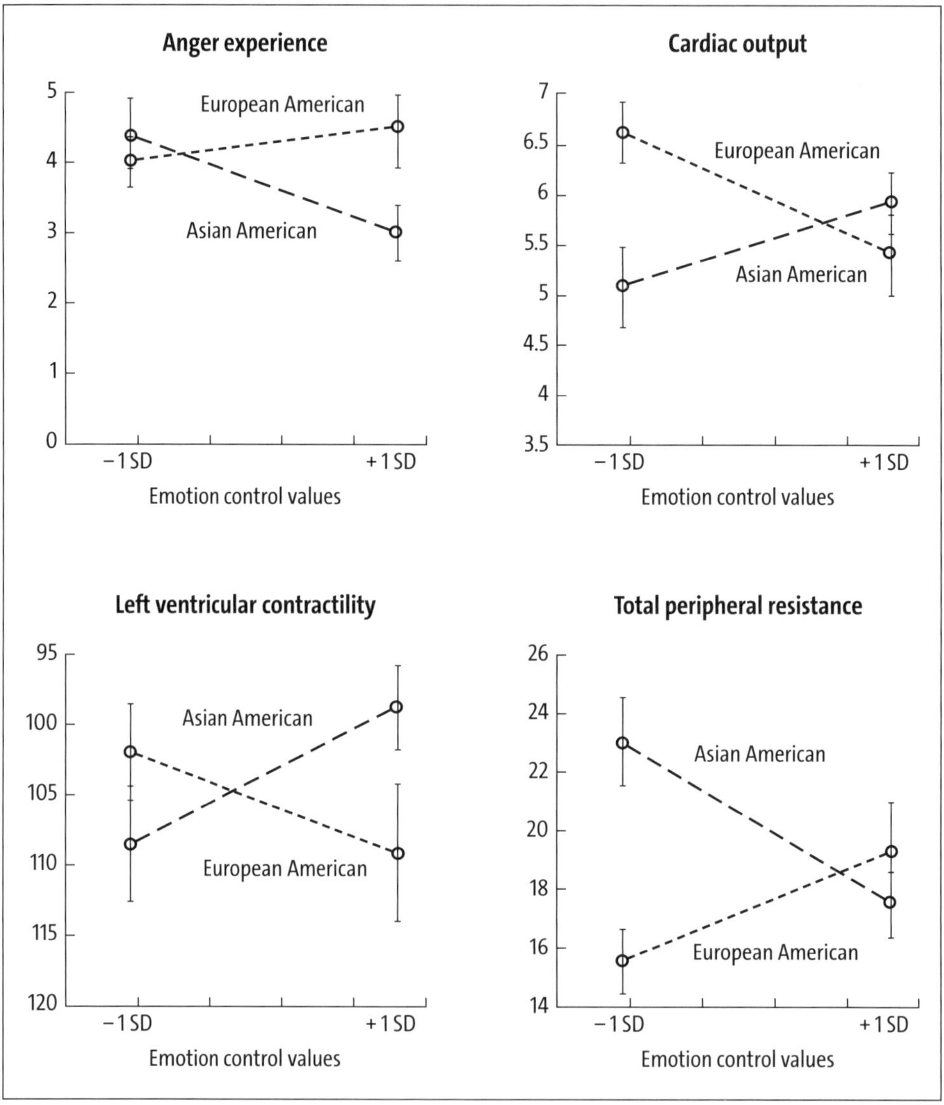

Figure 5.4. The interaction of ethnic background (Asian American versus European American) and emotion control values on anger experience, cardiac output, left ventricular contractility, and total peripheral resistance. The Asian Americans with higher emotion control values show reduced anger experience and a challenge pattern of cardiovascular response, but the European Americans with higher emotion control values show increased anger experience and a threat pattern of cardiovascular response.

ously described anger induction study (Mauss & Butler, 2010). As predicted and shown in Figure 5.4, we found that ethnic background interacted with emotion control values in predicting individuals' emotional and cardiovascular responses to an anger provocation. In line with the hypotheses, we found that in the Asian American group, emotion control values were associated with reduced anger experience and behavior, and a challenge pattern of cardiovascular responding (marginally greater cardiac output (CO) , greater venous capacity (VC), and lower total peripheral resistance (TPR)), a pattern consistent with relatively effective emotion control. In contrast, for European American participants emotion control values were associated with reduced anger behavior but not with anger experience, and a threat pattern of physiological responding (lower CO, no association with VC, and greater TPR), a pattern consistent with less effective emotion control.

Emotion Regulation in Cultural Context: Individual Versus National Level

Much of the research reviewed here focuses at the level of the individual, but other work shows that the associations between emotion components and regulatory strategies can also differ at the national level (Matsumoto et al., 2008). In a large cross-national study, countries valuing social order (long-term orientation, hierarchy, embeddedness) were found to be higher on reports of emotion suppression than those valuing affective autonomy and egalitarianism. In addition, suppression and reappraisal were positively correlated in high social-order countries but negatively correlated in high affective autonomy countries. Interestingly, the countries reporting higher suppression reported lower happiness, but also lower maladjustment (depression, anxiety, alcohol, etc.), and happiness at the country level was positively correlated with maladjustment. One possible explanation for these findings is that countries valuing affective autonomy present a cultural context that promotes high levels of happiness in some individuals, but also high maladjustment in others. Such variability within cultures is sometimes overlooked, but the match between an individual's emotional tendencies or temperament and the dominant cultural norms may be particularly important for illness and wellness. Cultural consonance has been defined as the degree to which a person is able to approximate in their own behavior the prototypical behaviors shared as cultural models (Dressler, Balieiro, Ribeiro, & Dos Santos, 2005). Higher cultural consonance is associated with lower blood pressure, suggesting that we must consider characteristics of both the individual and the cultural context to fully understand the interplay of emotion regulation and well-being.

Clinical Implications

The research reviewed here also has implications for identifying the presence of disease and diagnosis. Interventions for physical and psychological dysfunction must begin with an individual seeking help, but cultural shaping of emotions implies that the presentation of distress will differ based on cultural emotion norms (Ryder et al., in press). Cultural differences in emotional expression and support seeking suggest that individuals from cultures that discourage these behaviors are less likely to be willing to seek help. For example, Asian Americans are less likely to seek social support, largely due to concerns about negative relationship effects (Kim et al., 2006; Kim, Sherman, & Taylor, 2008). In addition, once a person does seek help the problem is likely to be presented differently, depending upon cultural meanings and practices surrounding illness. For example, research shows that Chinese are more likely to report somatic symptoms, rather than psychological ones, possibly because psychological symptoms are stigmatized (Ryder et al., in press). Clinicians will need to be sensitive to these issues if they are to be effective in reaching the people who need help and in providing appropriate interventions once they have made contact.

Concluding Comment

Any instance of emotion regulation occurs within a particular sociocultural context (Frijda & Mesquita, 1994; Kitayama et al., 2004; Matsumoto et al., 2008; Raver, 2004). These contexts differ both at the micro-level (eating dinner with your parents versus attending a football game with your friends) and a macro-level (living in the United States versus Japan). Sensitivity to these contexts and the flexible use of different emotion regulation strategies in different situations is critical for well-being (Bonnano et al., 2004; Bridges, Denham, & Ganiban, 2004; Gratz & Roemer, 2004; Kashdan & Steger, 2006; Rivers, Brackett, Katulak, & Salovey, 2007; Thompson, 1994; Valiente & Eisenberg, 2006). The research reviewed here suggests that every link between emotion regulation and well-being is modified by culture. The fact that many of the differences in emotion regulation reviewed here were observed in samples of European American and Asian American college students serves as a reminder that cultural differences can exist within very small geographic areas, such as a single university population. When we ignore cultural influences we risk drawing erroneous conclusions about a large portion of the world. Ultimately we would like to have the ability to harness our knowledge to answer the question, "How can we help individuals to enhance their emotion regulatory abilities in ways that promote their well-being?" The fact that the answer is "it depends on cultural context" means that we still have a lot of work to do in order to provide answers with enough precision to accomplish that goal.

References

Adam, H., Shirako, A., & Maddux, W. W. (2010). Cultural variance in the interpersonal effects of anger in negotiations. *Psychological Science, 21*, 882–889.

Adams, G., & Markus, H. R. (2004). Toward a conception of culture suitable for a Social Psychology of Culture. In M. Schaller & C. S. Crandall (Eds.), *The psychological foundations of culture* (pp. 335–360). Mahwah, NJ: Erlbaum.

Bagozzi, F. P., Verbeke, W., & Gavino, J. C. (2003). Culture moderates the self-regulation of shame and its effects on performance: The case of salespersons in the Netherlands and the Philippines. *Journal of Applied Psychology, 88*, 219–233.

Barrett, L. F., Ochsner, K. N., & Gross, J. J. (2007). Automaticity and emotion. In J. Bargh (Ed.), *Social psychology and the unconscious* (pp. 173–218). New York: Psychology Press.

Baumeister, R. F., Bratslavsky, E., Muraven, M., & Tice, D. M. (1998). Ego depletion: Is the active self a limited resource? *Journal of Personality and Social Psychology, 74*, 1252–1265.

Baumeister, R. F., Zell, A. L., & Tice, D. M. (2007). How emotions facilitate and impair self-regulation. In J. J. Gross (Ed.), *Handbook of emotion regulation* (pp. 408–426). New York: Guilford.

Berking, M., Wupperman, P., Reichardt, A., Pejic, T., Dippel, A., & Znoj, H. (2008). Emotion-regulation skills as a treatment target in psychotherapy. *Behavior Research and Therapy, 46*, 1230–1237.

Berlin, I. (1976). *Vico and Herder: Two studies in the history of ideas*. London: Hogarth Press.

Bonnano, G. A., Papa, A., O'Neill, K., Westphal, M., & Coifman, K. (2004). The importance of being flexible: The ability to enhance and suppress emotional expression as a predictor of long-term adjustment. *Psychological Science, 15*, 482–487.

Borrell-Carrio, F., Suchman, A. L., & Epstein, R. M. (2004). The Biopsychosocial Model 25 years later: Principles, practice, and scientific inquiry. *Annals of Family Medicine, 2*, 576–582.

Bridges, L. J., Denham, S. A., & Ganiban, J. M. (2004). Definitional issues in emotion regulation research. *Child Development, 75*, 340–345.

Butler, E. A. (2011). Three views of emotion regulation and health. *Social and Personality Psychology Compass, 5*, 563–577.

Butler, E. A., Egloff, B., Wilhelm, F. H., Smith, N. C., Erickson, E. A., & Gross, J. J. (2003). The social consequences of expressive suppression. *Emotion, 3*, 48–67.

Butler, E. A., Lee, T. L., & Gross, J. J. (2007). Emotion regulation and culture: Are the social consequences of emotion suppression culture-specific? *Emotion, 7*, 30–48.

Butler, E. A., Lee, T. L., & Gross, J. J. (2009). Does expressing your emotions raise or lower your blood pressure? The answer depends on cultural context. *Journal of Cross-Cultural Psychology, 40*, 510–517.

Cacioppo, J. T., Uchino, B., Crites, S. L., Snydersmith, M. A., Smith, G., Bernston, G. G., et al. (1992). Relationship between facial expressiveness and sympathetic activation in emotion: A critical review, with emphasis on modeling underlying mechanisms and individual differences. *Journal of Personality and Social Psychology, 62*, 110–128.

Campos, J. J., Mumme, D. L., Kermoian, R., & Campos, R. G. (1994). A functionalist perspective on the nature of emotion. *Monographs of the Society for Research in Child Development, 59*, 284–303.

Camras, L. A., Chen, Y., Bakeman, R., Norris, K., & Cain, T. R. (2006). Culture, ethnicity, and children's facial expressions: A study of European American, Mainland Chinese, Chinese American, and adopted Chinese girls. *Emotion, 6*, 103–114.

Camras, L. A., Oster, H., Campos, J., Campos, R., Ujiie, T., Miyake, K., … Meng, Z. (1998). Production of emotional facial expressions in American, Japanese, and Chinese infants. *Developmental Psychology, 34*, 616–628.

Chentsova-Dutton, Y. E., Chu, J. P., Tsai, J. L., Rottenberg, J., Gross, J. J., & Gotlib, I. H. (2007). Depression and emotional reactivity: Variation among Asian Americans of East Asian descent and European Americans. *Journal of Abnormal Psychology, 116*, 776–785.

Chentsova-Dutton, Y. E., & Tsai, J. L. (2010). Self-focused attention and emotional reactivity: The role of culture. *Journal of Personality and Social Psychology, 98*, 507–519.

Chentsova-Dutton, Y. E., Tsai, J. L., & Gotlib, I. H. (2010). Further evidence for the cultural norm hypothesis: Positive emotion in depressed and control European American and Asian American women. *Cultural Diversity and Ethnic Minority Psychology, 16*, 284–295.

Cohen, D., & Gunz, A. (2002). As seen by the other: Perspectives on the self in the memories and emotional perceptions of Easterners and Westerners. *Psychological Science, 13*, 55–59.

Cole, P. M., Martin, S. E., & Dennis, T. A. (2004). Emotion regulation as a scientific construct: Methodological challenges and directions for child development research. *Child Development, 75*, 317–333.

Cooper, M. L., Flanagan, M. E., Talley, A. E., & Micheas, L. (2006). Individual differences in emotion regulation and their relation to risk taking during adolescence. In D. K. Snyder, J. A. Simpson, & N. J. Hughes (Eds.), *Emotion regulation in couples and families: Pathways to dysfunction and health* (pp. 183–203). Washington, DC: American Psychological Association.

Dressler, W. W., Balieiro, M. C., Ribeiro, R. P., & Dos Santos, J. E. (2005). Cultural consonance and arterial blood pressure in urban Brazil. *Social Science and Medicine, 61*, 527–540.

Eid, M., & Diener, E. (2001). Norms for experiencing emotions in different cultures: Inter- and intranational differences. *Journal of Personality and Social Psychology, 81*, 869–885.

Engel, G. L. (1977). The need for a new medical model: A challenge for biomedicine. *Science, 196*, 129–136.

Falk, C. F., Dunn, E. W., & Norenzayan, A. (2010). Cultural variation in the importance of expected enjoyment for decision making. *Social Cognition, 28*, 609–629.

Fava, G. A., Rafanelli, C., Cazzaro, M., Conti, S., & Grandi, S. (1998). Well-being therapy: A novel psychotherapeutic approach for residual symptoms of affective disorders. *Psychological Medicine, 28*, 475–480.

Friedlmeier, W., & Trommsdorff, G. (1999). Emotion regulation in early childhood: A cross-cultural comparison between German and Japanese toddlers. *Journal of Cross-Cultural Psychology, 30*, 684–711.

Friedman, B. H. (2007). An autonomic flexibility-neurovisceral integration model of anxiety and cardiac vagal tone. *Biological Psychology, 74*, 185–199.

Friedman, H. S., & Miller-Herringer, T. (1991). Nonverbal display of emotion in public and in private: Self-monitoring, personality, and expressive cues. *Journal of Personality and Social Psychology, 61*, 766–775.

Frijda, N. H., & Mesquita, B. (1994). The social roles and functions of emotions. In H. R. Markus & S. Kitayama (Eds.), *Emotion and culture* (pp. 51–87). Washington, DC: American Psychological Association.

Granic, I., O'Hara, A., Peplar, D., & Lewis, M. D. (2007). A dynamic systems analysis of parent–child changes associated with successful "real-world" interventions for aggressive children. *Journal of Abnormal Child Psychology, 35*, 845–857.

Gratz, K. L., & Roemer, L. (2004). Multidimensional assessment of emotion regulation and dysregulation: Development, factor structure, and initial validation of the difficulties in emotion regulation scale. *Journal of Psychopathology and Behavioral Assessment, 26*, 41–54.

Gross, J. J. (1989). Emotional expression in cancer onset and progression. *Social Science Medicine, 28*, 1239–1248.

Gross, J. J. (1998). The emerging field of emotion regulation: An integrative review. *Review of General Psychology, 2*, 271–299.

Gross, J. J. (1999). Emotion and emotion regulation. In L. A. Pervin & O. P. John (Eds.), *Handbook of personality: Theory and research* (2nd ed., pp. 525–552). New York: Guilford.

Gross, J. J., & Levenson, R. W. (1993). Emotional suppression: Physiology, self-report, and expressive behavior. *Journal of Personality and Social Psychology, 64*, 970–986.

Gross, J. J., & Munoz, R. F. (1995). Emotion regulation and mental health. *Clinical Psychology: Science and Practice, 2*, 151–164.

Gross, J. J., & Thompson, R. A. (2007). Emotion regulation: Conceptual foundations. In J. J. Gross (Ed.), *Handbook of emotion regulation* (pp. 3–24). New York: Guilford.

Hoeksma, J. B., Oosterlaan, J., & Schipper, E. M. (2004). Emotion regulation and dynamics of feelings: A conceptual and methodological framework. *Child Development, 75*, 354–360.

Hoeksma, J. B., Oosterlaan, J., Schipper, E. M., & Koot, H. (2007). Finding the attractor of anger: Bridging the gap between dynamic concepts and empirical data. *Emotion, 7*, 638–648.

Hollenstein, T., Granic, I., Stoolmiller, M., & Snyder, J. (2004). Rigidity in parent-child interactions and the development of externalizing and internalizing behavior in early childhood. *Journal of Abnormal Child Psychology, 32*, 595–607.

Imada, T., & Ellsworth, P. C. (2011). Proud Americans and lucky Japanese: Cultural differences in appraisal and corresponding emotion. *Emotion, 11*, 329–345.

Izquierdo, C. (2005). When "health" is not enough: Societal, individual, and biomedical assessments of well-being among the Matsigenka of the Peruvian Amazon. *Social Science and Medicine, 61*, 767–783.

Kashdan, T. B., & Rottenberg, J. (2010). Psychological flexibility as a fundamental aspect of health. *Clinical Psychology Review, 30*, 865–878.

Kashdan, T. B., & Steger, M. F. (2006). Expanding the topography of social anxiety. *Psychological Science, 17*, 120–128.

Keller, H., & Otto, H. (2009). The cultural socialization of emotion regulation during infancy. *Journal of Cross-Cultural Psychology, 40*, 996–1011.

Kim, H. S., & Markus, H. R. (2002). Freedom of speech and freedom of silence: An analysis of talking as a cultural practice. In R. Shweder, M. Minow, & H. R. Markus (Eds.), *Engaging cultural differences: The multicultural challenge in liberal democracies.* (pp. 432–452). New York: Russell Sage Foundation.

Kim, H. S., & Sherman, D. K. (2007). "Express yourself": Culture and the effect of self-expression on choice. *Journal of Personality and Social Psychology, 92*, 1–11.

Kim, H. S., Sherman, D. K., Ko, D., & Taylor, S. E. (2006). Pursuit of comfort and pursuit of harmony: Culture, relationships, and social support seeking. *Personality and Social Psychology Bulletin, 32*, 1595–1607.

Kim, H. S., Sherman, D. K., Mojaverian, T., Sasaki, J. Y., Park, J., Suh, E. M., & Taylor, S. E. (2011). Gene–culture interaction: Oxytocin receptor polymorpism (OXTR) and emotion regulation. *Social Psychological and Personality Science, 2, 665–672.*

Kim, H. S., Sherman, D. K., Sasaki, J. Y., Xu, J., Chu, T. Q., Ryu, C., … Taylor, S. E. (2010). Culture, distress, and oxytocin receptor polymorphism (OXTR) interact to influence emotional support seeking. *Proceedings of the National Academy of Sciences of the United States of America, 107*, 15717–15721.

Kim, H. S., Sherman, D. K., & Taylor, S. E. (2008). Culture and social support. *American Psychologist, 63*, 518–526.

Kitayama, S. (2002). Culture and basic psychological processes – Toward a system view of culture: Comment on Oyserman et al. (2002). *Psychological Review, 128*, 89–96.

Kitayama, S., Karasawa, M., & Mesquita, B. (2004). Collective and personal processes in regulating emotions: Emotion and self in Japan and the United States. In P. Philippot & R. S. Feldman (Eds.), *The regulation of emotion* (pp. 251–273). Mahwah, NJ: Erlbaum.

Kitayama, S., Markus, H. R., & Kurokawa, M. (2000). Culture, emotion, and well-being: Good feelings in Japan and the United States. *Cognition & Emotion, 14*, 93–124.

Kitayama, S., Mesquita, B., & Karasawa, M. (2006). Cultural affordances and emotional experience: Socially engaging and disengaging emotions in Japan and the United States. *Journal of Personality and Social Psychology, 91*, 890–903.

Kleinman, A. (1988). *Rethinking psychiatry: From cultural category to personal experience.* New York: The Free Press.

Kroeber, A. L., & Kluckholm, C. K. (1952). *Culture: A critical review of concepts and definitions.* New York: Random House.

Lepore, S. J., Allen, K. A. M., & Evans, G. W. (1993). Social support lowers cardiovascular reactivity to an acute stressor. *Psychosomatic Medicine, 55*, 518–524.

Leu, J., Want, J., & Koo, K. (2011). Are positive emotions just as "positive" across cutures? *Emotion, 11*, 994–999.

Lewis, M. D. (2005). Bridging emotion theory and neurobiology through dynamic systems modeling. *Behavioral and Brain Sciences, 28*, 169–245.

Lindau, S. T., Laumann, E. O., Levinson, W., & Waite, L. J. (2003). Synthesis of scientific disciplines in pursuit of health: The Interactive Biopsychosocial Model. *Perspectives in Biological Medicine, 46*, S74–S86.

Markus, H. R., & Kitayama, S. (1991). Culture and the self: Implications for cognition, emotion, and motivation. *Psychological Review, 98*, 224–253.

Markus, H. R., & Kitayama, S. (1994). The cultural shaping of emotion: A conceptual framework. In H. R. Markus & S. Kitayama (Eds.), *Emotion and culture* (pp. 339–351). Washington, DC: American Psychological Association.

Mathews, A. (1990). Why worry? The cognitive function of anxiety. *Behavior Research and Therapy, 28*, 455–468.

Matsumoto, D. (1990). Cultural similarities and differences in display rules. *Motivation and Emotion, 14*, 195–214.

Matsumoto, D. (1993). Ethnic differences in affect intensity, emotion judgements, display rule attitudes, and self-reported emotional expression in an American sample. *Motivation and Emotion, 17*, 107–123.

Matsumoto, D., Yoo, S. H., & Nakagawa, S. (2008). Culture, emotion regulation, and adjustment. *Journal of Personality and Social Psychology, 94*, 925–937.

Mauss, I. B., & Butler, E. A. (2010). Cultural context moderates the relationship between emotion control values and cardiovascular challenge versus threat responses. *Biological Psychology, 84*, 521–530.

Mauss, I. B., Butler, E. A., Roberts, N. A., & Chu, A. (2010). Emotion control values and responding to an anger provocation in Asian-American and European-American individuals. *Cognition and Emotion, 24*, 1026–1043.

Mendes, W. B., Blascovich, J., Lickel, B., & Hunter, S. (2002). Challenge and threat during social interactions with white and black men. *Personality and Social Psychology Bulletin, 28*, 939–952.

Mendes, W. B., Reis, H. T., Seery, M. D., & Blascovich, J. (2003). Cardiovascular correlates of emotional expression and suppression: Do content and gender context matter? *Journal of Personality and Social Psychology, 84*, 771–792.

Mesquita, B. (2001). Emotions in collectivist and individualist contexts. *Journal of Personality and Social Psychology, 80*, 68–74.

Mesquita, B., & Frijda, N. H. (1992). Cultural variations in emotions: A review. *Psychological Bulletin, 112*, 179–204.

Mesquita, B., & Karasawa, M. (2002). Different emotional lives. *Cognition and Emotion, 16*, 127–141.

Miller, J. G. (2002). Bringing culture to basic psychological theory – Beyond individualism and collectivism: Comment on Oyserman et al. (2002). *Psychological Bulletin, 128*, 97–109.

Miyamoto, Y., & Ryff, C. D. (2011). Cultural differences in the dialectical and non-dialectical emotional styles and their implications for health. *Cognition and Emotion, 25*, 22–39.

Moses, E. B., & Barlow, D. H. (2006). A new unified treatment approach for emotional disorders based on emotion science. *Current Directions in Psychological Science, 15*, 146–150.

Muraven, M., Tice, D. M., & Baumeister, R. F. (1998). Self-control as limited resource: Regulatory depletion patterns. *Journal of Personality and Social Psychology, 74*, 774–789.

Ochsner, K. N., & Gross, J. J. (2007). The neural architecture of emotion regulation. In J. J. Gross (Ed.), *Handbook of emotion regulation* (pp. 87–109). New York: Guilford.

Oyserman, D., Coon, H. M., & Kemmelmeier, M. (2002). Rethinking individualism and collectivism: Evaluation of theoretical assumptions and meta-analyses. *Psychological Bulletin, 128*, 3–72.

Raver, C. C. (2004). Placing emotional self-regulation in sociocultural and socioeconomic contexts. *Child Development, 75*, 346–353.

Rivers, S. E., Brackett, M. A., Katulak, N. A., & Salovey, P. (2007). Regulating anger and sadness: An exploration of discrete emotions in emotion regulation. *Journal of Happiness Studies, 8*, 393–427.

Rottenberg, J., & Gross, J. J. (2003). When emotion goes wrong: Realizing the promise of affective science. *Clinical Psychology Science and Practice, 10*, 227–232.

Ryder, A. G., Ban, L. M., & Dere, J. (in press). Culture, self, and symptom: Perspectives from cultural psychology. In T. Hansen, K. Berliner, & J. de Lopez (Eds.), *Culture in self and mind: Conceptual and applied approaches*. Aalborg, Denmark: Aalborg University Press.

Scherer, K. R. (1987). Toward a dynamic theory of emotion: The component model of affective states. *Geneva Studies in Emotion and Communication, 1*, 1–96.

Scherer, K. R. (1997). The role of culture in emotion-antecedent appraisal. *Journal of Personality and Social Psychology, 73*, 902–922.

Scherer, K. R. (2000). Emotions as episodes of subsystem synchronization driven by non-linear appraisal processes. In M. D. Lewis & I. Granic (Eds.), *Emotion, development and self-organization: Dynamic systems approaches to emotional development* (pp. 70–99). Cambridge: Cambridge University Press.

Schimmack, U., Oishi, S., & Diener, E. (2002). Cultural influences on the relation between pleasant emotions and unpleasant emotions: Asian dialectic philosophies or individualism-collectivism? *Cognition and Emotion, 16*, 705–719.

Shiota, M. N., Campos, B., Gonzaga, G. C., Keltner, D., & Peng, K. (2010). I love you but…: Cultural differences in complexity of emotional experience during interaction with a romantic partner. *Cognition and Emotion, 24*, 786–799.

Shweder, R. A. (2007). An anthropological perspective: The revival of cultural psychology; Some premonitions and reflections. In S. Kitayama & D. Cohen (Eds.), *Handbook of cultural psychology* (pp. 821–836). New York: Guilford.

Soto, J. A., Levenson, R. W., & Ebling, R. (2005). Cultures of moderation and expression: Emotional experience, behavior, and physiology in Chinese Americans and Mexican Americans. *Emotion, 5*, 154–165.

Stipeck, D. (1998). Differences between Americans and Chinese in the circumstances evoking pride, shame, and guilt. *Journal of Cross-Cultural Psychology, 29*, 616–629.

Suh, E., Diener, E., Oishi, S., & Triandis, H. C. (1998). The shifting basis of life satisfaction judgements across cultures: Emotions versus norms. *Journal of Personality and Social Psychology, 74*, 482–493.

Tamir, M., Mitchell, C., & Gross, J. J. (2008). Hedonic and instrumental motives in anger regulation. *Psychological Science, 19*, 324–328.

Tavris, C. (1984). On the wisdom of counting to ten: Personal and social dangers of anger expression. *Review of Personality & Social Psychology, 5*, 170–191.

Thayer, J. F., & Brosschot, J. F. (2005). Psychosomatics and psychopathology: Looking up and down from the brain. *Psychoneuroendocrinology, 30*, 1050–1058.

Thayer, J. F., & Lane, R. D. (2000). A model of neurovisceral integration in emotion regulation and dysregulation. *Journal of Affective Disorders, 61*, 201–216.

Thayer, J. F., & Lane, R. D. (2007). The role of vagal function in the risk for cardiovascular disease and mortality. *Biological Psychology, 74*, 224–242.

Thayer, J. F., & Sternberg, E. (2006). Beyond heart rate variability: Vagal regulation of allostatic systems. *Annals of the New York Academy of Science, 1088*, 361–372.

Thompson, R. A. (1994). Emotion regulation: A theme in search of definition. *Monographs of the Society for Research in Child Development, 59*(2-3), 25–52.

Tomaka, J., Blascovich, J., Kelsey, R. M., & Leitten, C. L. (1993). Subjective, physiological, and behavioral effects of threat and challenge appraisal. *Journal of Personality and Social Psychology, 65*, 248–260.

Tomaka, J., Palacios, R., Schneider, K. T., Colotla, M., Concha, J., & Herrald, M. M. (1999). Assertiveness predicts threat and challenge reactions to potential stress among women. *Journal of Personality and Social Psychology, 76*, 1008–1021.

Tsai, J. L., Knutson, B., & Fung, H. H. (2006). Cultural variation in affect valuation. *Journal of Personality and Social Psychology, 90*, 288–307.

Tsai, J. L., & Levenson, R. W. (1997). Cultural influences on emotional responding: Chinese American and European American dating couples during interpersonal conflict. *Journal of Cross-Cultural Psychology, 28*, 600–626.

Valiente, C., & Eisenberg, N. (2006). Parenting and children's adjustment: The role of children's emotion regulation. In D. K. Snyder, J. A. Simpson, & N. J. Hughes (Eds.), *Emotion regulation in couples and families: Pathways to dysfunction and health* (pp. 123–142). Washington, DC: American Psychological Association.

Wang, Q. (2001). "Did you have fun?" American and Chinese mother–child conversations about shared emotional experiences. *Cognitive Development, 16*, 693–715.

Wierzbicka, A. (1993). A conceptual basis for cultural psychology. *Ethos, 21*, 205–231.

Wierzbicka, A. (1994). Emotion, language, and cultural scripts. In S. Kitayama & H. R. Markus (Eds.), *Emotion and culture* (pp. 133–196). Washington, DC: American Psychological Association.

Witherington, D. C., & Crichton, J. A. (2007). Frameworks for understanding emotions and their development: Functionalist and dynamic systems approaches. *Emotion, 7*, 628–637.

Emily A. Butler
Norton School Family and Consumer Sciences
Family Studies & Human Development
University of Arizona
McClelland Park, Room 301 D
650 N Park Ave.
Tucson, AZ 85721-0078
USA
E-Mail: eabutler@u.arizona.edu

Chapter 6

Unpacking Cultural Differences in Emotion Regulation

The Role of Flexibility

Elisabeth A. Arens

Department of Clinical Psychology and Psychotherapy, Institute of Psychology, University of Heidelberg, Germany

Abstract

A cultural perspective suggests that the consequences of emotional suppression on mental health are moderated by cultural values: Whereas in Western individualistic cultures suppression is related to worse mental health, the reverse is found in Eastern collectivistic individuals. The aim of this chapter is to understand the mechanism behind this cultural variation, that is, what causes better effects in one culture and worse in the other? For this, an instrumental approach of emotion regulation was used in order to differentiate between short- and long-term benefits of suppression. It is demonstrated that more positive consequences of suppression are not caused by cultural background per se, but by a higher flexibility in the use of this strategy. Collectivistic individuals may suppress their emotions for the sake of long-term benefits (e.g., to maintain group harmony) and shift to other strategies where these benefits are not given. The importance of flexibility as well as context- and goal-dependent effects of emotion regulation is highlighted above and beyond culture.

Keywords: emotion regulation, flexibility, suppression, adaptive strategies, maladaptive strategies

Blessed are the flexible,
for they shall not be bent out of shape.
(Author Unknown)

Introduction

Entering the phrase "express yourself" in the European or North American Google web search engine leads to a list of 162 million results. These sites range from blogs to music videos, cosmetics, therapy approaches, fashion styles, art graphics, and song lyrics. In most articles, self-expression and the expression of emotions is closely associated with positive concepts such as mental well-being, individuality, success, freedom, self-discovery, creativity, and courage. North American and European proverbs such as "the squeaky wheel gets the grease," or "laughter is the best medicine" also emphasize the benefits of a free and open expression of one's own emotions and needs. Thus, in our daily effort to handle and regulate our emotions, we learn about the benefits of expressing our joy, anger, worries, and wishes. Or in other words, suppressing our emotions is thought to have negative consequences, including the accumulation of negative feelings, deindividuation, and groupthink.

Nevertheless, many studies in cultural psychology have shown that the cultural values and norms endorsed by a society might guide which emotional regulatory styles we actually apply and how these might impact our personal and social functioning. The Asian proverbs "conquer your passions and you conquer the world" or "the nail that stands out gets pounded down" might give an idea that the beneficial role of open emotion expression is not equally evident across ethnic groups. For instance, things might be different in collectivistic cultures where in-group harmony and social order are highly valued, and the needs and well-being of the group are considered more important than those of the individual. Here, one would have to carefully consider the consequences of emotion expression, since strong emotions and emotional expression could disrupt intragroup relations and harmonious social functioning. Thus, in some social situations individuals might benefit from the use of suppression (since it contributes to the fulfillment of prosocial goals), whereas in other situations different ways of emotion regulation might be more adaptive. This raises the question whether the use of suppression might be beneficial under particular circumstances. Does it matter how and in which situation it is used?

The goal of this chapter goes beyond demonstrating cultural differences in the link between emotion suppression and mental health. Rather, the aim is to understand the mechanism behind this cultural variation by considering the role of flexibility in the use of suppression; that is, to what extent it is used in accord with situational demands and in combination with other strategies. It is about the consideration of how, why, when, and for whom emotion suppression might relate to health.

Conceptualizing Emotion Regulation

In a busy metropolitan airport, a traveler angrily threw his briefcase into a plate glass window when he learned that his flight was canceled. Within moments, airport security guards wrestled him to the ground, handcuffed him, and led him away (example taken from Golemann, 1995).

In everyday life we are confronted with a variety of situations, thoughts, and memories that generate emotions, but occasionally emotions become too intense or maladaptive. What caused this man (in the example above) to display such a dramatic explosion when his flight was canceled? What did this outburst of emotion accomplish for the traveler? What could he have done differently? These questions take us to what Gross and Thompson (2007) have called the "fabric of civilization," namely, the fundamental human capacity to control and regulate our emotions. Richards and Gross (2000) considered the capacity to self-regulate the cornerstone of adaptive success, whereas Muraven, Tice, and Baumeister (1998) considered self-regulation one of the "most impressive" functions of adulthood. Indeed, emotion regulation has been related to such important outcomes as mental health (Gross & Muñoz, 1995), physical health (Greenberg, Wortman, & Stone, 1996; Sapolsky, 2007), relationship satisfaction (Murray, 2005), and work performance (Diefendorff, Hall, Lord, & Strean, 2000; Newman, Joseph, & McCann, 2010). But what does it mean to regulate emotions?

Emotion regulation research has been characterized by extensive debates over how emotion regulation should be defined. Following Golemann (1995), when people try to control or regulate their emotions they try to not be carried away or "hijacked by their emotions"; that is, they seek to redirect the spontaneous flow of their emotions (Koole, 2009). Gross and Thompson (2007) highlight that "emotion regulatory processes may be automatic or controled, conscious or unconscious, and may have their effects at one or more points in the emotion generative process" (p. 10). Accordingly, changes in emotional responding may occur in the *kinds of emotions* that people have, *when* they have their emotions, and *how* they experience and express them (Gross, 1999). During the regulation process, people may increase, maintain, or decrease positive and negative emotions. But what do people exactly do to regulate emotions? Are some ways of regulating emotions more successful than others?

Are There "Good" and "Bad" Emotion Regulation Strategies?

Since the beginning of emotion regulation research, there has been a strong temptation to categorize strategies as adaptive or maladaptive. The notion that suppressing emotions has negative physical and mental health consequences has a long history. This assumption is central to psychodynamic theory, where repression and avoidance were conceptualized as strangulating the affect, while the healing and cleansing effect of catharsis was highlighted; that is, the recalling of affects to the conscious awareness and to allow for their expression (Freud, 1923/1961). Similar ideas on inhibited emotion and the desirability of expression were pursued within the field of psychosomatic medicine earlier in the last century (Consedine, Magai, & Bonanno, 2002). In the study of personality and health, individuals who chronically fail to express emotions have been categorized as being alexithymic, having a repressive coping style, having a

Type C personality, or being high in constraint and self-control (Consedine et al., 2002; Grossarth-Maticek, Bastiaans, & Kanazir, 1985; Leventhal & Patrick-Miller, 2000; Fox, Temoshok, & Dreher, 1988). Although conceptualizations of inhibition are gradually becoming more moderate and complex, the general view that suppression brings more costs than benefits remains a popular notion in contemporary (Western) theories of emotion regulation, personality, and health (Greenberg & Stone, 1992; Gross & Levenson, 1993; Pennebaker & Seagal, 1999). More recently, in a paper entitled "Healthy and Unhealthy Emotion Regulation," John and Gross (2004) state that *response-focused* emotion regulation strategies (i.e., inhibiting ongoing emotions *after* they have been generated), for example, expressive suppression, are less functional than *antecedent-focused* emotion regulation strategies (i.e., alteration of the emotional response *before* it arises), for example, cognitive reappraisal (i.e., the reframing or recontextualization of a negative stimulus in less emotional terms) (Campbell-Sills, Barlow, Brown, & Hofmann, 2006; Gross, 2002; Gross & John, 2003; John & Gross, 2004).

Indeed, results from numerous studies indicate that the use of cognitive reappraisal leads to far better psychological functioning than the use of expressive suppression (John & Gross, 2004; Richards, Butler, & Gross, 2003). Expressive suppression has been repeatedly linked to poor physical (Kune, Kune, Watson, & Bahnson, 1991), social (Butler et al., 2003), affective (Gross & Levenson, 1997; Stepper & Strack, 1993), and cognitive conditions (Richards & Gross, 2000), whereas the reverse has been true for cognitive reappraisal. In addition, cognitive reappraisal as a putatively adaptive strategy is an important component of a variety of treatment modalities, ranging from traditional cognitive-behavioral therapy to newer third-wave approaches (e.g., Beck, Rush, Shaw, & Emery, 1979; Hayes, 2008; Hofmann & Asmundson, 2008; Roemer, Orsillo, & Salters-Pedneault, 2008).

But does suppression entail the same kinds of costs for everyone? A careful reading of the more recent literature suggests that the link between emotion regulation styles and health may be more complex and open to a high degree of moderation effects (see Consedine et al., 2002). A major problem lies in the fact that current empirical work understands emotion regulation as an *intrapersonal* process and gives scant attention to *contextual* factors, that is, *who* regulates *how* under *which circumstances*. For instance, an examination of the samples out of which most of the aforementioned results have emerged shows that they are immensely homogeneous: Participants typically have been highly educated Europeans/European Americans (e.g., samples of European/American students). Given the known cultural differences in emotional experience, expression, and control (Mesquita & Frijda, 1992), we must not assume, however, that demonstrations of suppression–health relations will generalize across ethnic groups (Consedine et al., 2002).

The following sections outline why emotion regulation research cannot avoid discussion of the sociocultural context that elicited the need for regulation in the first place and that specifies the rules of proper conduct (Campos, Mumme, Kermoian, & Campos, 1994).

What Is "Adaptive" in One Context May Be "Maladaptive" in Another: An Instrumental Approach to Emotion Regulation

As shown earlier, research on emotion regulation has focused on *how* people modify their feelings and which strategies are adaptive or maladaptive. However, little research has examined *why* people do so. Is the goal of emotion regulation necessarily to feel good? In fact, people want to maximize immediate pleasure. Therefore, they want to feel pleasant emotions and avoid unpleasant ones (Tamir, 2011). However, there might be goals of emotion regulation other than short-term pleasure. It has been shown that people also want to maximize utility (i.e., long-term pleasure; Bentham, 1823/1968). Therefore, they may also want to feel emotions that are useful (not merely pleasurable) (see Figure 6.1, Tamir, 2009). When immediate benefits (i.e., immediate pleasure) outweigh long-term benefits (i.e., delayed pleasure derived from successful goal pursuit), people should prefer pleasant emotions. When long-term benefits outweigh immediate ones, people should prefer useful emotions. The balance between immediate and long-term benefits in turn depends on the goals people pursue (Tamir, 2009).

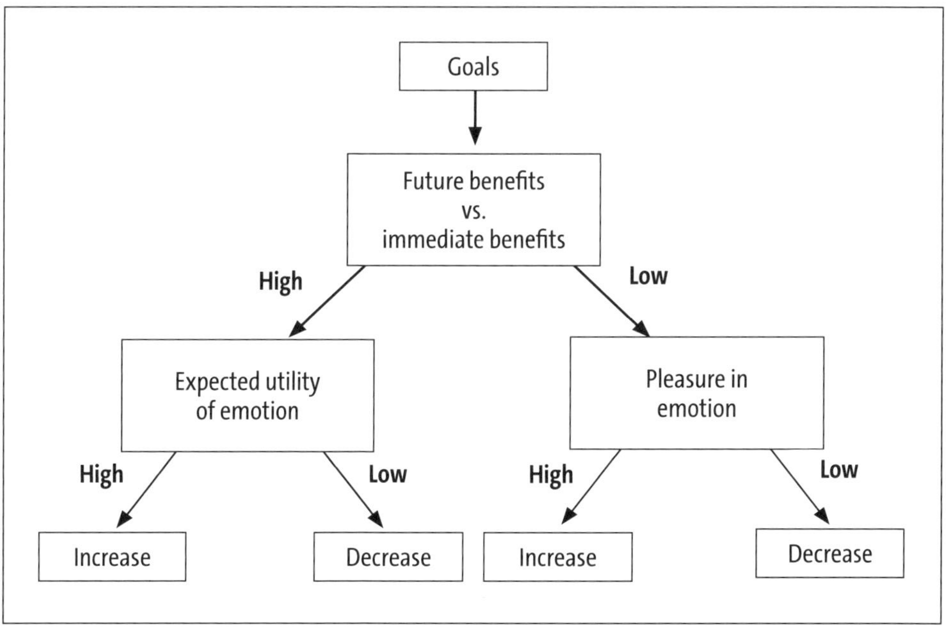

Figure 6.1. The role of pleasure and utility in determining emotional preferences (adapted from Tamir, 2009).

Virtually all definitions of emotion regulation emphasize its crucial role in adaptive functioning. Following Gross and Thompson (2007), civilization is defined by coordinated social interchanges that require us to regulate how emotions are experienced and expressed. Thus, the goal in emotion regulation is not necessarily to feel good. Rather, emotion regulation is sometimes undertaken in the service of higher-order instrumental goals, for example, to fulfill prosocial goals (Izard et al., 2011; Thompson, 2011). Accordingly, this instrumental approach to emotion regulation argues that any assessment of emotion regulation and its consequences must take into account the goals of the individual in the context in which emotions are regulated. In this light, strategies of emotion regulation are rarely inherently "good" or "bad." They are rather more or less adaptive in the context of specific goals in particular circumstances and their effectiveness will be a function of a person-situation-strategy fit.

Imagine that you have been struggling to find a parking space for 30 minutes. You drive around and drive around without any luck. Finally, you miraculously find the space you need. While positioning your car beside the vehicle you will park behind in order to reverse into the parking space, another car comes in from behind and steals the space before you can do anything. Most likely, your blood pressure will rise within seconds, your heart beat will increase, and your muscles tense, or, in other words, you will feel intense anger. This is a situation that could probably happen all over the world. Yet whether your emotional response/regulation style in that moment is adaptive or maladaptive might be heavily dependent on the cultural context in which this event takes place. According to the cultural norms of a Western European or North American city, rolling down the window and making a scathing comment to the other driver would probably be a socially acceptable reaction. Although aggressive anger expression is not promoted in Western cultures (Eisenberg et al., 2007), honesty and directness in communication are highly appreciated so as to serve instrumental goals such as self-assertion and autonomy. If one imagines this scenario in a culture with Eastern collectivistic norms, however, things might be different. For example, in Asian cultures, it is considered unwise to show emotions toward strangers, and expressing anger shows that you have lost control. In Eastern cultures, the same behavior might therefore be rated as highly embarrassing and socially inadequate. In this case, anger suppression might be more adaptive in order to attain the long-term goal of not losing face and following social norms.

This example highlights that emotion regulation strategies and their consequences cannot be understood without reference to the cultural and interpersonal context. But what causes these cultural differences? The following section will provide a theoretical basis for understanding cultural differences in emotion regulation.

A Theoretical Basis for Understanding Cultural Differences in Emotion Regulation

Although the concept of emotion regulation is encompassed within the framework of emotional display rules (Saarni, 1989, 1992), which are quintessentially a product of culture, there has been remarkably little research on how cultural origin might influence the way in which people regulate their emotions and what impact this might have on mental health (Consedine et al., 2002).

According to Markus and Kitayama (1991) one way to understand cultural differences in the regulation of emotions lies within the theoretical framework of individualistic and collectivistic cultural models. They assert that differences in emotion regulation styles exist because both cultural models contain differences in the meaning of social relations and the self. In individualistic cultures such as in Western Europe and North America, expressive suppression may clash with values such as independence and open emotion expression (Hofstede, 2001; Markus & Kitayama, 1991). In such contexts, individuals are seen as separate from one another and societies are expected to promote the well-being of the individual. In these cultures people are likely to prefer emotion-regulation styles that emphasize personal wishes and desires over and above relational harmony.

In collectivistic cultures such as in East Asia and North Africa, individuals are seen as fundamentally connected through relationships and they must fit into the group or society (Oyserman & Lee, 2008). Consequently, in these cultures people are likely to prefer emotion regulation styles that consider social group norms, preserve interpersonal harmony, and maintain one's face or honor in the eyes of the group. It has been argued, therefore, that in collectivistic cultures expressive suppression may be encouraged more than in individualistic cultures, so as to fulfill prosocial goals (e.g., suppression of anger to preserve group harmony) (Hui, Triandis, & Yee, 1991). This interdependence might lead to first, a higher frequency of applied suppression and second, to less negative consequences or even benefits from suppression. As the next section shows, these assumptions have received considerable empirical support.

Research Documenting Cultural Differences in Emotion Regulation

Indeed, there is recent evidence that frequency and psychological consequences of emotion regulation strategies differ in ethnic groups, depending on different cultural values (Barnow, Arens, & Balkir, 2011; Butler, Lee, & Gross, 2007; Chentsova-Dutton, Chu, Tsai, & Rottenberg, 2007; Butler, Lee, & Gross, 2009; Gross & John, 2003; Keller & Otto, 2009; Miyamoto & Ma, in press) (see chapters 4 and 5). It was shown that the use of suppression is applied more frequently in Eastern collectivistic cultures (Gross & John, 2003), more automatized (Butler et al., 2007; Soto, Levenson, & Eberling, 2005), related to lower levels of negative emotion (Butler et al., 2007), less negative social consequences (Butler et al., 2007), and better health (Butler et al., 2009; Consedine, Magai, & Horton, 2005) than in Western individualistic cultures. For instance, a study of Soto, Perez, Kim, Lee, and Minnick (2011) has shown that the habitual use of expressive suppression was associated with adverse psychological functioning for European Americans, but not for Chinese participants. Cheung and Park (2010) found that the suppression-depression link was moderated by cultural origin and self-construal of the participants in such a way that Asian American status (vs. European American) and a stronger interdependent (vs. independent) self-construal attenuated the relation between anger suppression and depressive symptoms.

In a study of our own (Arens, Balkir, & Barnow, in press; Barnow et al., 2011) we compared frequency of expressive suppression and cognitive reappraisal and their implications for subjective well-being between Turkish immigrants living in Germany and German women. Measurement of well-being included positive and negative affectivity, loneliness, and dysfunctional attitudes, all of which have been cited as common problems experienced by immigrants (Ponizovsky & Ritsner, 2004; Vedder & Virta, 2005) and hence might be crucial areas impacted by emotion regulation. Since the Turkish culture has often been described as high in collectivism (Hofstede, 1980; Schwartz, 1994), it was hypothesized that Turkish immigrants would show higher levels of emotional suppression and that this emotion regulation strategy would be associated with better mental well-being in Turkish women compared to German counterparts. Results provided support for this assumption. First, Turkish women reported to apply suppression more frequently. Second, in this group a higher level of suppression was linked to lower levels of negative affect, loneliness, and dysfunctional attitudes, while the reverse was true for German women (see Figures 6.2, 6.3, and 6.4).

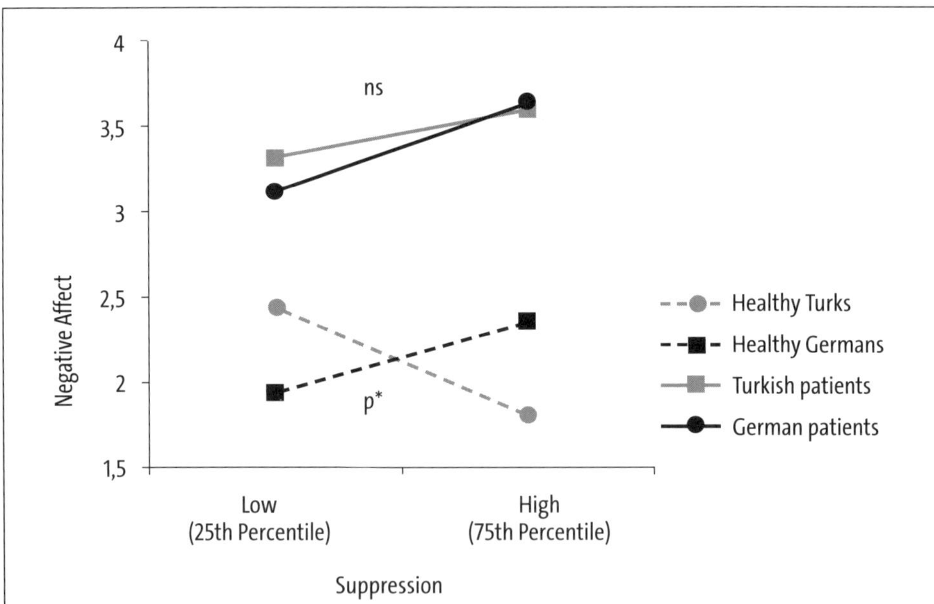

Figure 6.2. Negative affect depending on expressive suppression and culture in healthy Turkish and German women and depressed Turkish and German patients, assessed with the Positive and Negative Affect Schedule (PANAS) (Watson, Clark, & Tellegen, 1988); ns = not significant; $^*p \leq .05$.

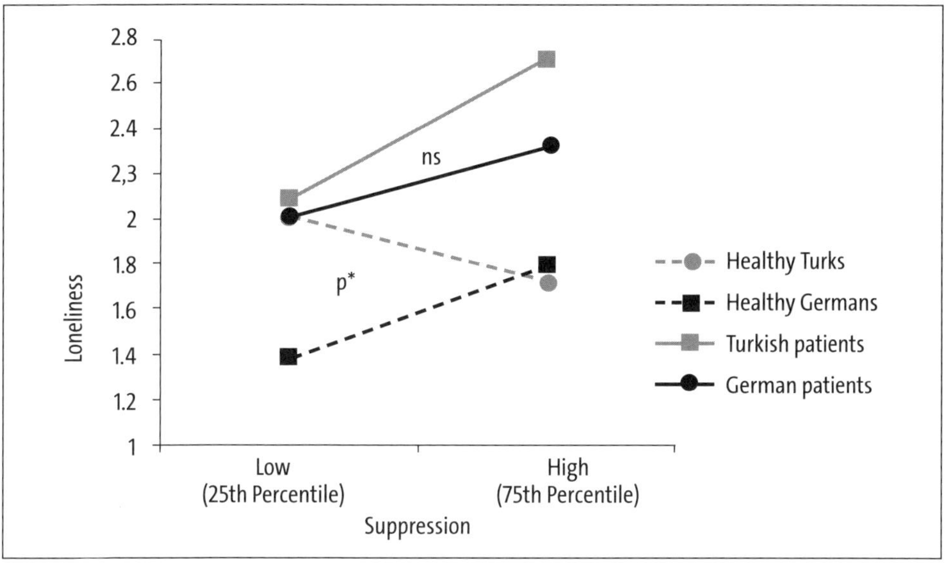

Figure 6.3. Loneliness depending on expressive suppression and culture in healthy Turkish and German women and depressed Turkish and German patients, assessed with the UCLA-Loneliness Scale (Russell, Peplau, & Ferguson, 1978); ns = not significant; $^{*}p \leq .05$

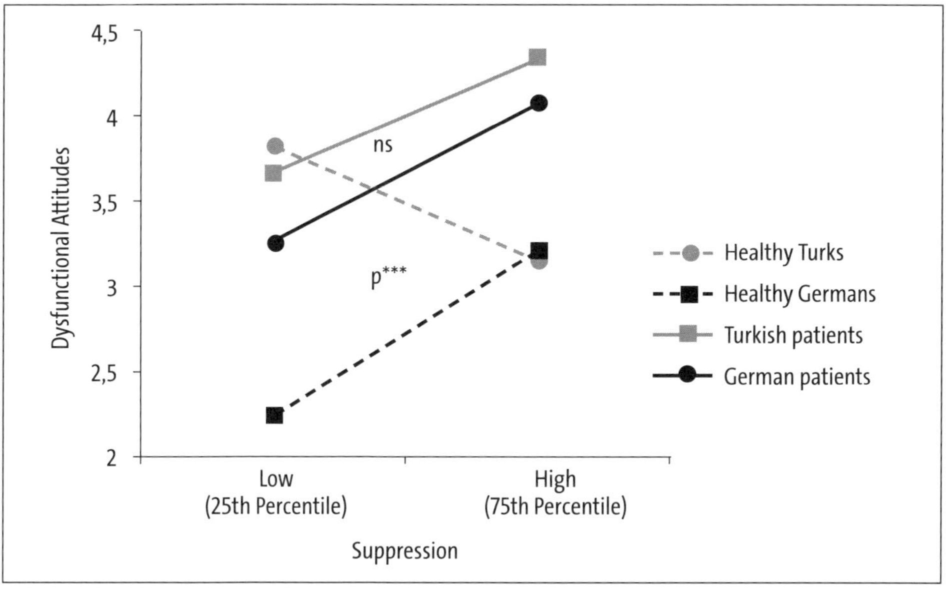

Figure 6.4. Dysfunctional attitudes depending on expressive suppression and culture in healthy Turkish and German women and depressed Turkish and German patients, total score calculated for all subscales of the Dysfunctional Attitude Scale (DAS) (Weissman & Beck, 1978); ns = not significant; $^{***}p \leq .001$

As these studies call into question whether emotion regulation strategies can be uniformly labeled as adaptive or maladaptive strategies, one might ask *how* culture causes the beneficial effect of emotional suppression; that is, what is the mechanism behind cultural variation in the suppression–health link?

Unpacking Cultural Differences: The Role of Flexibility

As individuals with a collectivistic cultural origin seem to benefit more from emotion suppression, the question arises whether they might have a somewhat different use of suppression. Following the instrumental approach to emotion regulation, the benefit of emotion regulation strategies is a function of the person-situation-strategy fit. This in turn would mean that collectivistic individuals might be more able to use suppression in accordance with the situation, that is, they may use suppression more flexibly. It can be hypothesized that individuals with a collectivistic cultural orientation use suppression when there is a long-term benefit (e.g., preserving group harmony) and that this might change when other strategies are more adaptive to the situation.

Indeed, there is recent evidence that the positive consequences of expressive suppression in individuals with a collectivistic background may rest on their not using suppression exclusively and rigidly, but that they shift to other emotion regulation strategies (e.g., cognitive reappraisal), whenever suppression would have a negative impact (Butler et al., 2007). In a recent study, Butler and colleagues (2007) (see chapter 5) found that among Asian and European Americans, those individuals holding Eastern values showed less negative consequences of emotional suppression. The authors suggest that one of the reasons that emotional suppression was associated with high levels of negative emotion for women with high European values was a tendency to use suppression rigidly, without sensitivity to contextual constraints. In contrast, it is assumed that the emphasis Asian cultures place on accommodating social demands and adjusting to others (Morling, Kitayama, & Miyamoto, 2002) enables women with bicultural Asian and European values to avoid using suppression in situations where it would have a negative social impact.

In line with these assumptions, a study of Cheng, Wang, and Golden (2011) showed that Chinese participants generally reported greater interpersonal flexibility than their Caucasian American counterparts. The authors suggest that the Chinese displayed greater discriminative responding across interpersonal situations, because they favor interdependent self-construal. For individuals with an interdependent self-construal, information processing operates in a "we" frame of mind that diverts their attention toward the group and social context (Gardner, Gabriel, & Lee, 1999). Such an encoding tendency facilitates greater sensitivity to subtle cues embedded in social situations and greater responsiveness to meet specific situational demands (Cheng et al., 2011), which in turn might ease the flexible application of suppression. Similarly, intercultural studies carried out by Bonanno and colleagues (Bonanno, 2005; Bonanno, Papa, Lalande, Nanping, & Noll, 2005) have shown that in contrast to subjects with Western individualistic cultural values (e.g., in the US), individuals from collectivistic cultures (e.g., China) are characterized by a more balanced repertoire of coping strategies, enabling them to flexibly move between expressing and suppressing emotions. Similarly, Miyamoto and colleagues (Miyamoto & Ma, in press; Miyamoto & Ryff, 2010) have shown in several studies, first, that Easterners combine both up and down regulation strategies in order to experience a balance between positive and negative emotions, and second, that this dialectical regulation is related to a better health profile in Eastern than in Western cultures.

In line with these findings, it has been demonstrated that the correlation between expressive suppression and cognitive reappraisal is higher in Eastern than in Western countries (Matsumoto, Yoo, & Nakagawa, 2008). This indicates that individuals with collectivistic cultural values may have a more balanced use of both strategies and thus may benefit more from the use of expressive suppression. This might be especially true for immigrants who "live at the juncture between two cultures" (LaFromboise, Coleman, & Gerton, 1993, p. 395) and thus may need to adopt various forms of emotional expression in order to flexibly shift between contrasting culture-specific communication styles (i.e., those of their heritage culture and those of the host culture) (Eng, Kuiken, Temme, & Sharma, 2005). Accordingly, immigrants with a heightened flexibility and an extended repertoire of emotion regulation strategies were shown to be less depressive and better integrated (Eng et al., 2005; Matsumoto, Hirayama, & LeRoux, 2006). It has been argued that regulating/controlling one's emotions might be important for positive adjustment, since it allows one not to be overly influenced by stress and negative emotions, which are inevitable in the acculturation process. Instead, emotion regulation and control allows one to think clearly and rationally, paving the way for using other psychological skills important for intercultural adjustment (e.g., openness, critical thinking, etc.). Thus, functional emotion regulation, flexibly applied suppression in particular, might mediate the link between mental health and integration of these immigrants.

Indeed, in our own study (Arens et al., in press) we found that Turkish immigrants, as compared to German women, exhibited a more balanced use of emotion regulation strategies (see Figure 6.5). As expected, German women reported a more frequent use of reappraisal compared to suppression. Turkish women reported a comparable use of reappraisal but additionally exhibited a frequent use of emotional suppression, thus having a greater repertoire of strategies. As mentioned before, emotional suppression was associated with better mental well-being in this group. To test the hypothesis of whether this beneficial effect of suppression can be attributed to their more flexible use of suppression, a mediated moderation model was computed. When entering flexibility scores (i.e., the higher the score the more balanced the use of reappraisal and suppression) into the model, the interaction of culture and emotional suppression was no longer significant, suggesting that the associations between suppression and more positive mental well-being in Turkish women can be attributed to their more balanced use of emotion regulation strategies.

Interestingly, these differences were absent when we compared Turkish and German depressed samples. Depressed women, regardless of their culture, showed a rigid use of suppression and in both groups, emotional suppression was associated with negative mental well-being. These results are in accordance with previous research, relating psy-

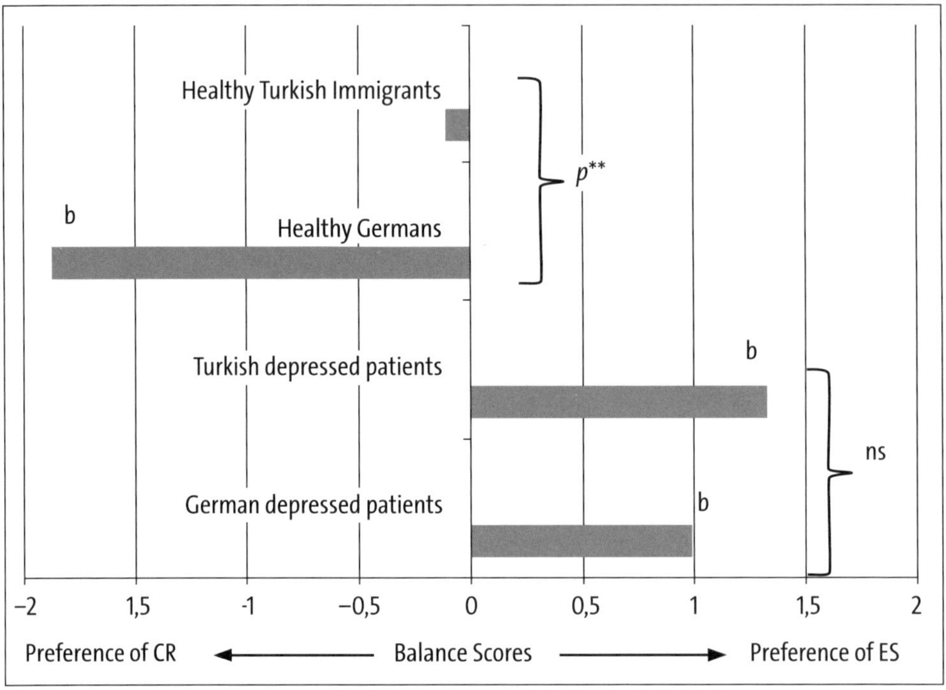

Figure 6.5. Balance scores between expressive suppression (ES) and cognitive reappraisal (CR) in Turkish ($n = 28$) and German healthy controls ($n = 26$) and Turkish ($n = 29$) and German depressed patients ($n = 25$). Scores were calculated by subtracting mean values of cognitive reappraisal from mean values of expressive suppression, positive values indicate relative preference for expressive suppression, negative values indicate relative preference for cognitive reappraisal; b = difference score significantly different from zero; ns not significant; $^{**}p \leq .01$

chopathology to a rigid and contextually insensitive application of emotion regulation strategies (Mennin, Holaway, Fresco, Moore, & Heimberg, 2007), in particular to the inflexible use of emotional suppression (Aldao & Nolen-Hoeksema, 2010; Joormann & Gotlib, 2010). This raises the question, whether all individuals, regardless of their culture, might benefit from emotion regulation flexibility. Is there a universal superiority of flexibility?

Above and Beyond Culture: The Importance of Being Flexible

There is mounting evidence that emotion regulation strategies can have very different outcomes in different contexts (e.g., Cheng, 2001), emphasizing the importance of flexible choice among emotion-regulation strategies in the face of different situational demands (Kashdan & Rottenberg, 2010; Watkins, 2011). Interestingly, a recent study of Sheppes, Scheibe, Suri, and Gross (2011) has demonstrated that the choice of emotion regulation strategy is dependent on the intensity of emotions: Healthy individuals manage their emotions by flexibly switching between a relative preference for engagement reappraisal (which allows emotional processing) when the intensity of negative emotion is low and for disengagement distraction (which blocks emotional processing at an early stage) when the intensity of negative emotion is high.

Thus it might be more important to vary emotional responses rather than to apply the same "adaptive" strategy across changing contexts. Likewise, Joormann and D'Avanzato (2010, p. 920) have concluded that "psychopathology may not so much be associated with the use of emotion regulation strategies that differ dramatically from strategies employed by other people but rather that it is the inflexible use of certain strategies, the poor fit of the regulation strategy with the situation, and differences in the ability to implement effective strategies that are important." A recently published study of Aldao and Nolen-Hoeksema (2012) yielded consistent results. The authors found that adaptive strategies had a negative association with psychopathology symptoms *only* at high levels of maladaptive strategies. This suggests that the effectiveness of adaptive strategies might depend on the other regulation strategies present in an individual's repertoire, allowing them to switch between strategies that might be differentially adaptive for varying contexts.

Similarly, Bonanno, Papa, Lalande, Westphal, and Coifman (2004, p. 483) assert that "successful adaptation depends on the ability to both enhance and suppress emotional expression and to do so flexibly in accord with situational demands." In a study designed to examine this assertion, the authors examined whether expressive flexibility predicts long-term adjustment in the aftermath of highly aversive or demanding life circumstances. The authors investigated undergraduate students shortly after the 9/11 terrorists attacks in New York City. The results showed that students who were best able to both enhance and suppress their emotion expression were less distressed two years later. Importantly, clear ability in only one facet of expressive regulation, either enhancement or expression but not both, failed to predict long-term adjustment. In another study Gupta and Bonanno (2011) measured expressive flexibility among a sample of widowed adults and a control sample of married adults. Bereaved adults suffering from complicated grief, as compared with asymptomatic bereaved and married adults, were less able to flexibly enhance and suppress their expressions of emotion when instructed to do so. The authors suggest that, after loss, some situational contexts will pull for greater expression of emotion, whereas others will tend to require dampening or suppression of grief-related emotions. For example, bereaved adults who have difficulties suppressing their emotional expressions may wallow in sad, painful emotions in inappropriate contexts that would usually require them to be alert and present in the moment. Similarly, such adults may have difficulties enhancing their emotional expression when they try to communicate their deep sadness and seek help from others.

Implications for Clinical Practice

In conclusion, this chapter demonstrates that we must be cautious in generalizing the consequences of suppression for all ethnic groups and in every instance. It is a mistake to believe that suppression is inherently unhealthy; rather, a more nuanced unpacking is required, asking under which circumstances suppression is related to costs and benefits. Following the instrumental approach, emotion regulation typically involves not only hedonic goals but also attaining instrumental goals. Individuals from a collectivistic cultural background might fulfill important prosocial goals through suppressing their emotions in a situation where it is required and hence benefit from that strategy.

That is why clinicians should be aware of their client's cultural background, which may differentially influence the impact of suppression on mental health outcomes. Mösko, Schneider, Koch, and Schulz (2008) have shown that after inpatient treatment, Turkish patients living in Germany had worse treatment effects compared to German patients. The authors suggest that existing psychotherapeutic strategies and techniques common to Western approaches are not adapted to the work with immigrant patients. Sometimes, these strategies may even be counterproductive and work against the well-being of the client. Since traditional Western approaches primarily focus on the *intra*-personal development, fostering independence and autonomy of the individual (e.g., self-efficacy, self-acceptance, self-management, etc.), the expression of one's own needs and emotions is majorly encouraged (see chapter 14). However, suppression of personal goals and emotions for the sake of *inter*personal goals might be more suitable for immigrant patients, an insight that might lead to different therapeutic interventions (e.g., interventions that secure cohesiveness of the family, defining the social role of the client, conflict avoidance, etc.). Further, the clinician should be aware that such immigrant patients often do express emotions and feelings, not verbally, but through somatic symptoms. Thus, training strategies that regulate emotions through bodily processes might be especially helpful for this patient group, since they might be socially more acceptable than verbal expression (see chapters 8 and 14).

However, it is also clear that better consequences of suppression are not related to culture per se but to a more flexible use of this strategy in combination with other strategies. Hence, despite the aforementioned culturally sensitive therapeutic interventions, promoting a more flexible use of emotion regulation strategies seems to be the silver bullet in psychotherapy, regardless of which cultural background the client has. Emotion regulation flexibility may be increased by promoting counter-regulation processes in patients (Rothermund, Voss, & Wentura, 2008). According to this principle, people are equipped with attentional biases that prevent the perseveration of current motivational or emotional states. Attentional counter regulation presumably helps to restore a balanced receptiveness to positive and negative information despite currently active affective-motivational states. Counter-regulation thus fosters contextual sensitivity, an important component of flexible emotion regulation. Indeed, it has been shown that counter-regulation is markedly stronger among individuals disposed toward flexible action control (Jostmann, Koole, Van der Wulp, & Fockenberg, 2005; Koole & Coenen,

2007), and markedly weaker among individuals suffering from emotional disorders (Mathews & MacLeod, 2005). Additional therapeutic techniques might be derived from mindfulness- and acceptance-based approaches. Since these trainings encourage people to perceive their emotions, thoughts, and body sensations in a more mindful manner, they may also increase a sensitivity of which regulation strategy best fits to their actual internal state.

Implications for Research

Between 2001 and 2011, 564 peer-reviewed empirical articles have been published about emotion regulation in adults and adolescents; of these, only 66 (11.7%) studied emotion regulation in a social/cultural context (Campos, Walle, Dahl, & Main, 2011). This shows that previous research has long been dominated by conceptualizing emotion regulation as an intrapersonal process. Future studies are needed considering contextual factors in emotion regulation. This chapter contributes to this avenue of research examining the impact of cultural context on emotion regulation processes: The context of collectivistic cultural norms might bring individuals to renounce their short-term pleasure through suppression of their emotions, if this can lead to the long-term pleasure of attaining group harmony and fulfilling social norms. These individuals may use suppression when it is beneficial for them and switch to other strategies when suppression is harmful, thereby highlighting the important function of a flexible use of emotion regulation strategies. Future research using more ecologically valid methods is needed to explicate the limits and bounds of the deleterious and beneficial effects of particular emotion regulation strategies and to investigate the flexibility of emotion regulation. For instance, investigations employing experience-sampling methodologies would allow for the examination of fluctuations in an individual's daily use of different strategies and their consequences.

The presented findings point out that, conceptually, we need to move beyond the term emotion regulation as a mere description of *how* we regulate emotions and whether this is adaptive or maladaptive. Rather, we need to integrate the concept of *emotion context sensitivity* (Coifman & Bonanno, 2010), the ability to flexibly adapt emotional responses to situational demands and in accordance with short- and long-term goals. Consider a student trying to maintain a moderately high level of anxiety about a test in order to work harder, get a better grade, and ultimately gain the approval of his parents or the favorable impression of an admissions committee for a medical school. In this example, the student is attempting to motivate himself to work harder, as opposed to "feel better" by repeatedly telling himself that he will do just fine without any effort (Campos et al., 2011). Tamir and Ford (2009) have conducted a series of studies showing how people sometimes choose exposure to anger or fear stimuli, when anger or fear is thought more conducive to success on a computer task or during a negotiation. Additional research is needed, shedding more light on context-dependent effects of emotion regulation, which may go far beyond culture.

References

Aldao, A., & Nolen-Hoeksema, S. (2010). Specificity of cognitive emotion regulation strategies: A transdiagnostic examination. *Behaviour Research and Therapy, 48*, 974–983.

Aldao, A., & Nolen-Hoeksema, S. (2012). When are adaptive strategies most predictive of psychopathology? *Journal of Abnormal Psychology, 121*, 276–281.

Arens, E. A., Balkir, N., & Barnow, S. (in press). Ethnic variation in emotion regulation: Do cultural differences end where psychopathology begins? *Journal of Cross-Cultural Psychology*.

Barnow, S., Arens, E. A., & Balkir, N. (2011). Emotion regulation and psychopathology taking cultural influences into account. *Psychotherapie in Psychiatrie, Psychotherapeutischer Medizin und Klinischer Psychologie, 16*, 7–17.

Beck, A. T., Rush, A. J., Shaw, B. F., & Emery, G. (1979). *Cognitive therapy of depression*. New York: Guilford.

Bentham, J. (1968). An introduction to the principles of morals and legislation. In A. L. Page (Ed.), *Utility Theory: A book of readings* (pp. 3–29). New York: Wiley. (Original work published 1823)

Bonanno, G. A. (2005). Resilience in the face of potential trauma. *Current Directions in Psychological Science, 14*, 135–138.

Bonanno, G. A., Papa, A., Lalande, K., Nanping, Z., & Noll, J. G. (2005). Grief processing and deliberate grief avoidance: A prospective comparison of bereaved spouses and parents in the United States and China. *Journal of Consulting and Clinical Psychology, 73*, 86–98.

Bonanno, G. A., Papa, A., Lalande, K., Westphal, M., & Coifman, K. (2004). The importance of being flexible: The ability to both enhance and suppress emotional expression predicts long-term adjustment. *Psychological Science, 15*, 482–487.

Butler, E. A., Egloff, B., Wilhelm, F. H., Smith, N. C., Erickson, E. A., & Gross, J. J. (2003). The social consequences of expressive suppression. *Emotion, 3*, 48–67.

Butler, E. A., Lee, T. L., & Gross, J. J. (2007). Emotion regulation and culture: Are the social consequences of emotional suppression culture-specific? *Emotion, 7*, 30–48.

Butler, E. A., Lee, T. L., & Gross, J. J. (2009). Does expressing your emotions raise or lower your blood pressure?: The answer depends on cultural context. *Journal of Cross-Cultural Psychology, 40*, 510–517.

Campbell-Sills, L., Barlow, D. H., Brown, T. A., & Hofmann, S. G. (2006). Effects of suppression and acceptance on emotional responses of individuals with anxiety and mood disorders. *Behaviour Research and Therapy, 44*, 1251–1263.

Campos, J. J., Mumme, D. L., Kermoian, R., & Campos, R. (1994). Commentary: A functionalist perspective on the nature of emotion. *Monographs of the Society for Research in Child Development, 59*, 2–3.

Campos, J. J., Walle, E., Dahl, A., & Main, A. (2011). Reconceptualizing emotion regulation. *Emotion Review, 3*, 26–35.

Chentsova-Dutton, Y. E., Chu, J. P., Tsai, J. L., & Rottenberg, J. (2007). Depression and emotional reactivity: Variation among Asian Americans of East Asian descent and European Americans. *Journal of Abnormal Psychology, 116*, 776–785.

Cheng, C. (2001). Assessing coping flexibility in real-life and laboratory settings: A multimethod approach. *Journal of Personality and Social Psychology, 80*, 814–833.

Cheng, C., Wang, F., & Golden, D. L. (2011). Unpackaging cultural differences in interpersonal flexibility: Role of culture-related personality and situational factors. *Journal of Cross-Cultural Psychology, 42*, 425–444.

Cheung, R. Y. M., & Park, I. J. K. (2010). Anger suppression, cultural orientation, and depression among Asian American and European American college students. *Cultural Diversity and Ethnic Minority Psychology, 16*, 517–525.

Coifman, K. G., & Bonanno, G. A. (2010). Emotion context sensitivity in adaption and recovery. In A. M. Kring & D. M. Sloan (Eds.), *Emotion regulation and psychotherapy* (pp. 157–173). New York: Guilford.

Consedine, N. S., Magai, C., & Bonanno, G. A. (2002). Moderators of the emotion inhibition-health relationship: A review and research agenda. *Review of General Psychology, 6*, 204–228.

Consedine, N. S., Magai, C., & Horton, D. (2005). Ethnic variation in the impact of emotion and emotion regulation on health: A replication and extension. *Journal of Gerontology: Psychological Sciences, 60*, 165–173.

Diefendorff, J. M., Hall, R. J., Lord, R. G., & Strean, M. L. (2000). Action-state orientation: Construct validity of a revised measure and its relationship to work-related variables. *Journal of Applied Psychology, 85*, 250–263.

Eisenberg, N., Ma, Y., Chang, L., Zhou, Q., West, S. G., & Aiken, L. (2007). Relations of effortful control, reactive undercontrol, and anger to Chinese children's adjustment. *Development and Psychopathology, 19*, 385–409.

Eng, T. C., Kuiken, D., Temme, K., & Sharma, R. (2005). Navigating the emotional complexities of two cultures: Bicultural competence, feeling expression, and feeling change in dreams. *Journal of Cultural and Evolutionary Psychology, 3*, 261–279.

Fox, B. H., Temoshok, L., & Dreher, H. (1988). Mind-body and behavior in cancer incidence. *Advances, 5*, 41–56.

Freud, S. (1961). *The ego and the id* (J. Strachey, Trans.). New York: W.W. Norton. (Original work published 1923)

Gardner, W. L., Gabriel, S., & Lee, A. Y. (1999). "I" value freedom, but "we" value relationships: Self-construal priming mirrors cultural differences in judgment. *Psychological Science, 10*, 321–326.

Goleman, D. (1995). *Emotional intelligence*. New York: Bantam Books. Greenberg, M. A., & Stone, A. A. (1992). Emotional disclosure about traumas and its relation to health: Effects of previous disclosure and trauma severity. *Journal of Personality and Social Psychology, 63*, 75–84.

Greenberg, M. A., Wortman, C. B., & Stone, A. A. (1996). Emotional expression and physical health: Revising traumatic memories or fostering self regulation? *Journal of Personality and Social Psychology, 71*, 588–602.

Grossarth-Maticek, R., Bastiaans, J., & Kanazir, D. T. (1985). Psychosocial factors as strong predictors of mortality from cancer, ischaemic heart disease and stroke: The Yugoslav prospective study. *Journal of Psychosomatic Research, 29*, 167–176.

Gross, J. J. (1999). Emotion regulation: Past, present, future. *Cognition and Emotion, 13*, 551–573.

Gross, J. J. (2002). Emotion regulation: Affective, cognitive, and social consequences. *Psychophysiology, 39*, 281–291.

Gross, J. J., & John, O. P. (2003). Individual differences in two emotion regulation processes: Implications for affect, relationships, and well-being. *Journal of Personality and Social Psychology, 85*, 348–362.

Gross, J. J., & Levenson, R. W. (1993). Emotional suppression: Physiology, self-report, and expressive behavior. *Journal of Personality and Social Psychology, 64*, 970–986.

Gross, J. J., & Levenson, R. W. (1997). Hiding feelings: The acute effects of inhibiting positive and negative emotions. *Journal of Abnormal Psychology, 106*, 95–103.

Gross, J. J., & Muñoz, R. F. (1995). Emotion regulation and mental health. *Clinical Psychology: Science and Practice, 2*, 151–164.

Gross, J. J., & Thompson, R. A. (2007). Emotion regulation: Conceptual foundations. In J. J. Gross (Ed.), *Handbook of emotion regulation* (pp. 3–24). New York: Guilford.

Gupta, S., & Bonanno, G. A. (2011). Complicated grief and deficits in emotional expressive flexibility. *Journal of Abnormal Psychology, 120*, 635–647.

Hayes, S. C. (2008). Climbing our hills: A beginning conversation on the comparison of acceptance and commitment therapy and traditional cognitive behavioral therapy. *Clinical Psychology: Science & Practice Reviews, 15*, 286–295.

Hofmann, S. G., & Asmundson, G. J. G. (2008). Acceptance and mindfulness-based therapy: New wave or old hat. *Clinical Psychology Review, 28*, 1–16.Hofstede, G. (1980). *Culture's consequences: International differences in work-related values*. Thousand Oaks, CA: Sage.
Hofstede, G. (2001). *Culture's Consequences, Comparing Values, Behaviors, Institutions, and Organizations across Nations*. Thousand Oaks, CA: Sage.
Hui, C. H., Triandis, H. C., & Yee, C. (1991). Cultural differences in reward allocation: Is collectivism the explanation? *British Journal of Social Psychology, 30*, 145–157.
Izard, C. E., Woodburn, E. M., Finlon, K. J., Krauthamer-Ewing, S., Grossman, S. R., & Seidenfeld, A. (2011). Emotion knowledge, emotion utilization, and emotion regulation. *Emotion Review, 3*, 44–52.
John, O. P., & Gross, J. J. (2004). Healthy and unhealthy emotion regulation: Personality processes, individual differences, and life span development. *Journal of Personality, 72*, 1301–1333.
Joormann, J., & D'Avanzato, C. (2010). Emotion regulation in depression: Examining the role of cognitive processes. *Cognition and Emotion, 24*, 913–939.
Joormann, J., & Gotlib, I. H. (2010). Emotion regulation in depression: Relation to cognitive inhibition. *Cognition and Emotion, 24*, 281–298.
Jostmann, N., Koole, S. L., Van der Wulp, N., & Fockenberg, D. (2005). Subliminal affect regulation: The moderating role of action versus state orientation. *European Psychologist, 10*, 209–217.
Kashdan, T., & Rottenberg, J. (2010). Psychological flexibility as a fundamental aspect of Health. *Clinical Psychology Review, 30*, 865–878.
Keller, H., & Otto, H. (2009). The cultural socialization of emotion regulation during infancy. *Journal of Cross-Cultural Psychology, 40*, 996–1011.
Koole, S. L. (2009). The psychology of emotion regulation: An integrated review. *Cognition and Emotion, 23*, 4–41.
Koole, S. L., & Coenen, L. H. M. (2007). Implicit self and affect regulation: Effects of action orientation and subliminal self priming in an affective priming task. *Self and Identity, 6*, 118–136.
Kune, G., Kune, S., Watson, L., & Bahnson, C. (1991). Personality as risk factor in large bowel cancer: Data from the Melbourne Colorectal Cancer Study. *Psychological Medicine, 21*, 29–41.
LaFromboise, T., Coleman, L. K. H., & Gerton, J. (1993). Psychological impact of biculturalism: Evidence and theory. *Psychological Bulletin, 114*, 395–412.
Leventhal, H., & Patrick-Miller, L. (2000). Emotions and physical illness: Causes and indicators of vulnerability. In J. Haviland & M. Lewis (Eds.), *Handbook of emotions* (pp. 523–537). New York: Guilford.
Markus, H. R., & Kitayama, S. (1991). Culture and the self: Implications for cognition, emotion, and motivation. *Psychological Review, 98*, 224–253.
Mathews, A., & MacLeod, C. (2005). Cognitive vulnerability to emotional disorders. *Annual Review of Clinical Psychology, 1*, 167–195.
Matsumoto, D., Hirayama, S., & LeRoux, J. (2006). Psychological skills related to intercultural adjustment. In Paul T. P. Wong and Lilian C. J. Wong (Eds.), *Handbook of multicultural perspectives on stress and coping* (pp. 387–408). New York: Kluwer Academic/Plenum Publishing.
Matsumoto, D., Yoo, S. H., & Nakagawa, S. (2008). Culture, emotion regulation, and adjustment. *Journal of Personality and Social Psychology, 94*, 925–937.
Mennin, D. S., Holaway, R., Fresco, D. M., Moore, M. T., & Heimberg, R. G. (2007). Delineating components of emotion and its dysregulation in anxiety and mood psychopathology. *Behavior Therapy, 38*, 284–302.
Mesquita, B., & Frijda, N. H. (1992). Cultural variations in emotions: A review. *Psychological Bulletin, 112*, 179–204.
Miyamoto, Y., & Ma, X. (in press). Dampening or savoring positive emotions: A dialectical cultural script guides emotion regulation. *Emotion*.

Miyamoto, Y., & Ryff, C. D. (2010). Cultural differences in the dialectical and non-dialectical emotional styles and their implications for health. *Cognition & Emotion, 25*, 22–39.

Mösko, M., Schneider, J., Koch, U., & Schulz, H. (2008). Beeinflusst der Türkische Migrationshintergrund das Behandlungsergebnis? Ergebnisse einer prospektiven Versorgungsstudie in der stationären Rehabilitation von Patienten mit psychischen/psychosomatischen Störungen [Does a Turkish migration background influence treatment outcome? Results of a prospective care provision study in the rehabilitation of in-patients with mental/psychosomatic complaints]. *Psychotherapie Psychosomatik Medizinische Psychologie, 58*, 176–182.

Morling, B., Kitayama, S., & Miyamoto, Y. (2002). Cultural practices emphasize influence in the U.S. and adjustment in Japan. *Personality and Social Psychology Bulletin, 28*, 311–323.

Muraven, M., Tice, D. M., & Baumeister, R. F. (1998). Self-control as a limited resource: Regulatory depletion patterns. *Journal of Personality and Social Psychology, 74*, 774–789.

Murray, S. L. (2005). Regulating the risks of closeness: A relationship-specific sense of felt security. *Current Directions in Psychological Science, 14*, 74–78.

Newman, D. A., Joseph, D. L., & MacCann, C. (2010). Emotional intelligence and job performance: The importance of emotion regulation and emotional labor context. *Industrial and Organizational Psychology, 3*, 1–6.

Oysermann, D., & Lee, S. W. S (2008). Does culture influence what and how we think? Effects of priming individualism and collectivism. *Psychological Bulletin, 134*, 311–342.

Pennebaker, J. W., & Seagal, J. D. (1999). Forming a story: The health benefits of narrative. *Journal of Clinical Psychology, 55*, 1243–1254.

Ponizovsky, A. M., & Ritsner, M. S. (2004). Patterns of loneliness in an immigrant population. *Comprehensive Psychiatry, 45*, 408–414.

Richards, J. M., Butler, E. A., & Gross, J. J. (2003). Emotion regulation in romantic relationships: The cognitive consequences of concealing feelings. *Journal of Social and Personal Relationships, 20*, 599–620.

Richards, J. M., & Gross, J. J. (2000). Emotion regulation and memory: The cognitive costs of keeping one's cool. *Journal of Personality and Social Psychology, 79*, 410–424.

Roemer, L., Orsillo, S. M., & Salters-Pedneault, K. (2008). Efficacy of an acceptance-based behavior therapy for generalized anxiety disorder: Evaluation in a randomized control trial. *Journal of Counseling and Clinical Psychology, 76*, 1083–1089.

Rothermund, K., Voss, A., & Wentura, D. (2008). Counter-regulation in affective attentional bias: A basic mechanism that warrants flexibility in motivation and emotion. *Emotion, 8*, 34–46.

Russell, D., Peplau, L. A., & Ferguson, M. L. (1978). Developing a measure of loneliness. *Journal of Personality Assessment, 42,* 290–294.

Saarni, C. (1989). Children's understanding of strategic control of emotional expression in social transaction. In C. Saarni & P. Harris (Eds.), *Children's understanding of emotion* (pp. 181–208). New York: Cambridge University Press.

Saarni, C. (1992). Children's emotional-expressive behaviors as regulators of others' happy and sad emotional states. In N. Eisenberg & R. A. Fabes (Eds.), *Emotion and its regulation in early development* (pp. 91–106). San Francisco, CA: Jossey-Bass.

Sapolsky, R. M. (2007). Stress, stress-related disease, and emotional regulation. In J. J. Gross (Ed.), *Handbook of emotion regulation* (pp. 606–615). New York: Guilford.

Schwartz, S. H. (1994). Cultural dimensions of values: Towards an understanding of national differences. In U. Kim, H. C. Triandis, C. Kagitcibasi, S. C. Choi, & G. Yoon (Eds.), *Individualism and collectivism: Theoretical and methodological issues* (pp. 85–119). Thousand Oaks, CA: Sage.

Sheppes, G., Scheibe, S., Suri, G., & Gross, J. J. (2011). Emotion-regulation choice. *Psychological Science, 22*, 1391–1396.

Soto, J. A., Levenson, R. W., & Eberling, R. (2005). Cultures of moderation and expression: Emotional experience, behavior, and physiology in Chinese Americans and Mexican Americans. *Emotion, 5*, 154–165.

Soto, J. A., Perez, C. R., Kim, Y.-H., Lee, E. A., & Minnick, M. R. (2011). Is expressive suppression always associated with poorer psychological functioning? A cross-cultural comparison between European Americans and Hong Kong Chinese. *Emotion, 11*, 1450–1455.

Stepper, S., & Strack, F. (1993). Proprioceptive determinants of emotional and nonemotional feelings. *Journal of Personality and Social Psychology, 64*, 211–220.

Tamir, M. (2009). What do people want to feel and why? Pleasure and utility in emotion regulation. *Current Directions in Psychological Science*, *18,* 101–105.

Tamir, M. (2011). The maturing field of emotion regulation. *Emotion Review, 3*, 3–7.

Tamir, M., & Ford, B. Q. (2009). Choosing to be afraid: Preferences for fear as a function of goal pursuit. *Emotion, 9*, 488–497.

Thompson, R. A. (2011). Emotion and emotion regulation: Two sides of the developing coin. *Emotion Review, 3*, 53–61.

Vedder, P., & Virta, E. (2005). Language, ethnic identity, and the adaption of Turkish immigrant youth in the Netherlands and Sweden. *International Journal of Intercultural Relations, 29*, 317–337.

Watkins, E. (2011). Dysregulation in level of goal and action identification across psychological disorders. *Clinical Psychology Review, 31*, 260–278.

Watson, D., Clark, L. A., & Tellegen, A. (1988). Development and validation of brief measures of positive and negative affect: The PANAS scales. *Journal of Personality and Social Psychology, 54,* 1063–1070.

Weissman, A., & Beck, A. (1978, November). *Development and validation of the Dysfunctional Attitude Scale.* Paper presented at the meeting of the Association for Advancement of Behavior Therapy, Chicago, IL, USA.

Elisabeth A. Arens
Department of Clinical Psychology and Psychotherapy
Institute of Psychology
University of Heidelberg
Hauptstraße 47–51
69117 Heidelberg
Germany
E-mail: elisabeth.arens@psychologie.uni-heidelberg.de

IV. Diagnosis

Culture and Psychiatric Disorders

Chapter 7

Culturally Informing Diagnostic Systems

Juan E. Mezzich

Mount Sinai School of Medicine, New York University, New York, NY, USA

Abstract

Culture as a key component of an adequate theoretical framework of illness and health in psychiatry and medicine has historically been largely ignored in the design of broad diagnostic systems, only recently beginning to receive some attention. The development of culturally-informed diagnostic systems is therefore still very much work in progress. This paper provides some general conceptual reflections and then organizes this work in progress in terms of the presence of culture in the Diagnostic and Statistical Manual of Mental Disorders (DSM-IV) and the International Classification of Diseases (ICD-10) as well as in various national and regional adaptations of these international classification standards, and then outlines some recent and evolving developments aimed at bringing culture to the core of diagnostic assessment.

Keywords: diagnostic formulation, diagnostic systems, culture, cultural formulation, culture-bound syndromes, person-centered integrative diagnosis

Along with biological, psychological, social and spiritual dimensions, culture represents a key component of an adequate theoretical framework of illness and health in psychiatry and medicine at large (Mezzich, Lewis-Fernandez & Ruiperez, 2008). One should expect, therefore, to see every crucial clinical activity, such as diagnosis, as culturally informed. However, only in the past two decades has culture been given pointed attention in the design of broad diagnostic systems. Such attention, while welcome and promising, has usually been rather marginal. Thus, the story of culturally-informed diagnostic systems is very much one of work in progress. After some general conceptual reflections, this paper organizes this work in progress in terms of the presence of culture in DSM-IV (American Psychiatric Association, 1994), ICD-10 (World Health Organization, 1992, 1993), and various national and regional adaptations of the international classification standard and then outlines some recent and evolving developments aimed at bringing culture to the core of diagnostic assessment.

As suggested above, psychiatric diagnosis, as an activity and as a formulation, is to be keenly informed by culture and other major domains of a broad theoretical framework. As an activity, diagnosis involves interviewing the patient and relevant others and consulting documentary sources in order to obtain information on the patient's history of psychiatric and general medical illnesses as well as on family, personal, and social histories. It also involves conducting examinations of psychopathology and physical status, and using supplementary diagnostic procedures, all aimed at substantiating a valid diagnostic formulation. At each step of this complex process, cultural factors may play a significant role as illustrated by the cultural sensitivity required to establish rapport among people with different ethnicities, dealing with variations in language knowledge and preferences between clinician and patient, appropriately engaging relatives and significant others, the manner of exploring intimate personal matters, the interpretation of patient reports concerning the significance and severity of emotional complaints, the evaluation of difficulties with social functioning and the extent and value of social supports, and the actual availability of culturally validated assessment instruments (Mezzich & Lewis-Fernandez, 1997).

Although the interaction between nosologists and cultural experts has not always been smooth, opportunities for some sort of rapprochement have appeared in recent decades. They initially focused on specific points of collaboration as it happened for the development of DSM-IV (American Psychiatric Association, 1994) and, to a lesser degree, for ICD-10. More recently, interest in the cultural framework of prospective diagnostic systems is becoming increasingly conspicuous, as reflected in wide international surveys (Mezzich, 2002). This chapter reviews the presence of culture in diagnostic systems of high international visibility and use, such as ICD-10 and DSM-IV, and in annotations or adaptations of the International Classification of Diseases, such as the Chinese Classification of Mental Disorders (Chen, 2002) and the Latin American Guide for Psychiatric Diagnosis (Berganza, Mezzich & Jorge, 2002). Developments advanced by the World Psychiatric Association as International Guidelines for Diagnostic Assessment (Mezzich et al., 2003) and by the International College of Person-centered Medicine as person-centered integrative diagnosis (Mezzich et al., 2010) are also relevant and are outlined here.

Cultural Developments in DSM-IV

In 1990, the leaders of the American Psychiatric Association's DSM-IV Task Force decided to explore the possibility of addressing culture in the DSM series for the first time. The demographic pressures represented by the growing presence of ethnic minorities in the US population seem to have been decisively influential. The emerging research on culture and mental health (Fabrega, 1989; Kirmayer, 1984; Kleinman, 1988a) made the enterprise feasible – and the Office for Special Populations of the National Institute of Mental Health funded it. A landmark conference on culture and psychiatric diagnosis in Pittsburgh in 1991 offered an opportunity for a meeting of minds between nosologists and cultural experts. Major conclusions of the conference included the identification of specific points for culturally enhancing DSM-IV (i.e., the introduction to the diagnostic manual, cultural considerations pertinent to the various diagnostic categories and the multiaxial schema, and a glossary of culture-bound syndromes). In the ensuing process, an effort was also made to design a pioneering cultural formulation to guide an ethnographic exploration of the experience of patients seen for psychiatric evaluation. The main elements of the presence of culture in DSM-IV are outlined in the following sections.

Introducing Culture Into the Manual

In order to alert clinicians to the challenge of using DSM-IV thoughtfully in a multicultural society, a statement was prepared for the manual's introduction touching on the concepts of culture and ethnicity and referring to the substantial anthropologic research underlying the specific recommendations offered. It encouraged clinicians to become aware of their ethnocentric biases and attend to the personal and cultural perspectives of each patient being assessed. The statement attempted to frame the entire DSM as a cultural document in that it reflects the values and perspectives of certain segments of US society (Fabrega, 1995). A shortened version of the proposed text was included in the last two pages of the 11-page introduction. This placement and the elimination of important distinctions reduced the cultural perspective to an addendum to the core of the introduction.

Cultural Considerations for Specific Disorders

Detailed proposals concerning modifications of diagnostic criteria, differential diagnosis, and accompanying text on cultural considerations were offered by the Culture and Diagnosis Work Group. Most of the proposed text was targeted at specific disorders but some important considerations applied to whole categories and their interconnections. Text was prepared for most disorders within all broad diagnostic classes, except factitious disorders. The cultural considerations summarized information on cultural variations in modes of describing distress, symptom patterns, dysfunctions, course, and sociodemographic correlates of the disorder. These remarks were intended to promote culturally sensitive application of the corresponding diagnostic criteria. Attention was called to the fact that, at a minimum, cultural sensitivity in diagnosis implies that an examiner is able to take into account the social and cultural context of the person being examined in order to ascertain whether specific diagnostic criteria are applicable in the present case and generate an appropriate differential diagnosis.

For the most part, simplified versions of the proposed cultural comments on diagnostic criteria and accompanying text were incorporated into DSM-IV. Except for the personality disorders, cultural considerations proposed for the introductory sections of the broad classes were not included. A total of 76 individual diagnostic categories within all 15 broad diagnostic classes have sections labeled "culture, age, and gender considerations." The extent to which proposed text was incorporated into DSM-IV varied markedly across its sections. Proposals involving cross-cultural variations in symptoms or prevalence rates tended to be included while those presenting challenges to the presumed universality of standard diagnostic categories and criteria tended to be ignored.

Cultural Comments on the Multiaxial Schema

Proposed text pointed out that application of the standardized axial typologies and scales requires careful attention to how cultural factors influence such assessments. This applies to the formulation of mental disorders in Axis I and, especially, Axis II, and to the general medical disorders in Axis III, which can be differentially distributed across social class and ethnic groups. Certain psychosocial stressors (Axis IV) are particularly frequent in minority, displaced, and economically disadvantaged populations. The accurate rating of levels of functioning (Axis V) can be enhanced by considering the collective experience of the individual's reference groups and demographic information.

Cultural annotations for the multiaxial assessment are virtually absent in the published manual. Exceptions are the inclusion of one cultural example within psychosocial problems related to social environment in Axis IV and a reference to the axes within the cultural statement in the general introduction and within the introduction to the cultural formulation.

Cultural Formulation

As mentioned above, the proposed cultural formulation emerged later than the other components of the cultural proposals for DSM-IV but was quickly recognized as a crucial innovation (Mezzich & Good, 1997). It supplements the nomothetic or standardized diagnostic ratings with an idiographic statement, emphasizing the patient's personal experience and the corresponding cultural reference group (Good & Good, 1986; Jones & Thorne, 1987; Kleinman, 1988b).

A literature review found several broad dimensions relevant to a cultural formulation that were distilled into a brief set of guidelines with the following five elements:

1. Cultural identity of the patient, including reference groups, language, spiritual and religious affiliation, and multicultural identity
2. Cultural explanations of the illness (i.e., idioms of distress, explanatory models, and popular and professional sources of care)
3. Cultural factors related to psychosocial environment and functioning (e.g., the meaning of social support and stigma)

4. Cultural aspects of the relationship between patient and clinician (e.g., attitudes toward authority, dependency, and relevance to transference and counter-transference)
5. Overall formulation, synthesizing elements critical to diagnosis and care.

Field trials of the guidelines with various ethnic groups (African American, American Indian, Asian American, and Latino) pointed out the value of their use and yielded illustrative case formulations, four of which were included in the proposed text to clarify the application of the cultural formulation. The introduction and the five elements of the proposed cultural formulation outline were included almost completely. The cultural formulation was, however, placed within the ninth appendix of the manual, not, as originally proposed, in the section immediately following the presentation of the multiaxial assessment. The illustrative cases, which the Work Group considered important to facilitate clinicians' use of the novel contribution, were omitted.

More recently, among a number of contributions appearing in several countries (Baarnhielm, 2008; Lewis-Fernandez, 1996; Rohlof, 2008), a set of guidelines for preparing a cultural formulation has been published (Mezzich, Caracci, Kirmayer & Fabrega, 2009). A cultural formulation reader assembling multi-authored contributions and case formulations has also appeared (Mezzich & Caracci, 2008).

Glossary of Culture-Bound Syndromes and Idioms of Distress

Culture-bound syndromes (CBS) used to be the mainstay of the consideration of culture in diagnosis (Simons & Hughes, 1985). They were, however, considered with a critical perspective for DSM-IV. This collation of terms and their meanings was intended to provide definitions of some of the folk or popular psychiatric syndromes and idioms of distress – that is, culturally shaped constellations of symptoms and culturally prescribed ways of describing distress that may or may not have psychopathologic significance and that are likely to be encountered in cross-cultural psychiatric work. It would provide a handy reference for terms used elsewhere in the DSM-IV text. By highlighting distinctive forms of illness experience and local approaches to describing, explaining, classifying, and responding to distress, the CBS glossary also illustrates the importance of an anthropologic framework to understand any disorder. In many cases, they are not syndromes at all but locally formulated descriptions and interpretations of illness and the title of this section reflects this diversity.

The glossary proposal began with a brief introduction and then presented 25 terms drawn from a much larger set, focusing on those that have been most studied and that are widely recognized in non-Western societies and in North America among African Americans (e.g., rootwork, falling out), American Indians and Alaska Natives (ghost sickness, pibloktoq), Asian Americans (shenjing shuairuo, taijin kyofusho), and Latinos (susto, ataque de nervios). Importantly, and in reference to DSM itself as a cultural document, Western culture-related syndromes (e.g., anorexia nervosa, multiple

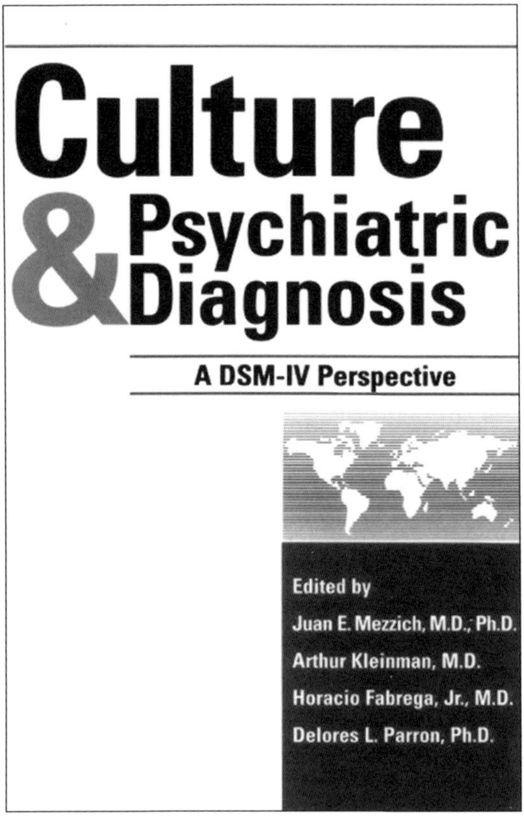

Figure 1. *Culture & Psychiatric Diagnosis: A DSM-IV Perspective*

personality disorder) were also identified and linked to specific features of Western countries or highly westernized segments of other societies. The CBS glossary is also contained in the ninth appendix and the title was shortened by eliminating the phrase "and idioms of distress." The section on Western CBS was excluded from the glossary. Many references to culture-specific terms in the cultural considerations sections of the text were cut, leaving the glossary as virtually the only place where several of these terms are mentioned in the DSM. The divorce of the glossary from the body of the text and the exclusion of Western CBS has the effect of rendering the glossary a museum of exotica.

A volume edited by the leaders of the Culture and Diagnosis Work Group presents and discusses the contributions outlined in the preceding sections (Mezzich, Kleinman, Fabrega & Parron, 1996). Further information, with a critical analysis of the cultural elements in DSM-IV, can be found in Mezzich et al. (1999).

Cultural Elements in ICD-10

The decennial revision of the ICD by the World Health Organization (WHO) would seem to offer a natural opportunity for the study of mental and general medical disorders in culture-informed ways. Curiously, and especially in comparison to DSM-IV, the

Table 1. Culture-bound syndromes included in DSM-IV and ICD-10

Culture-bound syndromes	DSM–IV	ICD–10
1. Amok	+	+
2. Ataque de Nervios	+	–
3. Bilis and Colera	+	–
4. Bouffee delirante	+	–
5. Brain Fag	+	–
6. Dhat	+	+
7. Falling-out or black-out	+	–
8. Ghost sickness	+	–
9. Hwa-byung	+	–
10. Koro	+	+
11. Latah	+	+
12. Locura	+	–
13. Ma1 de ojo	+	–
14. Nervios	+	+
15. Piblokto	+	+
16. Qi-gong psychotic reaction	+	–
17. Rootwork	+	–
18. Sangue dormido	+	–
19. Shenjing Shuariuo	+	–
20. Shen-K'uei	+	–
21. Shin-bvg	+	–
22. Spell	+	–
23. Susto, Espanto	+	+
24. Taijin Kyofu Sho	+	+
25. Zar	+	–
26. Pa-leng (frigophobia)	–	+
27. Ufufuyane, Saka	–	+
28. Uqamairineq	–	+
29. Windigo	–	+

presence of culture in the current ICD-10 is quite limited. This may reflect an effort to emphasize transcultural uniformities and convergence rather than attending to variations in clinical presentations and needs.

The most conspicuous cultural element in ICD-10 is the list of culture-specific disorders included in the Diagnostic Criteria for Research version of the ICD-10 Classification of Mental and Behavioral Disorders (World Health Organization, 1993). After a brief introduction to the concept of culture-specific disorders, it briefly presents 12 of these disorders. Included for each of these conditions is a brief connotative definition, suggested ICD-10 codes, related culture-bound syndromes, and some bibliographic references.

Table 1 presents a comparative listing of all culture-bound syndromes described in DSM-IV and ICD-10. It shows that eight of these syndromes are discussed in both diagnostic systems, 17 only in DSM-IV, and four only in ICD-10.

Other ICD-10 Components Relevant to Cultural Factors

These include, first, the Multiaxial Presentation of the ICD-10 (World Health Organization, 1997). It is composed of three axes: I. Clinical Diagnoses, II. Disablement, and III. Contextual Factors. Cultural information could, in principle, be accommodated under the above rubrics, especially Contextual Factors.

Second, the ICD-10 primary care version (World Health Organization, 1998) is a simple, brief classification arrangement compatible with and translatable into the ICD-10 standard classification of mental disorders. It is linked with management aids prepared for use by primary care practitioners. Its closeness to community information affords the possibility of identifying relevant cultural information.

Third, the ICD-10 chapter XXI on "Factors influencing health status and contact with health services" (World Health Organization, 1992) includes problems potentially related to *culture* and dealing with family or primary support group, general social environment, education, employment, housing and economic circumstances, legal issues, family history of illness, and personal life management and lifestyle.

Culture in National and Regional Adaptations of ICD-10

DSM-IV could be considered as the US version or adaptation of the ICD in the form of its Clinical (really meaning American) Modification. Other developments formally presented as ICD-10 adaptations or annotations are the Chinese Classification of Mental Disorders (CCMD-2-R and CCMD-3), the Japanese Clinical Modification of ICD-10 and other Asian developments, the Cuban Glossary of Psychiatry (GC-3), and the Latin American Guide for Psychiatric Diagnosis. They are culturally important because they represent attempts to adapt the international standard to local realities and needs.

Chinese Classification of Mental Disorders

China has over one fifth of the world's population, and Chinese people constitute one of the fastest growing ethnic minorities in Western societies. Therefore, knowledge of the Chinese Classification of Mental Disorders presented as adaptations of ICD-10 in CCMD-3 (Chinese Society of Psychiatry, 2001) may be helpful to understand the particularities of psychopathology in China and in patients of Chinese extraction. It contains a number of cross-culturally salient features, including additions, such as chi-gong-induced mental disorders and traveling psychosis, and variations in the concepts of neurasthenia, depressive neurosis, and anorexia nervosa.

Cuban Glossary of Psychiatry

The current third edition of the *Cuban Glossary of Psychiatry* (GC-3) (Otero, 2000) includes a number of contributions to the diagnosis of mental disorders as experienced and presented in Cuba. These encompass general psychiatry and child psychiatry. A basic principle in the development of GC-3 was to be similar to ICD-10, attempting to minimize differences. In line with this, the coding system of ICD-10 was closely followed. Contributions and changes were incorporated through the use of fifth digits in the diagnostic code or of codes not used in ICD-10. The ICD-10 diagnostic guidelines for the various psychiatric disorders were also largely respected. In some cases, supplemental text was added. References to DSM-IV and to the ICD-10 criteria for research were often made. Of note, GC-3 encourages diagnostic formulations based on the careful use of all information available and allows experienced clinicians to formulate diagnoses without strictly adhering to standard diagnostic criteria.

The cultural value of GC-3 is further attested by the broad participation of mental health professionals in its development and the wider opportunities this afforded for local needs to be considered. Its use of an extended multiaxial system allows substantial contextualization of clinical conditions.

Latin American Guide for Psychiatric Diagnosis

The Latin American Guide for Psychiatric Diagnosis (*Guía Latinoamericana de Diagnóstico Psiquiátrico*; GLADP) was prepared and published by the Latin American Psychiatric Association (APAL, 2004) as an adaptation of the ICD-10 for the use of psychiatrists and mental health professionals in Latin America. Its major motivations were, first, to make the classification of mental disorders in ICD-10 more relevant to the realities and needs of mental health care and life in Latin America – principally through Latin American annotations attached to the diagnostic criteria of pertinent mental disorders – and second, to personalize the diagnostic approach and include the assessment of positive health (quality of life). It was received warmly by mental health professionals

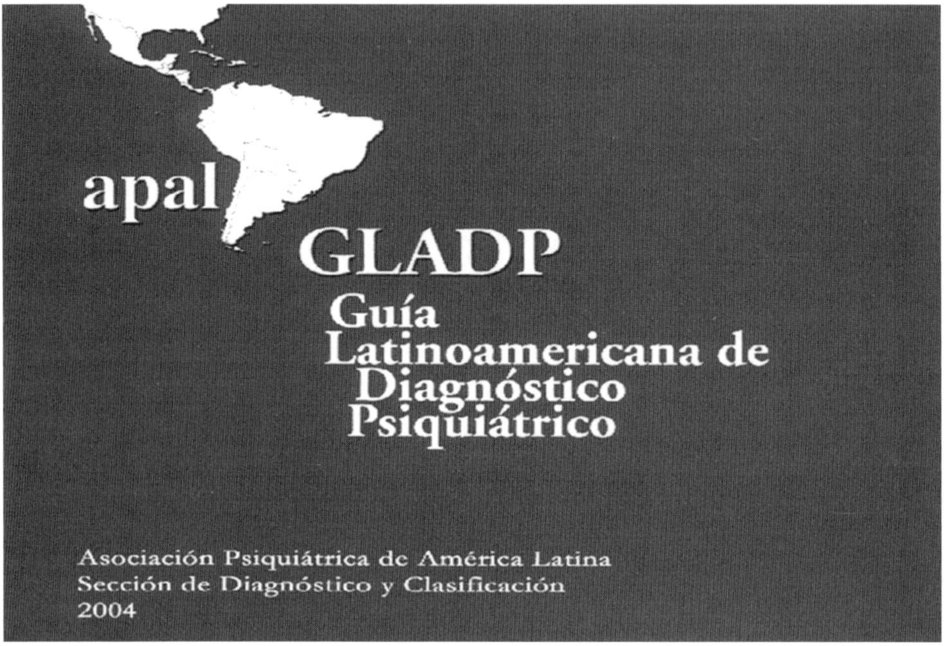

Figure 2. *Guía Latinoamericana de Diagnóstico Psiquiátrico* (GLADP), the Latin American Guide of Psychiatric Diagnosis)

in the region because of these features. Additionally, as it can be downloaded freely from the websites of APAL and other official bodies, it has become the main means of accessing the ICD-10 classification of mental disorders, the original version of which appears to be out of print.

In 2009, in view of the emerging revision of the ICD and DSM disease classification systems, APAL and its Diagnosis and Classification Section decided to update the GLADP to enhance further its cultural sensitivity and person-centeredness (Otero, Saavedra, Mezzich & Salloum, 2011). This effort was undertaken in association with the ongoing development of the person-centered integrative diagnosis model (Mezzich et al., 2010) by the World Psychiatric Association Classification Section and the International Network of Person-centered Medicine. Work groups have been established with experts from 15 Latin American countries dealing, respectively, with ten broad disorder categories as well as integrative diagnosis, cultural framework, and public health epidemiology. An initial survey of Latin American psychiatrists showed the GLADP was preferred over the ICD and DSM systems because of its integrative, personalized, and culturally sensitive features (Saavedra, Otero, Mezzich & Salloum, 2011). Work is advancing towards completing a GLADP revision (maintaining the still official ICD-10 categories and codes) to be followed by a full new edition of the GLADP to coincide with the finalization of ICD-11 in 2015.

Culture in Evolving Diagnostic Systems

Considerable advances have taken place in recent decades concerning the methodology for psychiatric diagnosis. These have included most prominently a more systematic and reliable description of disorders and the use of multiaxial schemas for covering the frequent plurality of a patient's clinical problems and their biopsychosocial contextualization. At the same time, compelling arguments have been made about the need to enhance the validity of these diagnostic formulations by attending to symbols and meanings that are pertinent to the patient's identity and personal perspectives (Tasman, 2002). Lain-Entralgo (1982) cogently argued that diagnosis is more than just identifying a disorder (nosologic diagnosis) and distinguishing one disorder from another (differential diagnosis); it is in fact understanding thoroughly what goes on in the mind and the body of the person who presents for care. This understanding must be additionally contextualized along the history, social situation, and culture of every patient for it to be adequately meaningful. Furthermore, in the increasingly multicultural world in which we live, it is essential when developing new diagnostic systems to strive for an effective balance between universalism (that facilitates professional communication across centers and continents) and local realities and needs (which address the person of the patient in its particular context).

WPA International Guidelines for Diagnostic Assessment

An innovative development on the interface between culture and psychiatric diagnosis was represented by the World Psychiatric Association (WPA) project on International Guidelines for Diagnostic Assessment (IGDA). Its roots can be found in the dedicated collaboration between the WHO and the WPA through its Executive Committee and its Section on Classification and Diagnostic Assessment towards the development of ICD-10 and related diagnostic systems. Another important root was the International Survey on Diagnostic Assessment Procedures (Mezzich, 1993) conducted by the WPA Section on Classification and Diagnostic Assessment, which revealed a widely perceived need for more comprehensive diagnostic approaches, which should be culturally informed and generated in a truly international manner.

A fundamental feature of the IGDA approach (Mezzich et al., 2003) involves the assessment of the psychiatric patient as a whole person, rather than just as a carrier of disease. Thus, it pointedly assumes in the clinician the exercise of scientific competence, humanistic concern, and ethical aspirations, and covers all key areas of information (biological, psychological, and social) pertinent to describing the patient's pathology, dysfunctions, and problems as well as the patient's positive aspects or assets. Another important feature involves basing the diagnostic assessment on the interactive engagement among the clinician, the patient, and his or her family, leading to a joint understanding of the patient's clinical condition and a joint development and monitoring of the treatment plan. Finally, IGDA uses ICD-10 for the first three axes of its multiaxial formulation (classification of mental and general medical disorders, disabilities, and contextual factors), to which it adds an axis on quality of life, an eminently culturally informed concept. The standardized multiaxial formulation is complemented by a personalized idiographic formulation to constitute a comprehensive diagnostic model. The idiographic formulation includes a contextualized (culturally framed) statement on clinical problems, patient's assets, and expectations on restoration and promotion of health.

The IGDA diagnostic formulation was incorporated into the Latin American Guide of Psychiatric Diagnosis (APAL, 2004) and this way it became available for clinical practice in a major area of the world.

Culture in the Ongoing DSM and ICD Revisions

As the door for the consideration of cultural issues in diagnostic system development was opened in DSM-IV and ICD-10, it can hardly be closed again. On the other hand, one must remember that these standard diagnostic systems are fundamentally classifications of illnesses where nosotaxia predominates over nosology, and that they have considerable internal and external institutional implications which render them rather traditional and difficult to change.

Preparations for DSM-5 started in 1999 with the development of a research agenda which led to the publication of a set of white papers (Kupfer, First, & Regier, 2002). This was followed between 2004 and 2008 by a set of research planning conferences (First, 2008), and then by the appointment of a task force and work groups that are carrying out the preparations for DSM-5 (Regier, Narrow, Kuhl, & Kupfer, 2009). This work is expected to be concluded in 2013. From a cultural viewpoint, the cultural elements of DSM-IV are being evaluated, and major attention is being given to the cultural formulation.

The design of ICD-11 started in earnest in 2007 under the coordination of the WHO Classifications Office (Ustun & Jakob, 2009). As its predecessor, it will cover mortality, morbidity, and related health problems in all areas of human disease through updated categories and definitions. As an innovation, the construction of the whole classification will emphasize formal terminologies and ontologies. Therefore, it will be suitable for emerging digital applications such as electronic health records. A web-based collaboration platform will support the overall revision process with semantic linkages to existing databases. The chapter on mental disorders is being drafted by a Topical Advisory Group (Saxena & Saraceno, 2009). For this chapter, particular attention is being paid to the definition of the disorders covered, to an efficient grouping of psychopathological syndromes, to the use of the classification in primary care and specialty settings, to harmonization with the evolving DSM-5 and other national and regional adaptations of the ICD, and to implications for public health. Many of these aspects need cultural attention. It remains to be seen how the ICD-10 cultural elements and others under consideration will fare in the final version of ICD-11. It is expected that work on the new ICD revision will be completed in 2015.

Person-centered Integrative Diagnosis

The conceptualization of person-centered integrative diagnosis (PID) started in 2005 within the WPA and its Institutional Program on Psychiatry for the Person (Mezzich, 2007; Mezzich & Salloum, 2007). It has unfolded in more recent years through extended collaboration with top global medical and health organizations participating in the International Network (now College) of Person-centered Medicine (Mezzich, Snaedal, van Weel, & Heath, 2009; Miles & Mezzich, 2011). It represents a key conceptual development in the process of building a psychiatry and medicine for the person.

The PID model (Mezzich et al., 2010) seeks to articulate science and humanism to obtain a diagnosis of the person (of the totality of the person's health, both ill and positive aspects), by the person (with clinicians extending themselves as full human beings), for the person (assisting the fulfillment of the person's health aspirations and life project), and with the person (in respectful and empowering relationship with the person who consults). This broader and more fundamental notion of diagnosis goes beyond the more restricted concepts of nosological and differential diagnoses. The PID model is defined by three keys: a) broad informational domains, covering both ill health and positive health on three levels: health status, experience of health, and contributors to health (see Table 2 displaying the PID informational domains), b) pluralistic descriptive procedures (categories, dimensions, and narratives), and c) evaluative partnerships among clinicians, patients and families.

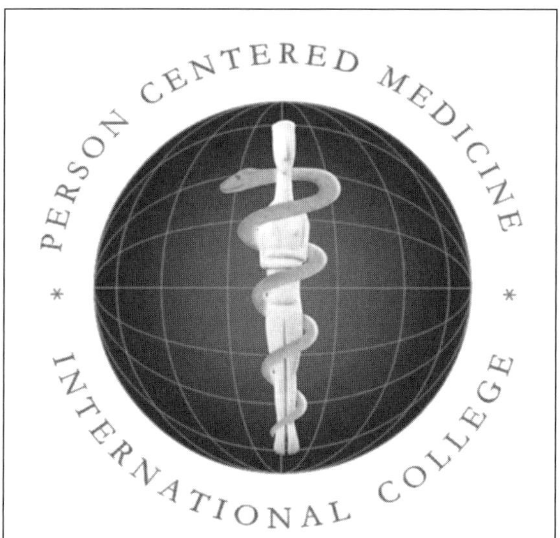

Figure 3. Logo of the *International College of Person-centered Medicine*

Table 2. Informational domains of Person-centered Integrative Diagnosis

Levels	Ill Health	Positive Health
1. Health status	Ill-being (a) Disorders (b) Disabilities	Well-being (a) Recovery (b) Functioning
2. Experience of health	Experience of illness	Expreince of positive health
3. Contributory factors	Risk factors (internal and external)	Protective factors (internal and external)

The conceptual bases and structural model of Person-centered Integrative Diagnosis call for an evaluation of the experience of illness and health as one of the three key domain levels of the diagnostic model. A major aspect of such domain levels involves a broad concept of culture with an emphasis on its experiential base. In line with this, a significant operational precedent would be the cultural formulation (Mezzich et al., 1996) proposed for and then included in the APA's DSM-IV. Another key element of person-centered medicine is attention to the values and needs of the patient who presents for evaluation and care. This is crucial to medicine's ethics commitment and the importance of individualization of care. In pointed reference to these aspirations, values-based medicine has been promoted (Fulford, 1999) and has been found conceptually consistent with person-centered care (Fulford, Christodoulou, & Stein, 2011). Procedurally, an efficient option to fulfill the objectives outlined above may be to combine the elements of the cultural formulation (expanded to address the experience of positive health in addition to that of illness) and a query on the person's needs and values.

Concluding Remarks

Pioneering attempts have taken place in the past two decades to introduce cultural considerations in psychiatric diagnostic systems. Most prominent in this respect has been the culture presence in DSM-IV, particularly in terms of a cultural formulation. Less substantial concerning culture has been the ICD-10 classification of mental disorders. Of high cultural interest are the national and international adaptations of ICD-10 because of their aim of articulating universality with local realities and needs. Among evolving innovative diagnostic systems, the WPA's IGDA introduced the combination of standardized multiaxial and personalized idiographic formulations, pointedly attending to culture issues; PID builds on IGDA concepts and experience to propose a bold new model in which health experience (culture and values), along with health status and health contributors, constitute the model's key informational domains.

References

American Psychiatric Association. (1994). *Diagnostic and statistical manual of mental disorders: DSM-IV* (4th ed.). Washington, DC: American Psychiatric Association.

APAL: Sección de Diagnostico y Clasificación de la Asociación Latinoamericana de Psiquiatría. (2004). *Guía latinoamericana de diagnóstico psiquiátrico* [Latin American guide of psychiatric diagnosis]. México: Editorial de la Universidad de Guadalajara.

Baarnhielm, S. (2008). Introducing the Cultural Formulation to mental health care in Stockholm, Sweden. In J. E. Mezzich, & G. Caracci (Eds.). *Cultural formulation: A Reader for psychiatric diagnosis*. New York: Rowman & Littlefield.

Berganza, C. E., & Mezzich, J. E., & Jorge, M. R. (2002). Latin American guide for psychiatric diagnosis (GLADP). *Psychopathology, 35*, 185–190.

Chen, Y. F. (2002). Chinese classification of mental disorders, third edition (CCMD-3). *Psychopathology, 35*, 171–175.

Chinese Society of Psychiatry. (2001). *The Chinese classification and diagnostic criteria of mental disorders, version 3* (CCMD-3). Jinan, China: Chinese Society of Psychiatry.

Fabrega, H. Jr. (1989). An ethnomedical perspective of Anglo-American psychiatry. *American Journal of Psychiatry, 146*, 588–596.

Fabrega, H. Jr. (1995). Cultural challenges to the psychiatric enterprise. *Comprehensive Psychiatry, 36*, 377–383.

First, M. (2008). Phase 2: Refining the research agenda for DSM-V: NIH conference series. Retrieved from http://www.psych.org/MainMenu/Research/DSMIV/DSMV/DSMRevisionActivities/ResearchPlanningatHigherMagnification.aspx

Fulford, K. W. M. (1999). *Moral theory and medical practice*. Cambridge: Cambridge University Press.

Fulford, K. W. M., Christodoulou, G. N., & Stein, D. J. (2011). Values and ethics: Perspectives on psychiatry for the person. *International Journal of Person Centered Medicine, 1*, 131–133.

Good, B., Good, & M.-J. D. (1986). The cultural context of diagnosis and therapy: A view from medical anthropology. In M. R. Miranda, & H. L. Kitano (Eds.). *Mental Health Research and Practice in Minority Communities*. Washington, DC: Government Printing Services.

Jones, E. E., & Thorne, A. (1987). Rediscovery of the subject: Intercultural approaches to clinical assessment. *Journal of Consulting and Clinical Psycho logy, 55*, 488–495.

Kleinman, A. (1988a). *Rethinking psychiatry: From cultural category to personal experience*. New York: Free Press.

Kleinman, A. (1988b). *The illness narratives*. New York: Basic Books.

Kirmayer, L. J. (1984). Culture, affect and somatization. *Transcultural Psychiatry Research Review, 23*, 159–188.

Kupfer, D., First, M., & Regier, D. (Eds.). (2002). *A research agenda for DSM-V*. Washington, D.C.: American Psychiatric Publishing, Inc.

Laín-Entralgo, P. (1982). El diagnóstico medico: Historia y teoría. Barcelona, Spain: Salvat.

Lewis-Fernandez, R. (1996). Cultural formulation of psychiatric diagnosis. *Culture, Medicine and Psychiatry 20*, 133–144.

Mezzich, J. E. (1993). An international survey on diagnostic assessment procedures. *Fortschritte der Neurologie und Psychiatrie, 61*, 13.

Mezzich, J. E. (2002). International surveys on the use of ICD-10 and related diagnostic systems. *Psychopathology, 35*, 72–75.

Mezzich, J. E. (2007). Psychiatry for the person: Articulating medicine's science and humanism. *World Psychiatry, 6*, 65–67.

Mezzich, J. E., Berganza, C. E., von Cranach, M., Jorge, M. R., Kastrup, M. C., Murthy, R. S., Okasha, A., Pull, C., Sartorius, N., Skodol, A., & Zaudig, M. (Eds.). (2003). Essentials of the World Psychiatric Association's International Guidelines for Diagnostic Assessment (IGDA). *British Journal of Psychiatry, 182*(45), 37–66.

Mezzich, J. E., Caracci, G. (2008). *Cultural formulation: A reader for psychiatric diagnosis.* New York: Rowman & Littlefield.

Mezzich, J. E., Caracci, G., Kirmayer, L., & Fabrega, H. (2009). *Cultural formulation guidelines. Transcultural Psychiatry, 46*, 383–405.

Mezzich, J. E., & Good, B. J. (1997). On culturally enhancing the DSM-IV multiaxial formulation. In T. Widiger, A. Frances, H. A. Pincus, et a1. (Eds.). (1997). *DSM-IV source book,* Vol 3. Washington, DC: American Psychiatric Press.

Mezzich, J. E., Kirmayer, I. J., Kleinman, A., Fabrega, H. Jr., Parron, D. L., Good, B. J., Lin, K. M., & Manson S. M. (1999). The place of culture in DSM-IV. *Journal of Nervous and Mental Disease, 187*, 457–464.

Mezzich, J. E., Kleinman, A., Fabrega, H., Parron, D. L. (Eds.). (1996). *Culture and psychiatric diagnosis: A DSM-IV perspective.* Washington, DC: American Psychiatric Press.

Mezzich, J. E., & Lewis-Fernandez, R. (1997). Cultural considerations in psychopathology. In A. Tasman, J. Kay, & J. A. Lieberman (Eds.). *Psychiatry*. Philadelphia, PA: WB Saunders.

Mezzich, J. E., Lewis-Fernandez, R., & Ruiperez, M. A. (2008). The cultural framework of psychiatric disorders. In A. Tasman, J. Kay, & J. A. Lieberman (Eds.). *Psychiatry* (3rd ed.). Chichester, UK: Wiley.

Mezzich, J. E., & Salloum, I. M. (2007). Towards innovative international classification and diagnostic systems: ICD-11 and Person-centered Integative Diagnosis. *Acta Psychiatrica Scandinavica, 116*, 1–5.

Mezzich, J. E., Salloum, I. M., Cloninger, C. R., Salvador-Carulla, L., Kirmayer, L., Banzato, C. E., Wallcraft J., Botbol, M. (2010). Person-centered Integrative Diagnosis: Conceptual bases and structural model. *Canadian Journal of Psychiatry, 55*, 701–708.

Mezzich, J. E., Snaedal, J., van Weel, C., & Heath, I. (2009) The International Network for Person-centered Medicine: Background and first steps. *World Medical Journal, 55*, 104–107.

Miles, A., & Mezzich, J. E. (2011). Advancing the global communication of scholarship and research for personalized healthcare: The International Journal of Person Centered Medicine. *International Journal of Person Centered Medicine, 1*, 1–5.

Otero, A. (2000). *Third Cuban glossary of psychiatry*. Havana, Cuba: Hospital Psiquiátrico de La Habana.

Otero, A., Saavedra, J. E., Mezzich, J. E., & Salloum, I. M. (2011). La guía latinoamericana de diagnóstico psiquiátrico y su proceso de revisión [The Latin American guide of psychiatric diagnosis and its revision process]. *Revista Latinoamericana de Psiquiatria, 11*, 18-25.

Regier, D., Narrow, W., Kuhl, E., & Kupfer, D. (2009). The conceptual development of DSM-V. *American Journal of Psychiatry, 166*, 645–50.

Rohlof, H. (2008). The cultural interview in the Netherlands: The cultural formulation in your pocket. In J. E. Mezzich, & G. Caracci. *Cultural formulation: A reader for psychiatric diagnosis.* New York: Rowman & Littlefield.

Saavedra, J. E., Otero, A., Mezzich, J. E., & Salloum, I. M. (2011). The revision of the Latin American guide for psychiatric diagnosis: A person-centered approach to international classification. *International Journal of Person Centered Medicine, 1*, 440–445.

Saxena, S., & Saraceno, B. (2009). The revision of the ICD classification of mental and behavioral disorders. In I. M. Salloum, J. E. Mezzich (Eds.). *Psychiatric diagnosis: Challenges and prospects.* Chichester, UK: Wiley-Blackwell.

Simons, R. C., & Hughes, C. C. (1985). *The culture-bound syndromes: Folk illnesses of psychiatric and anthropological interest.* Dordrecht, The Netherlands: Reidel.

Tasman, A. (2002). Lost in the DSM-IV check list: Empathy, meaning, and the doctor-patient relationship. *Academic Psychiatry, 26*, 38–44.

Ustun, T. B., & Jakob, R. (2009). The overall development of ICD-11. In I. M. Salloum, J. E. Mezzich (Eds.). *Psychiatric diagnosis: Challenges and prospects.* Chichester, UK: Wiley-Blackwell.

World Health Organization. (1992). *International statistical classification of diseases and related health problems. Tenth revision* (ICD-10). Geneva, Switzerland: WHO.

World Health Organization. (1993). *The ICD-10 classification of mental and behavioral disorders: Diagnostic criteria for research.* Geneva, Switzerland: WHO.

World Health Organization. (1997). *Multiaxial presentation of the ICD-10 for use in adult psychiatry.* Cambridge: Cambridge University Press.

World Health Organization. (1998). *Mental disorders in primary care.* Geneva, Switzerland: WHO.

Juan Mezzich
Department of Psychiatry
Mount Sinai School of Medicine
New York University
Fifth Avenue and 100th Street, Box 1093
New York, NY 10029
USA
E-mail: juanmezzich@aol.com
juan.mezzich@mssm.edu

Chapter 8

Depression and "Somatization" Among Two Divergent Cultural Groups

Sofie Bäärnhielm

Transcultural Centre, Stockholm County Council, S:t Görans' Hospital, Stockholm, Sweden

Abstract

Culture and context influence expression of distress. How a somatic language of distress can be used for depression and anxiety is illustrated with results from qualitative studies exploring meanings given to somatic symptoms among a group of ten Turkish and eight Swedish-born female patients in Sweden. The women encountered caregivers introducing a psychological and psychiatric conceptualization of their somatic symptoms. The women's understanding of the concepts of depression and anxiety are presented. The findings of the studies reflect the interactive nature of making meaning of illness and how important it is that caregivers actively try to understand what meanings patients give to their suffering. The results from these qualitative studies cannot be generalized, but argue for the importance of awareness of culture and context in clinical psychiatric diagnosing and will be discussed in relation to using the Outline for a Cultural Formulation in DSM-IV. The Cultural Formulation is an ethnographically-based method to attain an individualized understanding of patients' culture and context. As such, it may help clinicians to interpret patients' language of distress, as well as give information about the patient's life situation, including both stressful demands and supportive resources. Further, it may yield more knowledge about variety in the phenomenology of mental illnesses in multicultural milieus.

Keywords: culture, women, Turkish, somatization, depression, illness meaning

The challenge is not so much to find out who somatizes and who does not, but to incorporate an understanding of the meanings of somatization in all clinical work.
– Swartz (1998, p. 139)

Introduction

Mood, emotions, and sadness can be expressed in many ways and are influenced by culture and context. For instance, a predominantly somatic language can be used for expressing emotional distress, social problems, and for help-seeking in some ethnocultural groups. Still, critical examinations of the current concept of depression stress the problems of context-less evaluation of depression. Migration and globalization have increased the importance of awareness of culture and context in psychiatric assessment and treatment. From the results of research exploring the meaning given to somatic symptoms among a group of somatizing Turkish and Swedish-born female patients in Sweden, the variety in understandings of the concepts of depression and anxiety will be illustrated. The value of using narratives and ethnographic methods, such as the Cultural Formulation in DSM-IV, in psychiatric diagnostic practice for improving the understanding of the patient and the meaning of symptoms will be discussed.

Variety in Expressions of Distress

Culture may influence whether depression is expressed in psychological and emotional terms or in physical terms (Bhugra & Mastogrianni, 2004; Desjarlais, Eisenberg, Good, & Kleinman, 1996; Kirmayer, 2001). With regard to major depression, in the diagnostic system DSM-IV (APA, 2003), it is noted that culture influences the experience and communication of symptoms (see chapter 7). In some cultures, depression may be experienced in somatic terms rather than sadness and guilt; depression can be expressed by complaints of "nerves" and headaches, weakness, "imbalance," and problems of the "heart." Furthermore, cultures may differ in judgments about the seriousness of experiencing or expressing dysphoria.

In cross-cultural assessments of depression the variation in the language of affects is of significance. As an illustration, Manson (2005) identified some of the cross-cultural clinical difficulties in determining affects and the presence of dysphoria defined by Western experience. In the evaluation of mood and anxiety disorders, the author underscored the importance of taking into account the patient's social context and culture in addition to the consideration of symptoms. Similarly, in a history of ideas analyses, Johannisson (2001, 2004, 2009) demonstrated how the present, with its ideas and social discussions, influences the language of vulnerability that people use and how this language undergoes shifts in meanings. For instance, in his work of "Depression, Buddhism and the work of culture in Sri Lanka," Obeyesekere (1985) noted that, for a good Buddhist, life is suffering and sorrow; affects that are anchored to depression in the Western world are locked intrinsically into larger philosophical issues. Therefore, in such cultures in which personal efficacy is referred to as the acceptance of emotional distress, an open communication of emotional distress might be highly intolerable. Such rejection of some symptoms in a particular culture may influence the way in which people experience and express their distress. In these cultures, somatic language as cultural idioms of distress can be one of the alternative ways to communicate emotional or social problems (Kirmayer, 2001).

Using a Somatic Idiom of Distress

Somatization and psychologization can be seen as two culturally patterned styles of communication. White (1982) considered the psychological and psychosomatic mode of reasoning found in Western cultures unusual in the world's popular and traditional systems of beliefs. He also linked psychologization to the Western concept of the person and argued that investigations of somatization should proceed alongside investigations of psychologization. For instance, Mirdal (1985) investigated the expression of distress, and changes in expressions of distress over time, among Turkish immigrant women living in Denmark. In the study, these women were interviewed about their own evaluation of their physical, psychological, and social conditions. None of the women had any severe psychopathology. The author found that all complaints were of a somatic character, with the exception of "sıkıntı," meaning "tightness," which has both somatic and psychic components. Analyzing the women's formation of expression of distress Mirdal identified the significance of sex roles and language. She suggested that in a very restricted environment, focusing on illness may become a way to keep oneself alive and that illness may provide a socially approved way of obtaining relief from oppressing conditions, a culturally comprehensible alarm signal that alleviates oppression. Further, Mirdal has proposed that the structure of the Turkish language lends itself well to expressing somatic experiences. Twenty years later (2000–2001) follow-up interviews occurred with the same women. Also on this occasion, none of the women suffered from any severe psychopathology. The women still used the concept of "sıkıntı" but the concept of stress (pronounced "sitres" in Turkish) was introduced and used for describing their situation. When the women described their mood, this time they used concepts of sadness and depression; depression was preferred to anxiety (Mirdal, 2005).

In line with the previous demonstration, Swartz (1998, p. 136) formulated the question, "Somatization: patient problem or practitioner construction?" and identified the clinician's task as, "The challenge is not so much to find out who somatizes and who does not, but to incorporate an understanding of the meanings of somatization in all clinical work" (Swartz, 1998, p. 139). Similarly, Kirmayer (2001) also emphasized the importance of clinicians in decoding the meaning of somatic and dissociative symptoms as part of a language of distress with interpersonal and wider social meanings.

Lay Understandings of Symptoms of Depression

In the diagnostic systems, like DSM-IV and ICD-10, symptoms are organized, understood, and conceptualized according to current scientific knowledge and professional discussion (and politics). On the other hand, depressive symptoms can be grouped together and understood in different ways in different ethnocultural groups. For example, in their review of culture and anxiety, Lewis-Fernández et al. (2010) discussed the influence of local understandings of the workings of the body ("local ethnophysiologies") regarding the phenomenology of disorders. Looking at variation in panic attacks and in autonomic arousal symptoms, they showed how local understandings can influence the way in which symptoms "run together" in a specific culture. They gave several examples of the variety in the presentation of panic attacks; among them were *trung gió* (wind-related) attacks in Vietnam, *khyâl* (wind) attacks in Cambodia, and *ataque the nervios* (attack of nerves) among Latin Americans. Likewise, Dejman (2010) explored how women's depression was conceptualized in Iran among the three major ethnic groups, Fars, Kurds, and Turks. According to language (Farsi, Kurdish, and Turkish) the depressive symptoms were named differently. However, most of the women named depressive symptoms as *narahati asabi/narahati rohi*, [1] problems of nerves/soul. In all groups, depression was connected with an external stressor caused by a loss (death of relatives, job loss, etc.), environmental causes (including family conflict), gender-linked stressors, internal factors caused by emotional factors, cognition distortion, and hormonal factors. Their attributions for the causes of their depression affected their help-seeking behaviors as well (see chapter 14). Informal healers (family and friends, religious practices, and traditional healers) were preferred as an initial step in the treatment process. Furthermore, Okello (2006) explored the description and conceptualization of depressive symptoms by the Baganda population in Uganda. Among the Baganda, depression without psychotic features was regarded as illness of thoughts. Depression with psychotic symptoms was seen as a "clan illness," arising from poor relationships between the living and the dead. Both forms of illnesses were perceived as not requiring Western medication but traditional treatment, once again verifying the impact of lay models of attribution on help-seeking. However, psychiatric treatment was also seen as an option in the cases of severe depression or suicidal attempts, which was often stigmatized by social milieu.

Ascribing Lay Meaning to Depression

How laypersons ascribe meaning to their experience of distress has been described in various ways. Lay psychology, or folk psychology, creates an approximate understanding of phenomena that is often good enough in everyday situations. Young (1982) has introduced the concepts of "prototypes" and "chain complex" to describe how people organize the events and circumstances they are experiencing. "Prototypes" are described as a form of theoretical knowledge but without strong causal proposition. "Chain complex" is a string of empirical events, sensations, symptoms, and so forth

---

[1] In Persian, the meaning of the term *narahati* actually refers to discomfort, covertly meaning state of being ill. It is used to express undifferentiated feelings of physical and emotional discomfort. Languages such as Persian and Turkish, as a reflection of Eastern cultures, do not only lend themselves well to somatic experiences but also to covering up the state of being "mentally ill" as a result of sociocultural display rules (instead of "mental illness," it is expressed in everyday life as "mental discomfort") (see Pliskin, 1992).

that cohere and persist in the mind. Groleau, Young, and Kirmayer (2006) view prototypes to involve reasoning based upon salient episodes or events in one's own or others experiences. They give the example: "Last year, my uncle and aunt died of lung cancer, so I got scared and decided to quit smoking" (p. 676). They define "chain complex" as past experiences linked to present symptoms by a sequence of events but without causal connection. They give the example: "Around the time of my divorce, I starting having this pain in my chest. Then I got a cough that wouldn't go away" (Groleau et al., 2006, p. 676). Young (1982) considers informants' statements about sickness to be occasional products of a combination of loosely connected explanatory models, prototypical experiences, and chain complexes. Kleinman (1988) has defined explanatory models as "the notions that patients, families, and practitioners have about a specific illness episode" (p. 121). Kleinman gives emphasis to causality and attribution.

As laypersons, we know the world both through theory-laden participation and observations (Baer, Singer, & Susser, 2003). Discussing the difference in how laypersons and scientists create knowledge, the anthropologist Lévi-Strauss (1962/1995) used the French concept "bricoleur." This refers to someone working with his or her hands using diverse means, a sort of "handyman." The role of the bricoleur is to make do with whatever is at hand. Like a handyman or bricoleur, laypersons make sense of bodily and emotional sensations with what theory and experiences they have access to, this in contradiction to the professionals who try to work as the scientist. Similarly, the historian Shorter (1992) regarded psychosomatic illnesses as examples of the unconscious mind attempting to speak in a language of distress that will be understood in its time context; and that people at a given moment in history have a limited number of symptoms from which to choose when expressing their suffering; that is, a "symptom pool" (reference from Watters, 2010, p. 32).

Analyzing the role of culture in making meaning of illness, Angel and Thoits (1987) hypothesized the existence of learned cognitive structures, through which physical experiences are filtered and influence the interpretation of deviations from culturally-defined physical and mental health norms. Discussing this in relation to immigration, they propose that the specific situation for immigrants is one of having to restructure cognitive categorizations, to reorder their cognitive structures to conform to those that are consensually validated in the host society. For studying illness experiences, Hinton, Howes, and Kirmayer (2008) stress the importance of the cultural elaboration of sensation as a crucial complement to cognition and emotion. They used the concept of "sensation metaphor" to describe how sensation may be communicated and emphasize the importance of culturally-affected schemas for interpretation. Patients may complain of sensations that physicians classify as symptoms.

Decontextualizing the Concept of Depression

The professional conceptualization of psychiatric diagnostic categories, including depression, shifts over time. In her work, Johannisson (2009) analyzed how the use of the concepts of melancholia and depression have changed in history. She tied the once popular concept of melancholia to strong emotions and concluded that the concept of depression focuses primarily on the depressed mood. Johannisson also pointed out that the concept of depression hardly existed before 1900. Comparably, Shorter (1997) also suggested that the boundaries of what constitutes depression have been expanded relentlessly outward.

In their book *The Loss of Sadness – How Psychiatry Transformed Normal Sorrow into Depressive Disorder*, Horwitz and Wakefield (2007) raised a critical discussion of the current concept of depression in DSM-IV. The authors argued that according to the DSM classification system, a diagnosis of depression is made only in reference to the symptoms experienced by the patients. However, due to the lack of consideration of the context in which the symptoms occur, DSM fails to differentiate between normal sadness caused by external conditions and disordered sadness due to internal dysfunction. Accordingly the authors stated, "In attempting to characterize the kind of symptoms suffered in depressive disorders without reference to the context in which symptoms occur, contemporary psychiatry has also inadvertently characterized intense normal suffering as disease" (pp. 9–10). Moreover, Horwitz and Wakefield pointed to the importance of cultural and social values and meanings and the fact that culture plays a primary role in defining what sort of symptoms are considered harmful and what may be considered proportionate responses to loss. They regarded the consequences of the context-less definition of depression in DSM-IV as a factor behind epidemiological findings of an increased prevalence of depression. Decontextualization leads to the medicalization of sadness and to social problems being identified in medical terms. Likewise, the influence of the patient's context on symptoms is also illustrated in a study by Akbiyik, Sumbuloglu, Berksun, Senturk, and Priebe (2009). Symptoms among Turkish immigrant patients with depression in Germany (Berlin) were compared with those of patients in Turkey (Ankara). In the two cities the patients scored differently for several types of symptoms. Turkish patients who lived in Berlin had higher levels of depressive symptoms and patients who lived in Ankara reported higher levels of obsessive-compulsive symptoms, interpersonal sensitivity, anxiety, hostility, phobic anxiety, and paranoid ideation. In order to understand symptoms of depression Akbiyik and colleagues stress the importance of considering both the culture of origin and the actual cultural context of the immigrant patients. In the next section, the interconnections between patients' cultural background and their conceptualizations of illness and symptom presentation will be illustrated more in detail through the results of our recent studies conducted in Sweden.

Meanings Given to the Concepts of Depression and Anxiety Among Two Groups of "Somatizing" Women

The following section exemplifies how symptoms of depression can be understood in different manners among different ethnocultural groups. The data originated from a series of four qualitative interview studies conducted between 1997 and 2001 with a group of Turkish and Swedish-born female patients assessed as "somatizing" emotional distress (Bäärnhielm, 2000, 2003, 2004, 2005a, 2005b; Bäärnhielm & Ekblad, 2000). The studies were conducted with the aims of exploring how the women gave meaning to their illness and how meaning was changed and restructured in the clinical encounter. The studies were performed in a socioeconomically vulnerable suburban and multicultural area in Stockholm. To give an idea of the situation and context where the studies were carried out some information about immigration to Sweden, and in particular, Turkish immigration, is presented in the following.

Mental Health Care and Globalization in Sweden

Immigration to Sweden has taken place mainly during the postwar period. Until the mid-1970s this was primarily a matter of labor force immigration, mostly from Europe. Immigration varied with the needs of industry and commerce in Sweden (Bäärnhielm, Ekblad, Ekberg, & Ginsburg, 2005). In 1975, the character of immigration changed and labor migration almost ceased. Between 1975 and Sweden joining the EU in 1995, immigration to Sweden mainly consisted of refugees from conflict areas of the world seeking asylum and of family reunions. An exception was immigrants from the neighboring Nordic countries. With Swedish EU membership, immigration changed and emigration from other EU countries increased. In 2009, Sweden had a population of 9.3 million inhabitants, 14.3% of which were foreign-born (Statistics Sweden, 2011). Among foreign-borns, the most heavily represented country of origin was Finland (172,218 persons), followed by Iraq (117,919 persons).

Migration from Turkey

Turkish migration to Sweden began as labor migration but later continued mainly in the form of family reunions and marriage. In 1960 there were 168 Turkish-born persons in Sweden (Lundberg, 1991). Forty-seven years later, in 2009, the figure was 47,803 (Statistics Sweden, 2011). Migrants from Turkey constitute the tenth-largest national group of migrants in Sweden. Migration from Turkey to Sweden started as part of the Turkish exodus to Western Europe in the 1960s and 1970s. It began as a spontaneous chain-migration and many came from the Kulu area located north of Konya (Lundberg, 1991). The migration wave to Sweden was never as significant as in Germany and some other European countries. At the end of the seventies there was a peak in the migration of Syrian/Assyrians from Turkey due to religious oppression (Deniz, 1999). After the 1980 military coup in Turkey a period of refugee migration began. The Turkish migrants in Sweden today comprise different ethnic groups such as Turks, Kurds, Assyrians, and other groups, as well as various religious affiliations.

Challenges for Mental Health Care in Sweden

The increased cultural diversity in Sweden has put new demands on the health care system and on mental health care. One of the challenges is that of responding to the variety in expressions of distress and understanding of mental illness. The background to the start of the original studies, from which these data are taken, is the author's clinical experiences of difficulties in understanding patient's expressions of distress and illness meanings. At the time of the onset of these studies, I worked as a clinician in a considerably multicultural, segregated, poor, suburban area in Western Stockholm. It was my experience that patients often used a somatic mode of expressing emotional distress. Further, I often had the impression that patients gave their suffering and illness another meaning than that attributed by my colleagues and myself. This applied to both our professional assessments and our lay perspective. When the studies started, the major country of origin of the patients at the local psychiatric clinic where I worked was Sweden, followed by Turkey. Supporting our clinical experiences, a study examining the local psychiatric outpatient clinic by Al-Saffar, Borgå, Wicks, and Hällström (2004) found the diagnosis of "somatoform disorder" to be more common among immigrant patients than among Swedish-born patients. At the time of that study Al-Saffar et al. found the diagnosis for somatoform disorders particularly common among Greek patients (OR = 8.81, 95% CI = 4.41–17,59) compared with Swedish (OR = 0.18, 95% CI = 0.06–0.51).

Method and Overall Findings

In all four of the referred studies, data was collected by semi-structured interviews conducted with groups of Turkish- and Swedish-born female patients living in a multicultural area in western Stockholm. All the women were in contact with local health care services. Thirty-seven interviews were conducted with 10 Turkish-born women and 34 interviews with 8 Swedish-born women. All the interviews were carried out by the author, and data from the interviews were analyzed with a grounded theory approach.

All the women interviewed were evaluated by their caregivers as somatizing. The definition for somatization used in these studies refers to a tendency to experience and communicate psychological and social distress in the form of physical symptoms and to seek medical help for them (Lipowski, 1987). In the clinical encounter the patients in all studies were introduced to a "psychological language" of understanding their bodily distress and psychological and psychiatric attributions. Concepts such as depression, anxiety, and panic were introduced for defining and understanding their bodily distress. The clinical encounter entailed a restructuring of the meanings given to illness by all groups of women.

The restructuring of previous meanings involved a loss of earlier meanings given to illness, shifts in expressions and healing strategies, and a push toward restructuring illness and suffering into a psychological or psychiatric framework of understanding their distress. The patients tried to grasp the meanings of the caregivers but found difficulties in doing so. Restructuring of illness meanings was for many a complicated process where the possibilities of contextual support shifted between the Swedish and

Turkish-born women. The Turkish-born women, in general, did not have friends, family members, or others that could help them to understand the caregiver's view of their illness. This was in contradiction to the Swedish-born women who usually had a lot of resources such as family, friends, and colleagues, and used the media for understanding the caregiver's perspective. Data from these studies will be used to illustrate the variety in the understanding of depression and anxiety.

The Turkish-Born Women

Sample and Data Collection

The Turkish-born women interviewed were, at the time of the first interviews, between 31 and 48 years of age, with a mean age of 35. All came from rural areas or small towns in Turkey. Concerning ethnical affiliation, eight were Turkish, one Kurdish, and one Assyrian. The background reasons for immigration were diverse, including work, marriage, following the family, and refugee status. The duration of their stay in Sweden ranged from 4 to 29 years, with a mean duration of 19 years.

All the Turkish-born women interviewed had a low socioeconomic status. Among them, three were employed, four were receiving some form of sickness benefit, one was on social security, and two were without any income of their own. The years of schooling varied between 0 and 12 years, with a mean of 6.5 years. None had any higher education. Eight of the ten evaluated their language skills in Swedish as being good to fluent and two as having difficulties with the Swedish language; some preferred to have the interview in Swedish and others in Turkish with an interpreter.

A psychiatric diagnostic assessment was made, including a SCID-RV-1 (1994) interview. All the women had a psychiatric diagnosis according to the criteria of DSM-IV and several had more than one diagnosis. The following diagnoses were established (number of cases in parentheses): major depressive disorder (3); dysthymic disorder (5); panic disorder (7); generalized anxiety disorder (1); somatization disorder 300.81 (1); pain disorder associated with psychological factors (4).

Meaning Making

The women were first interviewed about making meaning of illness and later about meaning and restructuring of illness meanings. In the first interviews the women talked about their health situation in terms of pain, impairment, social loss, and emotional difficulties. Pain was prominent and often lateralized to one side of the body. For most of the women the right side was affected. The women often talked about heart problems and palpitations. One of the women, Sevgi (all the names used are pseudonyms and correspond with those used in previous publications), suffered from neck pain and heart palpitations. Sevgi's doctor had told her that she suffered from stress and anxiety. Sevgi was asked about how these words fit with her experience. Sevgi answered by talking about how her health status was expressed in Turkey:

> *Interviewer:* Is the heart getting bigger? Is that what you say in Turkey?
> *Sevgi:* Well it is like, one says, "heart worry" (*yürek kalkınması* –Turkish), not bigger but fear (*korku* –Turkish). (Bäärnhielm and Ekblad, 2000, p. 439)

Asked about her health situation, another woman, Fatma, responded:

> There is no peace and quiet in my body. I feel pain. That is my health. The pain never passes. It makes me very disappointed, feelings of pressure. I feel it during sleep too. It never passes. Every hour is different. Sometimes my blood pressure rises. I tire easily and the heart gets affected by this tiredness. When I feel it in my heart then I want to lie down. If I do not lie down there is a risk that I may fall down and perhaps faint. I feel like my heart is hanging somewhere and is dangling. I just want to lie, lie down, if I don't. I will fall and faint. It is that serious. (Bäärnhielm, 2003, pp. 75–76)

Bodily symptoms were often described parallel to problems, difficulties, and life events. Their stories included little description of causal attribution to distress but rich descriptions of links of coherence between health and their life. The health professionals had given the women's bodily symptoms psychiatric attributions and referred them to psychiatric care. Both these attributions and the referrals were difficult for the women to understand. One woman, Havva, formulated her thoughts in the following way:

> She (the psychiatrist) said that I had pain in my soul. I said that I did not have pain in my soul. She spoke my language (Turkish). It became a real conflict between us. I told her that she knew how we lived and how we worked and that it did not have anything to do with the soul. If it had been because of the soul I would have gone to Beckomberga (name of a local mental hospital). She asked me whether I heard voices, if I thought, if I did this and that. (Bäärnhielm, 2005b, p. 167).

The health professional's explanation of bodily symptoms in terms of psychiatric and psychological attribution was difficult for the women to make sense of and to accept. How the concept of depression was given different meaning among the women varied. At the time of the first interviews depression was for many of the Turkish-born women an unfamiliar word. In time it was given some sort of acceptance. Depression was given meanings such as: bad nerves, being nervous, sleeping difficulties, lack of patience, tensions in the body, shattered nerves, tired, being worn-out, pain, the gossiping of others. Fatma was asked about receiving the diagnosis and said:

> I had heard about it from others, they have had depression, become ill, got shattered nerves (*sinirleri bozulmuş* – Turkish), they said, for example,

> "that her nerves got shattered." I had heard something like that but when I got it myself I understood better what sort of illness it was. (Bäärnhielm, 2004, p. 50)

Sevgi told people in her surroundings about her depression diagnosis. She spoke about the reactions in her context:

> I got it accepted. Many friends phoned me. They had similar problems but they had hidden them. Later I explained and told them. They asked, "What sort of place is it? What happens there (referring to the psychiatric clinic)? What do you do there?" I told them. Several of my friends come here and get treatment (referring to the psychiatric clinic). It's like normal to have a depression. (Bäärnhielm, 2004, p. 52)

Words related to anxiety were used in various ways among the Turkish-born women. Panic was given a core of somatic meaning but also linked to emotional factors such as fear. In the first interviews anxiety was described as an unfamiliar word. Later on some women gave anxiety a mainly somatic meaning like heart palpitations, the legs giving away, a feeling of dying. As long as the concept of anxiety was given a somatic meaning it was accepted. Later on other women gave anxiety a mental meaning and connected anxiety with stigmatizing mental illnesses (Bäärnhielm, 2004).

In the clinical encounter the health professionals had renamed the women's, mainly bodily, expressions of distress using psychiatric and psychological words. Renaming illness and restructuring meaning given to illness were complicated for the women. Havva tried to understand the meaning of the concept "anxiety" and put it this way:

> I feel that I have something like a ball here, (points to her neck) that causes harm even in my neck and under the ears [...] They call it anxiety. I do not know. I believe that it is. As I do not have any other choice, I have to believe in (*tro på* – Swedish) what they say. Now I have the symptoms and I read about it in brochures and can see that they are symptoms of anxiety. But I did not have the symptoms earlier. (Bäärnhielm & Ekblad, 2000, p. 445)

Among the women in the initial interviews, there was sometimes a split between body and mind expressed in terms such as body/brain, body/head. The split may have been due to fear of stigmatizing psychiatric conceptualization but may also have been an adaptive strategy for protecting the capacity for good relations toward others, especially children (Bäärnhielm and Ekblad, 2000). For the Turkish-born women, the psychological and psychiatric attribution did not bridge the split, except for the concept of panic, which was given both a somatic and emotional meaning (Bäärnhielm, 2004).

Contextual Support

For the Turkish-born women, restructuring meaning was made with poor contextual support to facilitate understanding of the new information given by the health professionals. The women seldom had family members who could help them understand the information given in clinical care. They often avoided discussing their distress in psychiatric terms with friends and their social network. The women did not want to be stigmatized as having a mental illness.

These Turkish-born women did not follow the discussions in Swedish newspapers about illness, treatment, and medication. Nor did they participate in the social discussion on illness in their country of origin. At the time of the interviews a popular medical and lay discussion on the concept of burnout was taking place in Sweden. This discussion did not affect the Turkish-born women, as it did the Swedish- born women living in the same geographical area. The lack of contextual support to understand the medical information made the Turkish-born women dependent upon, and vulnerable to, the interaction with the clinicians and the health care system. In contrast to the lack of support to understand medical information many, but not all, of the Turkish-born women often had a great deal of social support from family members in their daily life situation, such as help running the household and taking care of the children.

The Swedish-Born Women

Sample and Data Collection

The ages of the Swedish-born women ranged from 30 to 55, with a mean age of 47 years at the start of the interviews. Four had less than 11 years of formal education and four had 12 years, with a mean of 8.2 years. Four had higher education. Three were working full-time, two had combined work and sick leave, and three had only some form of sickness benefit. A psychiatric diagnostic assessment was made and included a SCID-RV-I (1994) interview. All the women had a psychiatric diagnosis according to the criteria of DSM-IV and several of them had more than one diagnosis. The following diagnoses were established (number of cases in parentheses): major depressive disorder (3); dysthymic disorder (2); panic disorder (4); generalized anxiety disorder (1); somatization disorder (2); pain disorder associated with psychological factors (1).

Meaning Making

The interviews questioning illness meaning and restructuring of meaning were presented with the same questions in the same order and conducted parallel to the Turkish-born women. In the first interviews the Swedish-born women talked about their health situation by referring to bodily symptoms and emotions, but also psychiatric and psychological concepts. Their narratives included rich descriptions of causal attribution, reevaluation of earlier ideas, and of seeking new knowledge of the explanatory process of illness. They had often several noncompeting explanations for their illness (Bäärnhielm, 2000).

Health professionals had given the women psychiatric attributions for their bodily symptoms. For many of the Swedish-born women this idea had often already been introduced by friends and family. Most of the women considered depression as a mental illness with a risk of progression to more severe conditions. The concept of depression was usually accepted as a correct term for labeling distress by caregivers, family, and friends, but not used outside of this close circle. Lay terms used instead of depression were feeling down (*nedstämd* – Swedish) and being low (*låg* – Swedish), referring to the mood being pushed down. The participant Sonja expressed her view about depression this way:

> God preserve me from being depressed, that it, that it can really be bad. I think it seems to be very tough to become that apathetic and not have the energy for anything. (Bäärnhielm, 2005a, p. 352)

For these Swedish-born women the clinical encounter, at this time, involved renaming distress and a shift in expressions of distress. The concept of burnout was preferred instead of depression, which was not introduced by caregivers but by the surrounding context. Burnout was attributed to stressful working conditions and pushing oneself too hard. Burnout did not include the severity given to depression. To use the word "burnout" instead of "depression" was preferred in interactions with others outside the close family. Gerd, diagnosed as depressed, said:

> [...] for me in some way it feels worse to say depressed, because for many people depression is something else [....] I am afraid to say that I have or that I have had a depression. I am afraid that people will think that I am not able to take care of my children. I think this is something that I have inside me. (Bäärnhielm, 2005a, p. 353)

Gerd was asked why she preferred the term burnout instead of depression. She responded:

> [I] think that the fear has been a lot to do with my surroundings, what are they going to say, ... at work and people around me. Not my closest friends and so. I have been afraid that people will see me as mentally ill. (Bäärnhielm, 2005a, p. 353)

The Swedish-born women were very familiar with using the words panic and anxiety and used them in their ordinary language. Panic and anxiety were used interchangeably. Anxiety was linked to other lay words like "death anxiety," and so forth. Being distressed was labeled as anxiety and was appreciated and contributed to improved understanding for the women. Gerd said,"Some anxiety, you can say that, because in some way it's accepted" (Bäärnhielm, 2005a, p. 353). The women tried to understand the medical meaning of the word "anxiety." The Swedish-born women did not pronounce a clear split between body and mind.

Contextual Support

For the Swedish-born women, restructuring of illness meaning was made with rich contextual support by recourse to family, friends, network, television, newspapers, and other written information. The study was made before the wide public use of the Internet as a source of information. These Swedish-born women's ways of making sense of their distress and expressing themselves were quickly affected and influenced by the external medical discussion through the media. At the time of the last interviews the women talked about themselves as being burned out.

Concluding Remarks

Clinical Implications

Due to low sample size the results of our studies cannot be generalized, but the data provides some theoretical insights. The outcome of the in-depth interviews highlights the importance of considering patients' culture and context in evaluating their expressions of distress. Further, the findings reflect the interactive nature of meaning making. Meanings given to illness are influenced by a multitude of factors, including cultural traditions, personal experiences, sociocultural context, participation in ongoing medical discussions, and the interaction with clinicians and the health care system. Change in meaning making can have an impact on the experience of distress and contribute to changes in ways of expressing distress. The Swedish-born women in these studies were in a different situation than the Turkish-born ones as they had many resources to facilitate the understanding of new medical information given by health professionals. The Swedish-born women were in a more significant way taking part in, and affected by, the current sociomedical discussion, pointing out that patients in a socially and culturally marginalized position may need special support and attention for understanding new information given by health professionals.

Treatment of depression in patients with a mainly somatic idiom of distress often requires an introduction of a psychiatric or psychological conceptualization of their distress. This is facilitated if the clinician has some idea about patients' understanding of illness. The findings from these studies argue that a new understanding of illness needs to be introduced with a sense of coherence to patients' understanding in order to be helpful and not just intrusive (see chapter 15). The Swedish and Turkish-born patients' meanings given to illness were explored within the frame of a research project. However, there is a broader need for including shared clinical models into conventional clinical psychiatric assessments in community practice to explore patients' illness meaning, and the influence of culture and context on symptoms and expressions.

Using Ethnography and Narratives in Clinical Psychiatric Diagnosing

Ethnography is a useful method for attaining an individualized understanding of patients' culture, context, and to facilitate understanding of expressions and meanings. Ethnography aims to describe life in a local world at a specific place (Kleinman & Benson, 2006). It emphasizes the importance of trying to understand the other's point of view (Geertz, 1973). In clinical care, ethnography can contribute a personalized (ideographic) knowledge of the patient as a complement to the general (monothetic) knowledge. Ethnographic information can help to identify the patient's resources and possible supportive resources in the patient's context.

Ethnography has various manifestations and has always been marked with diversity (Atkinson, Coffey, Delamont, Lofland, & Lofland, 2001). Ethnographic fieldwork allows the researcher to attend to everyday interpretations of sensations as they are happening and offers prospective insights into the transformation process of sensations into symptoms (Hay, 2008). An ethnographic-based narrative interview is not as close to the situation as fieldwork but provides clinicians with a practical tool to include culture from an individualized (emic) perspective in the diagnostic process. For clinical care in multicultural milieus, ethnography is a new method to enhance the capacity to respond to cultural variety.

The Outline for Cultural Formulation in DSM-IV – A Practical Guideline

An interesting ethnographic approach for use in clinical psychiatric assessments is the Outline for Cultural Formulation in DSM-IV, in Appendix I (APA, 2003). The cultural formulation in DSM-IV is meant to supplement the multiaxial diagnostic assessment and to address difficulties that arise when DSM-IV criteria are applied in a multicultural environment. It provides a systematic review of the person's cultural background, the role of the cultural context for expressions of distress and dysfunction, and the effect that cultural differences may have on the relationship between the patient and the clinician. Culture and context are evaluated in an individualized way. The Outline for a Cultural Formulation was developed by the Group on Culture and Diagnosis of the National Institute of Mental Health (Mezzich, 1995) as a practical suggestion for a systematic review of culture and context in clinical psychiatric diagnosing (see chapter 7).

The Cultural Formulation includes the following categories: cultural identity of the individual; cultural explanations of the individual's illness; cultural factors related to the psychosocial environment and levels of functioning; cultural elements of the relationship between the individual and the clinician; and overall cultural assessment for diagnosis and care. A narrative approach to data collection and an overall cultural assessment documented as narrative summary is suggested. The Cultural Formulation is intended to be a standardized and structured model for cultural assessments (Lewis-Fernández & Díaz, 2002). It is also an idiographic statement emphasizing the patient's personal perspective and the corresponding cultural reference group.

The Cultural Formulation is described as a "mini-ethnographic" narrative assessment (Lewis-Fernández, 1996). The narrative approach originates from the growing importance of the study of narratives in anthropology and other social sciences (Lewis-Fernández & Díaz, 2002). To encourage clinical use of the Cultural Formulation, several interview guides have been developed (Mezzich, Carracci, Fabrega, & Kirmayer, 2009; Rohlof, Knipscheer, & Kleber, 2009; Bäärnhielm, Scarpinati, & Pattyi, 2007). Mezzich & Caracci (2008) have edited a textbook on the Cultural Formulation. In 1996 the journal *Culture, Medicine and Psychiatry* (CMP) started a series of Cultural Formulation case analyses. This has been followed by case presentations in books and several journals such as: *Indian & Alaska Native Mental Health Research*, *Israel Journal of Psychiatry & Related Sciences*, *Journal of Forensic Sciences*, *Journal of Muslim Mental Health*, *Psychiatric Quarterly*, *Social Work in Health Care*, and *Transcultural Psychiatry*.

As the Cultural Formulation in DSM-IV provides a structured tool for awareness of culture and context in psychiatric assessment it may contribute to improved reliability of the diagnostic process, validity of psychiatric categorizing, and more knowledge about variety in phenomenology of illness. For clinicians, an ethnographic approach may facilitate the challenge of decoding the patient's expressions of distress. The usefulness of a cultural analysis in the diagnostic process is formulated by Lewis-Fernández (1996, p. 135) as follows: "The fundamental challenge that cultural analysis brings to diagnostic thinking is its capacity to render visible the socially constructed context that mediates key features of a patient's presentation and subsequent course."

Acknowledgment

My thanks to Steve Wicks for help with the English.

References

Akbiyik, D., Sumbuloglu, V., Berksun, O. E., Senturk, V., & Priebe, S. (2009). Symptoms of Turkish patients with depression in Ankara and Berlin. *Culture, Medicine and Psychiatry*, 33, 412–420.

Al-Saffar, S., Borgå, P., Wicks, S., & Hällström, T. (2004). The influence of the patients' ethnicity, socio-demographic conditions and strain on psychiatric diagnoses given at an outpatient clinic. *Nordic Journal of Psychiatry, 58*, 421–427.

American Psychiatric Association. (2003). *Diagnostic and Statistical Manual of Mental Disorders* (4th ed., Text Revision). Washington, DC: American Psychiatric Association.

Angel, R., & Thoits, P. (1987). The impact of culture on the cognitive structures of illness. *Culture, Medicine and Psychiatry,* 11, 465–494.

Atkinson, P., Coffey A., Delamont, S., Lofland, J., & Lofland L. (2001). Editorial Introduction. In P. Atkinson, A. Coffey, S. Delamont, J. Lofland, & L. Lofland (Eds.), *Handbook of Ethnography* (pp. 1–7). London: Sage.

Bäärnhielm, S. (2000). Making sense of suffering. Illness meaning among somatizing Swedish women in contact with local health care services. *Nordic Journal of Psychiatry, 54*, 423–430.

Bäärnhielm, S. (2003). *Clinical encounters with different illness realities. Qualitative studies of illness meaning and restructuring of illness meaning among two cultural groups of female patients in a multicultural area of Stockholm.* Doctoral thesis, Division of Psychiatry, Neurotec Department, Karolinska Institutet, Stockholm, Sweden.

Bäärnhielm, S. (2004). Restructuring illness meaning through the clinical encounter: A process of disruption and coherence. *Culture, Medicine and Psychiatry,* 28, 41–65.

Bäärnhielm, S. (2005a). Making sense of different illness realities. Restructuring of illness meaning among Swedish-born women. *Nordic Journal of Psychiatry,* 59, 350–356.

Bäärnhielm, S. (2005b). Seeking health care: Practical steps by a women in an immigration context. In R. Bibace, J. Laird, K. Noller, & J. Valsiner, (Eds.), *Science and medicine in dialogue: Thinking through particulars and universals* (pp. 161–172). Westport, CT: Greenwood.

Bäärnhielm, S., & Ekblad, S. (2000). Turkish migrant women encountering health care in Stockholm. A qualitative study of somatization and illness meaning. *Culture, Medicine and Psychiatry, 24,* 431–452.

Bäärnhielm, S., Ekblad, S., Ekberg, J., & Ginsburg, B. E. (2005). Historical reflections on mental health care in Sweden. The welfare state and cultural diversity. *Transcultural Psychiatry, 42,* 394–419.

Bäärnhielm, S., Scarpinati Rosso, M., & Pattyi. (2007). *Kultur, kontext och psykiatrisk diagnostik. Manual för intervju enligt kulturformuleringen i DSM-IV* [Culture, context and psychiatric diagnostics. Manual for interviewing according to the Cultural Formulation in DSM-IV]. Stockholm, Sweden: Transkulturellt Centrum, Stockholms läns landsting.

Baer, H. A., Singer M., & Susser, I. (2003). *Medical anthropology and the world system* (2nd ed.). Westport, CT: Greenwood.

Bhugra, D., & Mastrogianni, A. (2004). Globalisation and mental disorders. Overview with relation to depression. *British Journal of Psychiatry, 184,* 10–20.

Dejman, M. (2010). *Cultural explanatory model of depression among Iranian women in three ethnic groups (Fars, Kurds and Turks).* Doctorial thesis, Karolinska Institutet, Stockholm, Sweden.

Deniz, F. (1999). *En minoritets odyssé. Upprätthållande och transformation av etnisk identitet i förhållande till moderniseringsprocesser* [The odyssey of a minority. Maintenance and transformation of ethnic identity in response to processes of modernization – the Assyrian case]. Dissertation, Uppsala University, Department of Sociology, Uppsala, Sweden.

Desjarlais, R., Eisenberg, L., Good, B., & Kleinman, A. (1996). *World mental health. Problems and priorities in low-income countries.* New York: Oxford University Press.

Geertz, C. (1973). *The interpretation of cultures. Selected essays.* New York: Basic Books.

Groleau, D., Young, A., & Kirmayer, L. J. (2006). The McGill Illness Narrative Interview (MINI): An interview schedule to elicit meanings and modes of reasoning related to illness experience. *Transcultural Psychiatry, 43,* 671–691.

Hay, M. C. (2008). Reading sensations: Understanding the process of distinguishing "fine" from "sick." *Transcultural Psychiatry, 45,* 198–229.

Horwitz, A. V., & Wakefield, J. C. (2007). *The loss of sadness – How psychiatry transformed normal sorrow into depressive disorder.* Oxford: Oxford University Press.

Hinton, D. E, Howes, D., & Kirmayer, L. J. (2008). Toward a medical anthropology of sensations: Definitions and research agenda. *Transcultural Psychiatry, 45*(2), 142–162.

Johannison, K. (2001). *Nostalgia. En känslas historia* [Nostalgia. Story of an emotion]. Smedjebacken, Sweden: Bonniers förlag.

Johanisson, (2004). *Tecknen. Läkaren och konsten att läsa kroppar* [The signs. The physician and the art of reading bodies]. Stockholm, Sweden: Nordsedts förlag.

Johannisson, K. (2009). *Melankoliska rum. Om ångest, leda och sårbarhet i förfluten och nutid [Melancholic spaces. About anxiety, suffering and vulnerability in the past and present].* Falun, Sweden: Bonniers förlag.

Kirmayer, L. J. (2001). Cultural variations in the clinical presentation of depression and anxiety: Implications for diagnosis and treatment. *Journal of Clinical Psychiatry, 62*(suppl. 13), 22–28.

Kleinman, A. (1988). *Illness narratives. Suffering, healing and the human condition*. New York: Basic Books.

Kleinman, A., & Benson, P. (2006). Anthropology in the clinic: The problem of cultural competency and how to fix it. *Public Library of Science – Medicine, 3*, 1673–1676.

Lévi-Strauss, Claude. (1995). *The savage mind*. Oxford: Oxford University Press. (Original work published 1962).

Lewis-Fernández, R. (1996). Cultural formulation of psychiatric diagnosis. *Culture, Medicine and Psychiatry, 20*(2), 132–144.

Lewis-Fernández, R., & Díaz, N. (2002). The cultural formulation: A method for assessing cultural factors affecting the clinical encounter. *Psychiatric Quarterly, 73*(4), 271–295.

Lewis-Fernández, R., Hinton, D. E., Laria, A. J., Pattersson, E., Hofman, S.G., Craske., ... Liao, B. (2010). Culture and the anxiety disorders: Recommendations for DSM-V. *Depression and Anxiety, 27*, 212–229.

Lipowski, Z. J. (1987). Somatization: The experience and communication of psychological distress as somatic symptoms. *Psychother Psychosom, 47*, 160–167.

Lundberg, I. (1991). *Kulubor i Stockholm. En svensk historia* [People from Kulu living in Stockholm. A Swedish history]. Stockholm, Sweden: Invandarminnesarkivet.

Manson, S. M. (2005). Culture and DSM-IV: Implications for the diagnosis of mood and anxiety disorders. I. J. Mezzich, A. Kleinman, H. Fabrega, & D. Parron (Eds.), *Culture & psychiatric diagnosis: A DSM-IV perspective* (pp. 99–113). Washington, DC: American Psychiatric Press.

Mezzich, J. E. (1995). Cultural formulation and comprehensive diagnosis: Clinical and research perspectives. *Psychiatric Clinics of North America, 18*, 649–657.

Mezzich, J. E., & Carracci, G. (2008). *Cultural formulation: A reader for psychiatric diagnosis*. Lanham, MD: Rowman & Littlefield.

Mezzich, J. E., Caracci, G., Fabrega, H., Jr., & Kirmayer, L. J. (2009). Cultural formulation guidelines. *Transcultural Psychiatry, 46*, 383–405.

Mirdal, G. M. (1985). The condition of "tightness": The somatic complaints of Turkish migrant women. *Acta Psychiatrica Scandinavica, 71*, 287–296.

Mirdal, G. M. (2005). Tyrkiska kvinders somatiske klager: Tyve år efter [Turkish women's somatic complaints]. *Månedsskr Prakt Lægern, 83*, 877–993.

Obeysekere, G. (1985). Depression, Buddhism, and the work of culture in Siri Lanka. In A. Kleinman, & B. Good (Eds.). *Culture and depression. Studies in the anthropology and cross-cultural psychiatry of affect and disorder* (pp. 134–152). Berkeley, CA: University of California Press.

Okello, E. S. (2006). *Cultural explanatory models of depression in Uganda*. Doctoral thesis, Makerere Univestity, Kampala, Uganda, and Karolinska Institutet, Stockholm, Sweden.

Pliskin, K. L. (1992). Dysphoria and somatization in Iranian culture. *Western Journal of Medicine, 157*, 295–300.

Rohlof, H., Knipscheer, J. W., & Kleber, R. J. (2009). Use of the cultural formulation with refugees. *Transcultural Psychiatry, 46*, 487–505.

SCID-RV. (1994). *Structured clinical interview for DSM-IV Axis I disorders – research version*. New York: Biometrics Research Department, New York State Psychiatric Institute.

Shorter, E. (1992). *From paralysis to fatigue. A history of psychosomatic illness in the modern era.* New York: Free Press.

Shorter, E. (1997). *A history of psychiatry: from the era of the asylum to the age of Prozac*. Hoboken, NJ: Wiley.

Statistics Sweden. (2011). *Statistical yearbook of Sweden.*

Swartz, L. (1998). *Culture and mental health. A southern African view*. Cape Town, South Africa: Oxford University Press.

Watters, E. (2010). *Crazy like us. The globalization of the American psyche.* New York: Free Press.
White, G. M. (1982). The role of cultural explanations in "somatization" and "psychologization." *Social Science and Medicine, 16*, 1519–1530.
Young, A. (1982). The anthropologies of illness and sickness. *Annual Review of Anthropology, 11*, 257–285.

Sofie Bäärnhielm
Transcultural Centre
Stockholm County Council
S:t Görans' Hospital, Floor 13
112 81 Stockholm
Sweden
E-mail: sofie.baarnhielm@sll.se

Chapter 9

Cultural Influences on Perceptions of Pain

Herta Flor

Department of Cognitive and Clinical Neuroscience, Central Institute of Mental Health, Medical Faculty Mannheim, Heidelberg University, Germany

Abstract

This chapter presents evidence that cultural variables modify both the experience of pain and the ability to modulate it, including brain processes involved in pain perception and pain control. Prior experience and social learning are important mechanisms in the development of the response to nociceptive stimulation. We also discuss that emotional pain and physical pain share similar substrates and that emotional pain can impact, enhance, or reduce physical pain. The high levels of generalized pain seen in migrant workers and their inability to profit from psychological pain management programs might be related to such emotional variables. We make suggestions about future research on cultural variables in pain and how they might be incorporated in treatment.

Keywords: chronic pain, social, learning, immigrants, ethnic, pain modulation, modeling, treatment

Cultural Differences in Pain Perception and Pain Modulation

Chronic pain has been defined as an unpleasant sensory and emotional experience associated with actual or potential tissue damage or described in terms of such damage (Merskey & Bogduk, 1994). This definition by the International Association for the Study of Pain implies that pain, and especially chronic pain, is not only a sensory experience but also includes emotional and cognitive factors and thus also cultural influences. Pain beliefs and expectations about pain are thought to be determined by many factors related to social interaction. In their biocultural model of pain perception, Bates, Edwards, and Anderson (1993) proposed that pain perception and pain responses are greatly determined by social comparison and social learning processes within ethno-cultural group situations that are influenced by prior pain experiences as well as attitudes toward pain and modulate cognitive control mechanisms as well as pain inhibition. A number of studies have shown that there are substantial differences between ethnic groups related to pain perception. Bates et al. (1993) compared persons of older American, Hungarian, Italian, French-Canadian, Irish, and Polish descent and found significant differences between those six ethnic groups in pain intensity ratings as well as in locus of control related to pain experiences. For example, persons of Polish descent had the highest internal locus of control whereas Hungarians tended to have a more external locus of control. A further study by Wang et al. (2010) examined the response to capsaicin, which induces a sharp pain, in Hispanic, African American, Caucasian, and East Asian subjects and found the highest pain response in East Asian persons, followed by Hispanics and very low values in Caucasian and African American people. In a study of pain thresholds and intolerance, Campbell, Edwards, and Fillingim (2005) observed differences in pain tolerance and pain thresholds in African American and Caucasians depending on a type of nociceptive stimulation procedure that was used. Whereas African Americans had in general lower pain thresholds and pain tolerance in heat and cold pain stimulation, the picture was different for ischemic pain, where African Americans had a higher threshold. Further, ischemic pain tolerance was lower in African Americans compared to Caucasians. It is therefore important to realize that different types of painful stimulation may yield very different results for various ethnic groups.

Not only pain perception, but also the ability to control pain differs among ethnic groups. For example, medication use and the efficacy of analgesics are different in Caucasians and African Americans across ethnic groups (Tan et al., 2008). Campbell et al. (2008) compared non-Hispanic whites with African Americans in their ability to control pain by counterstimulation in a so-called diffuse noxious inhibitory control experiment, where one attempts to inhibit pain by the application of noxious input in a another body region. These authors observed that African Americans were much less likely to successfully control pain compared to non-Hispanic whites in this paradigm. In addition, Riley et al. (2002) assessed types of dealing with pain and identified higher pain unpleasantness, pain behaviors, and emotional responses to pain. Behavioral and emotional variables (fear, depression) were both significantly more associated with pain in African Americans. It is at this point not known to what extent genetic factors or cultural experience contribute to these differences. However, it is most likely that there is an interaction of these variables.

The Role of Prior Pain Experiences

As noted above, the biocultural model of pain perception by Bates et al. (1993) puts a special focus on the role of prior pain experiences. In a recent study we were interested to see how predictability of pain and an ongoing painful experience can influence how pain is processed on the subjective and the neurophysiological level. For this experiment, we asked healthy subjects to participate in ten sessions of repetitive painful stimulation and divided these subjects into two groups. Group 1 received a predictable painful stimulation; that is, the painful stimulus was preceded by a visual signal and the absence of a painful stimulus was signaled as well. Group 2 received the same visual signals and the same nociceptive stimulation but in random order so that no prediction of pain was possible. When we examined pain thresholds, pain tolerance, and pain-related brain responses before and after the ten days of training we found substantial differences between the two groups to the identical nociceptive stimulation. The group that was able to predict pain had higher pain tolerance and higher pain thresholds (see Figure 9.1). These subjects also activated brain regions that are involved in prediction of pain and fear, the cognitive control of pain as well as areas involved in emotion regulation such as the dorsolateral prefrontal cortex, the striatum, and the amygdala. In contrast, the group that was not able to predict pain had substantially more activation in the anterior cingulate cortex, the hippocampus, and the periaqueductal gray, all indicative of a more affective processing of pain and higher anxiety levels. These brain activation differences and differences in subjective ratings emerged as a consequence of the training to the identical physical stimulus, indicating that it is the prior experience with pain that shapes current pain processing. The pain-related learning history must thus be considered when acute and chronic pain patients are examined.

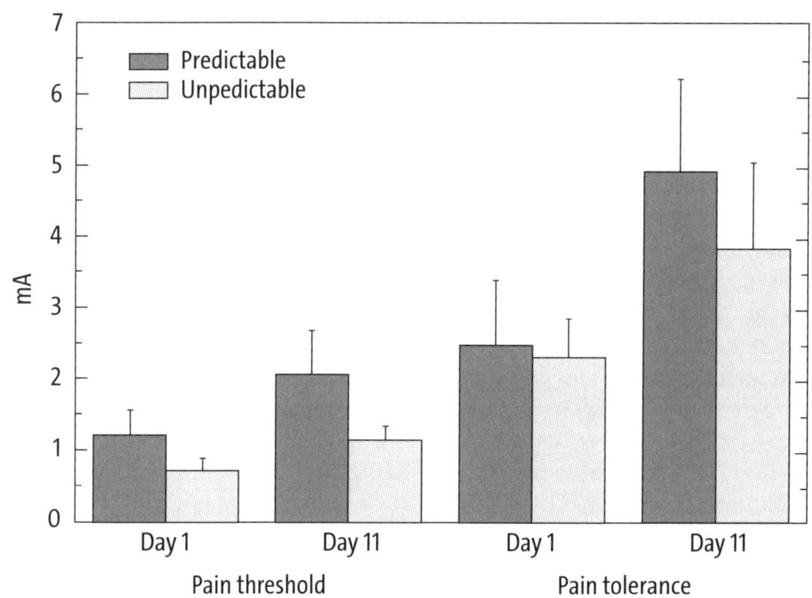

Figure 9.1. Pain threshold and pain tolerance levels pre (day 1) and post (day 11) the 10 sessions with painful stimulation. "Predictable" refers to the group with signaled pain presentation and "unpredictable" refers to the group with random painful stimulation.

A further variable that may impact on pain processing in adults are pain experiences early in life. Both an overexposure and an underexposure to pain may result in later hyperreactivity to nociceptive input and deficient pain modulation. There is evidence from early studies that dogs and monkeys that were not exposed to painful stimulation were relatively insensitive to pain stimuli and unable to learn avoidance responses to nociceptive stimuli later in life (Lichstein & Sackett, 1971; Melzack & Scott, 1957). This is also evident in ethnomedical observations. Early sensitization to traumatic injury through rituals such as the severing of the ear lobes or nose at a young age seem to leave the young less susceptible to later trauma. For example, Schiefenhövel's (1980) observations of pain tolerance and pain behaviors among the Eipo tribe in New Guinea or Sargent's (1984) studies of the Bariba in Benin and Nigeria suggest that early experience with tolerant role models who cope successfully with painful stimulation reduces the expression and possibly the experience of pain and suffering in adults as compared to Western cultures.

The converse, sensitization, may also be true. Uncontrolled pain in young children or neonates seems to have a sensitizing effect later in life (Hermann, Hohmeister, Demirakca, Zohsel, & Flor, 2006; Wollgarten-Hadamek et al., 2009). In addition to leading to perceptual sensitization, early uncontrollable pain experiences also alter how the brain processes nociceptive input and it was shown that there is an overactivation in areas related to the more affective processing of pain and that there is an underactivation in areas that are involved in pain control. Since pain is also greatly determined by cognitive variables, it is important to note that catastrophizing was also influenced by early life experiences (Hohmeister, Demirakca, Zohsel, Flor, & Hermann, 2009). It was also reported that early life experience reduces the positive effect of the presence of others on pain. Hohmeister et al. (2009) showed that the soothing effect of the presence of a mother is absent in children who were exposed to early pain experiences, suggesting that early pain experiences and social variables greatly interact (see the following).

As another example of the priming effect of prior experiences, Fearon, McGrath, and Achat (1996) observed the play behavior of 3- to 7-year-old children in a day care center. They noted that, on average, children in this age range experienced 2–3 painful incidents each day, with the most common location being head and neck, face, hands, and knees. Thus, for young children painful episodes are extremely common. The authors noted that children who experienced incidents of pain most often showed the strongest responses to the pain, suggesting that increased exposure to acute pain may sensitize the children to pain and thereby reduce their threshold for labeling noxious stimuli as painful.

A specific relationship of early sexual abuse and chronic pelvic pain in women has been reported in several studies and this relationship has been confirmed for several pain syndromes (Paras et al., 2009). Riley, Robinson, Kvaal, and Gremillion (1998) suggest that physical and sexual abuse may lead to overly high attentiveness to and overinterpretation of bodily symptoms, a view that is compatible with higher vulnerability due to excessive stimulation. The results of a study by Morpurgo, Gavazzi, Pollin, Amsallem, and Lombard (1983) provide experimental evidence supporting this assumption. These authors showed that the brains of kittens exposed to noxious stimuli showed larger representations of the affected body part in thalamus and cortex. This might provide a physiological basis for the vulnerability of certain body parts based on early trauma and is in accordance with the vast literature on cortical reorganization related to injury and environmental changes (cf., Flor & Turk, 2011).

The results on neonatal pain exposure and physical abuse seemingly contradict the assumption that early exposure to painful stimulation may be necessary for adequate pain responses to develop. It is, however, possible that these conflicting results are related to the controllability and intensity of the noxious stimulation. Moderate levels of noxious stimulation in a controllable situation combined with social disapproval for the expression of pain behaviors and approval for coping as reported for the children of the Eipo tribe may result in positive and adaptive physiological and psychological consequences as compared to the uncontrollable noxious stimulation to which battered and sexually abused children are exposed. Buchner et al. (1999) have shown that reorganizational changes in primary somatosensory (S1) cortex are modulated by attention. Focusing of attention leads to an expansion of anesthetized fingers in S1 cortex, distraction of attention to the opposite effect – a reduced interdigital distance. Thus reorganizational changes in the brain and nociceptive system in general related to early childhood experience may vary, depending on psychological variables such as predictability and controllability of the stimulation.

Observing Pain in Others: The Role of Social Learning

Another important aspect of cultural modification of pain is social learning related to pain. Viewing pain in others elicits not only empathic responses but also activates the same brain regions that are involved in the processing of pain. Thus modeling and social influences can greatly impact on the experience of pain.

Many studies suggest that how pain is responded to by others, either within the person himself or herself or the responses to pain observed in others, will have an impact on subsequent interpretation and responses. Thus, prior experience, direct and observed, plays a role in influencing future responding such as stoicism, distress, or hyperreactivity. Perceived or actual controllability of the painful stimulus may be an important determinant of the direction of the response (see above).

Children acquire attitudes about health and health care, the perception and interpretation of physical symptoms and physiological processes as well as appropriate responses to injury and disuse from their parents and by observing others as well as through cultural rules and rituals. Thus, based on prior experience they may be more or less likely to ignore or overemphasize symptoms.

A large body of evidence has been reported for the importance of observational learning in pain tolerance, pain ratings, and nonverbal expressions of pain (for a review see Goubert, Vlaeyen, Crombez, & Craig, 2011). For example, Van Slyke and Walker (2006) observed mothers' responses to children's pain and found three different types of responses. Mothers prefer to protect, to minimize, or to encourage when their children experience pain. Such different responses by the mothers will likely influence future interpretations and responses to noxious stimulation in general.

There is also evidence that the observation of pain in other family members may predispose people to similar pain problems, thus implicating a learning process in the development of a diathesis that will serve as the template through which future stressful and painful circumstances will be filtered. This can be seen in the context of empathy and begins with the fact that babies start crying when they hear other babies crying – long before they develop a sense of a self separate from others (Singer & Lamm, 2009). Chambers, Craig, and Bennett (2002) showed that mothers' pain-promoting behaviors led to more pain expression in their daughters but not their sons, suggesting sex effects in modeling pain. Levy et al. (2004) examined patients with irritable bowel syndrome and their children and found clear evidence for an effect of parent behavior on the children's complaints and absence from school.

Avenanti, Bueti, Galati, and Aglioti (2005) showed that there are not only empathic responses to seeing pain in others but that there is also a site-specific muscular response that corresponds to the muscle where one sees the pain inflicted in another person. This anticipatory response, which is driven by central processes, is also highly correlated with the perception of pain. These changes in output to the muscle are mirrored by changes in somatosensory processing. Bufalari, Aprile, Avenati, Di Russo, and Aglioti (2007) provided evidence that seeing pain inflicted in another person leads to very early (P45 amplitude) changes in the pain-related electroencephalographic event-related

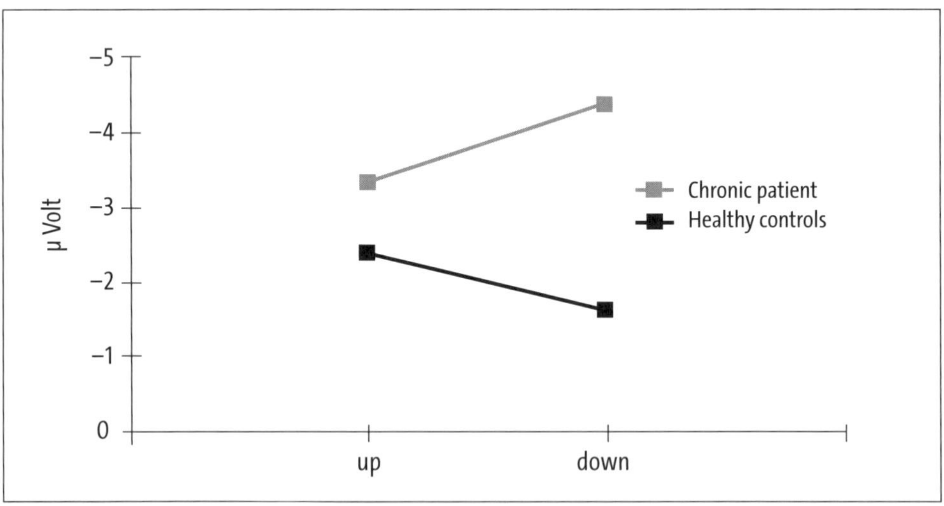

Figure 9.2. N150 component of the pain-related potential of the electroencephalogram in microvolts after the up- and down-training with the respective extinction session for the healthy controls and the chronic pain patients. Note that the patients do not show a reduction in the amplitude of the event-related response after extinction, as visible in the healthy controls.

potential located in primary somatosensory cortex that was again related to perceived pain intensity.

In addition to social modeling, operant conditioning variables related to other persons are also important modulators of the pain experience. Fordyce (1976) was the first to argue that positive or negative reinforcement of pain behaviors might greatly impact on the experience of pain and the development of a chronic pain problem. We used verbal and monetary feedback in chronic back pain patients and healthy controls and showed that patients and controls learn to increase or decrease their pain perception based on reinforcement equally well but that the chronic pain patients do not extinguish their response when the reinforcement is terminated (Flor, Knost, & Birbaumer, 2002; see Figure 9.2). This deficient extinction was also mirrored in die N150 amplitude of the electroencephalogram, which remained high after extinction and suggests that there are lasting central changes related to chronic pain that can be instigated by social variables, such as the response of others.

Emotional and Physical Pain

In his book *The Culture of Pain*, David Morris (1993) discussed the problematic dichotomy of physical and psychological pain and suggested that the emotional side of pain is increasingly neglected in Western cultures, whereas it is much more integrated in non-Western cultures. He also comments that pain experiences in a controlled context are lacking since pain is viewed as evil and that this enhances maladaptive emotional processing as suggested earlier.

Social pain has been shown to evoke similar brain responses as physical pain (Eisenberger, Lieberman, & Williams, 2003). These authors showed that anterior cingulate and right ventral prefrontal activation was present during social rejection and that this activation was highly correlated with the amount of social distress the subjects showed. Anterior cingulate cortex showed a positive and right ventral prefrontal cortex showed a negative correlation to social distress much in line with similar studies on physical pain. Along these lines Burgess et al. (2009) showed that perceived discrimination has an enhancing effect on bodily pain and this suggests that there may be a close interaction between emotional and physical aspects of pain. This might be especially important for the understanding of pain problems in groups of persons that are characterized by very high levels of chronic pain affliction. This is the case in migrant workers, who indicate substantially higher levels of pain problems than their non-migrant colleagues (von Ferber, Köster, & Celayir-Erdogan, 2003). An interesting feature of this is that these persons are especially afflicted by generalized pain problems (David, Braun, & Borde, 2004). It is very likely that difficult living conditions and stressful life experiences, for example, migration and adaptation to a new host culture, contribute to this elevated number of pain problems. There is, however, very little research to substantiate this assumption. The problem is increased by the fact that migrant or immigrant workers are less likely to participate in pain-related psychological treatments and also drop out in much higher rates (Keel & Calanchini, 1989). Sleptsova, Woessmer, and Langewitz (2009) introduced a culturally sensitive pain treatment for Turkish immigrant pain patients, which was adapted to specific cultural needs of these patients. Unfortunately, this program had no significant effect on pain and inference related to pain and it did not show significant changes in activity levels or use of the health care system. Contrary to expectations, it also showed a very high drop-out rate of 30%. Interestingly, these difficulties do not arise in cognitive behavioral treatment programs in Turkey and these negative treatment effects were also not observed in Swiss workers with the same type of social status. This suggests that the experience of immigration and the experience of living as a migrant may have special effects on pain processing and the acceptance of psychological pain treatment programs that need to be examined. Another mitigating factor in this context may be that there are differences also in treatment expectancy related to psychological versus somatic interventions in migrant workers compared to non-immigrant patients. For example, migrant workers do have higher expectancies in the efficacy of medical treatment and this might negatively impact on the efficacy of psychological treatments (von Ferber et al., 2003).

Conclusions and Outlook

We have reviewed evidence that suggests substantial impacts of cultural factors on both the perception and the ability to modulate pain. Prior experience and social learning are key mechanisms in the development of the response to nociceptive stimulation. These variables alter subjective pain experience, pain control, and brain processes involved in pain perception and pain control. There is also evidence that emotional pain and physical pain share similar substrates and that emotional pain can impact in physical pain. We suggested that the high levels of generalized pain seen in migrant workers and their inability to profit from psychological pain management programs might be related to such emotional variables. Based on these findings, it would be interesting to examine the relationship of emotional and physical pain in a larger population. It would specifically be interesting to determine to what extent discrimination related to the migrant status as well as the experience of distress in this status is predictive of physical pain and its neural correlates. We also need to consider to what extent an effective pain treatment should focus on the emotional pain component.

Acknowledgments

This research was supported by "Psychobiological analysis of musculoskeletal pain and development of mechanism-based modular treatment components" within the research network "Localized and generalized musculoskeletal pain: psychobiological mechanisms and implications for treatment" (LOGIN), funded by the Federal Ministry for Education and Research (01EC1010D); "Examination of a new transdisciplinary framework on pain and suffering by integrating philosophical, psychological, and neuroscientific perspectives" (PASCOM) funded by German Research Foundation (FL 156/34); and "Phantom phenomena: A window to the mind and the brain" (PHANTOM-MIND) project, which receives research funding from the European Community's Seventh Framework Programme (FP7/ 2007–2013)/ERC Grant Agreement No. 230249. This manuscript reflects only the author's views and the community is not liable for any use that may be made of the information contained therein.

References

Avenanti, A., Bueti, D., Galati, G., & Aglioti, S. M. (2005). Transcranial magnetic stimulation highlights the sensorimotor side of empathy for pain. *Nature Neuroscience, 8*, 955–960.

Bates, M. S., Edwards, W. T., & Anderson, K. O. (1993). Ethnocultural influences on variation in chronic pain perception. *Pain, 52*, 101–112.

Buchner, H., Reinartz, U., Waberski, T. D., Gobbele, R., Noppeney, U., & Scherg, M. (1999). Sustained attention modulates the immediate effect of de-afferentation on the cortical representation of the digits: Source localization of somatosensory evoked potentials in humans. *Neuroscience Letters, 260*, 57–60.

Bufalari, I., Aprile, T., Avenanti, A., Di Russo, F., & Aglioti, S. M. (2007). Empathy for pain and touch in the human somatosensory cortex. *Cerebral Cortex, 17*, 2553–2561.

Burgess, D. J., Grill, J., Noorbaloochi, S., Griffin, J. M., Ricards, J., van Ryn, M., & Partin, M. R. (2009). The effect of perceived racial discrimination on bodily pain among older African American men. *Pain Medicine, 10*, 1341–1352.

Campbell, C. M., Edwards, R. R., & Fillingim, R. B. (2005). Ethnic differences in responses to multiple experimental pain stimuli. *Pain, 113*, 20–26.

Campbell, C. M., France, C. R., Robinson, M. E., Logan, H. L., Geffken, G. R., & Fillingim, R. B. (2008). Ethnic differences in diffuse noxious inhibitory controls. *Journal of Pain, 9*, 759–766.

Chambers, C. T., Craig, K. D., & Bennett, S. M. (2002). The impact of maternal behavior on children's pain experiences: An experimental analysis. *Journal of Pediatric Psychology, 27*, 293–301.

David, M., Braun, T., & Borde, T. (2004). Schmerz und Ethnizität – Ergebnisse einer Befragung an drei internistisch/gynäkologischen Rettungsstellen in Berlin [Pain and ethnicity – results of a survey at three internal medicine/gynecology emergency units in Berlin]. *Zentralblatt der Gynäkologie, 126*, 81–86.

Eisenberger, N. I., Lieberman, M. D., & Williams, K. D. (2003). Does rejection hurt? An FMRI study of social exclusion. *Science, 302*, 290–292.

Fearon, I., McGrath, P. J., & Achat, H. (1996). "Booboos": The study of everyday pain among young children. *Pain, 68*, 55–62.

Fordyce, W. E. (1976). *Behavioral methods in chronic pain and illness*. St. Louis, MO: Mosby.

Flor, H., Knost, B., & Birbaumer, N. (2002). The role of operant conditioning in chronic pain: An experimental investigation. *Pain, 95*, 111–118.

Flor, H., & Turk, D. C. (2011). *Chronic pain: An integrated biobehavioral perspective.* Seattle, WA: IASP Press.

Goubert, L., Vlaeyen, J. W., Crombez, G., & Craig, K. D. (2011). Learning about pain from others: An observational learning account. *Journal of Pain, 12*, 167–174.

Hermann, C., Hohmeister, J., Demirakca, S., Zohsel, K., & Flor, H. (2006). Long-term alteration of pain sensitivity in school-aged children with early pain experiences. *Pain, 125*, 278–285.

Hohmeister, J., Demirakca, S., Zohsel, K., Flor, H., & Hermann, C. (2009). Responses to pain in school-aged children with experience in a neonatal intensive care unit: Cognitive aspects and maternal influences. *European Journal of Pain, 13*, 94–101.

Keel, P., & Calanchini, C. (1989). Chronische Rückenschmerzen bei Gastarbeitern aus Mittelmeerländern im Vergleich zu Patienten aus Mitteleuropa: demographische und psychosoziale Aspekte [Chronic back pain in migrant workers from Mediterranean countries compared to Middle European patients: Demographic and psychosocial aspects]. *Schweizer Medizinische Wochenschrift, 119*, 22–31.

Levy, R. L., Whitehead, W. E., Walker, L. S., Von Korff, M., Feld, A. D., Garner, M., & Christie, D. (2004). Increased somatic complaints and health-care utilization in children: Effects of parent IBS status and parent response to gastrointestinal symptoms. *American Journal of Gastroenterology, 99*, 2442–2451.

Lichstein, L., & Sackett, G. P. (1971). Reactions by differentially raised rhesus monkeys to noxious stimulation. *Developmental Psychobiology, 4*, 339–352.

Melzack, R. , & Scott, T. H. (1957). The effects of early experience on the response to pain. *Journal of Comparative Physiological Psychology, 50*, 155–161.

Merskey, H., & Bogduk, N. (Eds.). (1994). *Classification of chronic pain: Descriptions of chronic pain syndromes and definitions of pain terms*. Seattle, WA: IASP Press.

Morpurgo, C. V., Gavazzi, G., Pollin, B., Amsallem, B., & Lombard, M. C. (1983). Changes of somatic organization in thalamic ventrobasal nucleus of chronic awake cats associated with persistent nociceptive stimulation. In J. J. Bonica, U. Lindblom, & A. Iggo (Eds.), *Advances in pain research* (Vol. 5, pp. 179–184). New York: Raven Press.

Morris, D. (1993). *The culture of pain.* Berkeley and Los Angeles, CA: University of California Press.

Paras, M. L., Murad, M. H., Chen, L. P., Goranson, E. N., Sattler, A. L., Colbenson, K. M., . . . Zirakzadeh, A. (2009). Sexual abuse and lifetime diagnosis of somatic disorders: A systematic review and meta-analysis. *Journal of the American Medical Association, 302*, 550–561.

Riley, J. L., III, Robinson, M. E., Kvaal, S. A., & Gremillion, H. (1998). Effects of physical and sexual abuse in facial pain: Direct or mediated? *Cranio, 16*, 259–266.

Riley, J. L., III, Wade, J. B., Myers, C. D., Sheffield, D., Papas, R. K., & Price, D. D. (2002). Racial/ethnic differences in the experience of chronic pain. *Pain, 100*, 291–298.

–Sargent, C. (1984). Between death and shame: Dimensions of pain in Bariba culture. *Social Science and Medicine, 19*, 1299–1304.

Schiefenhövel, W. (1980). Verarbeitung von Schmerz und Krankheit bei den Eipo, Hochland von West-Neuguinea [Coping with pain and illness in the Eipo tribe in the highland of West-New Guinea]. *Medizinische Psychologie, 6*, 219–234.

Singer, T., & Lamm, C. (2009). The social neuroscience of empathy. *Annals of the New York Academy of Sciences, 1156*, 81–96.

Sleptsova, M., Woessmer, B., & Langewitz, W. (2009). Migranten empfinden Schmerzen anders [Migrants perceive pain differently]. *Schweizer Medizinisches Forum, 9*, 319–321.

Tan, E. C., Lim, Y., Teo, Y. Y., Goh, R., Law, H. Y., & Sia, A. T. (2008). Ethnic differences in pain perception and patient-controlled analgesia usage for postoperative pain. *Journal of Pain, 9*, 849–855.

Van Slyke, D. A., & Walker, L. S. (2006). Mothers' responses to children's pain. *Clinical Journal of Pain, 22*, 387–391.

Von Ferber, L., Köster, I., & Celayir-Erdogan, N. (2003). Türkische und deutsche Hausarztpatienten – Erkrankungen, Arzneimittelerwartungen und Verordnungen [Turkish and German patients of general practitioners – Diseases, drug expectations and drug prescriptions]. *Gesundheitswesen, 65*, 304–311.

Wang, H., Papoiu, A. D., Coghill, R. C., Patel, T., Wang, N., & Yosipovitch, G. (2010). Ethnic differences in pain, itch and thermal detection in response to topical capsaicin: African Americans display a notably limited hyperalgesia and neurogenic inflammation. *British Journal of Dermatology, 162*, 1023–1029.

Wollgarten-Hadamek, I., Hohmeister, J., Demirakca, S., Zohsel, K., Flor, H., & Hermann, C. (2009). Do burn injuries during infancy affect pain and sensory sensitivity in later childhood? *Pain, 141*, 165–172.

Herta Flor
Department of Cognitive and Clinical Neuroscience
Central Institute of Mental Health
Medical Faculty Mannheim
Heidelberg University
J5
68159 Mannheim
Germany
E-mail: herta.flor@zi-mannheim.de

Chapter 10
Embitterment in Cultural Contexts

Michael Linden

Charité Research Group Psychosomatic Rehabilitation, Berlin, Germany

Abstract

Embitterment is familiar to everyone and is a complex emotion at the end of an emotional hierarchy involving: (a) frustration when things do not go as expected; (b) disappointment since things could have gone otherwise; (c) anger when something could have been done about it; (d) aggression, as some other person is seen as guilty; (e) shame, since one has to admit that oneself is part of the cause; (f) humiliation, as one is disparaged by others; (g) despair, as repeated efforts to do something turned things even worse; (h) hopelessness, depression, and giving up since one can do nothing more to react; (i) embitterment, as injustice, infidelity, or feelings of having been let down are involved; (j) intense and grave embitterment, as this involves the violation of central basic beliefs; and (k) rampage, as the present state is unbearable. Embitterment is a last resort emotion and has been characterized as aggression by self-destruction. The clinical picture has been described as posttraumatic embitterment disorder (PTED). As violations of basic beliefs and the belief in a just world are important in the development of this disorder, the cultural context must be taken into account in its understanding and treatment, as this context determines what persons experience as injustice. Treatment must reconcile with what has happened. Wisdom psychology and wisdom therapy are ways of helping to overcome experiences of injustice and humiliation.

Keywords: embitterment, belief, injustice, culture

Introduction

All human beings know the emotion of embitterment (Linden & Maercker, 2011). It is a feeling of having been let down and humiliated, often associated with experiences of injustice combined with helplessness. Embitterment and concomitant actions can be understood as last resort emotions, similar to extreme anxiety (i.e., panic), which also is a last resort emotion. Panic is helpful in moments of serious endangerment of life, as it produces strength that would otherwise not be available. In a state of panic persons can run, fight, swim, or freeze to a degree that is only possible in panic. Similarly, severe embitterment is a helpful emotion in extreme situations. The psychoanalyst Alexander (1960) characterized embitterment as "aggression by self destruction." When persons are cornered and in a situation with no way out, where the enemy has full control and life is endangered, embitterment can be a last option, where you kill yourself rather than be killed. This type of reaction can already be observed in children who have dreams about leaving the house to die in the snow in order to punish their mother who has forced them to go to bed. This aggression by self-destruction is exactly what can be seen in severely embittered persons. They attack regardless of the consequences. They start legal fights without any prospect of success, they spend their last money on pointless actions, they even perform seemingly ridiculous actions such as keying someone's car. They can run amok and go on a rampage, they can kill their spouse and afterwards themselves (Felber, Lammel, Sutarski, & Lau, 2010).

This chapter aims to understand the nature of embitterment, how this might be dependent on the cultural orientation of an individual, and which treatment approaches might be effective.

Embitterment and Posttraumatic Embitterment Disorder

In order to understand the nature of embitterment and to put it in the context of culture it may be helpful to have a look at emotion psychology (Ekman, 1997; Merten, 2003; Plutchik, 1980). For example, Figure 10.1 shows a model of emotions from Plutchik (1980, 2001). This three-dimensional circumplex model describes basic emotions and their complex relation to each other. Analogous to colors, the order of emotions in the circle corresponds to the degrees of similarity between emotions and the vertical dimension from the outside to the inner circle reflects intensity. There are eight primary emotion dimensions, arranged as four pairs of opposites. Emotions that are mixtures of two emotions are primary dyads. Combinations of several emotions are complex emotions. All emotions result in emotion-congruent actions. If there are combinations of opposite emotions, such as anger and fear, this can lead to blockades of action.

According to cognitive theory, emotions are the product of cognitive appraisals (Lazarus, 1991; Scherer, 2004). Thus, embitterment can be described as a complex emotion with a blend of several contradictory and mutually inhibiting emotions, which can be understood as the result of a stepwise appraisal process and development:

- Frustration occurs when things do not go as expected
- Disappointment is added if things could have gone otherwise
- Anger is added if there is the impression that something could have been done about it
- Aggression is added if some other person is seen as guilty and should be punished
- Shame is added if one has to admit that one is oneself part of the cause
- Humiliation is added if one is disparaged by others

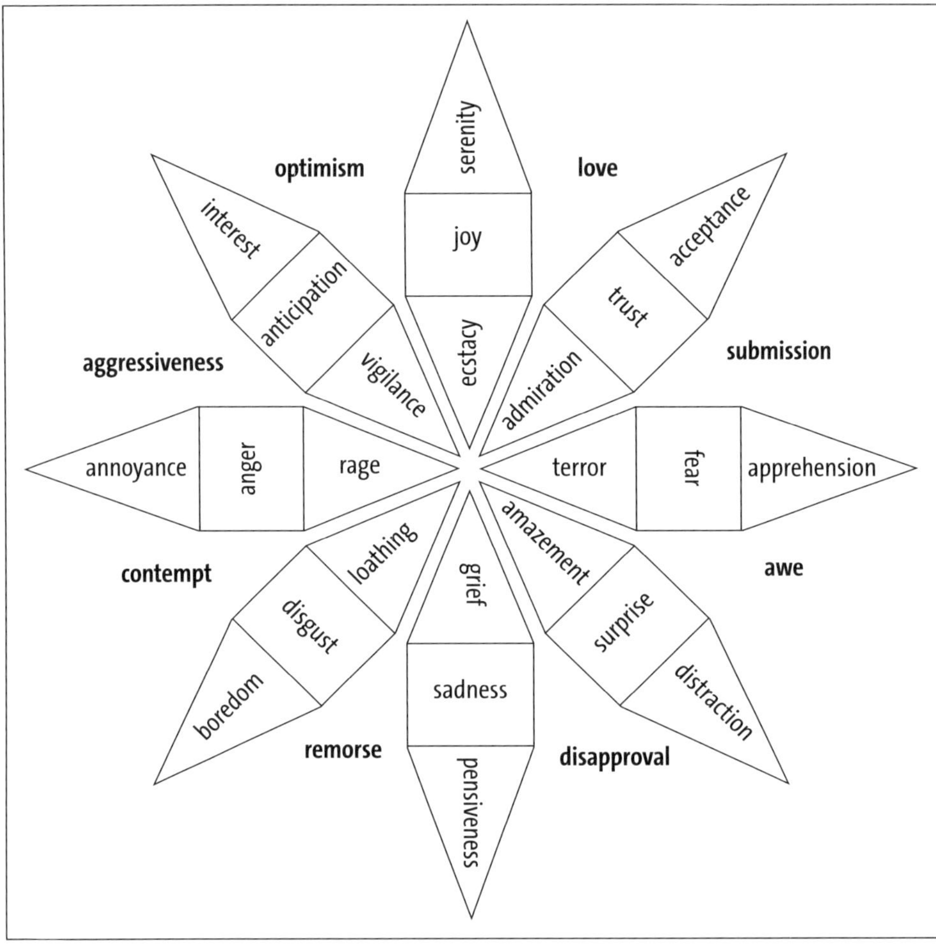

Figure 10.1. The spectrum and interrelation of emotions

- Despair is added if repeated efforts to do something turned things even worse
- Hopelessness, depression, and giving up is added if one can do nothing more to react
- Embitterment is added if injustice, infidelity, or feelings of having been let down are involved
- Intense and grave embitterment occurs if this involves the violation of central basic beliefs
- Rampage is added if the present state is unbearable

Thus, embitterment is a complex interplay of several diverse emotions. There is no simple way to react, and rampage is the next best thing to do. This complex emotion of embitterment can be measured with the Bern Embitterment Inventory (Znoj, 2008, 2011). The scale has 18 items with the subdimensions of lowered mood and bitterness, misanthropy and aggression, feelings of injustice, pessimism, and hopelessness. Embitterment is correlated with aggression, fatalistic attitudes, help- and hopelessness and the feeling of being attacked and persecuted. Znoj (2008) has defined embitterment as a feeling of having been let down, of anger, and injustice. Actions that arise from this emotion can be protest and open aggression, but also passiveness, isolation, and retreat. In contrast to depression, emotional modulation is unimpaired (Linden, Rotter, Baumann, & Lieberei, 2007).

Table 10.1. Diagnostic criteria for posttraumatic embitterment disorder

Core criteria

- A single exceptional negative life event precipitates the onset of the illness.
- Patients know about this life event and see their present negative state as a direct and lasting consequence of this event.
- Patients experience the negative life event as "unjust" and respond with embitterment and emotional arousal when reminded of the event.
- No obvious mental disorder present in the year before the critical event. The present state is no recurrence of a preexisting mental disorder.

Additional signs and symptoms

- Patients see themselves as victims and as helpless to cope with the event or the cause.
- Patients blame themselves for the event, for not having prevented it, or for not being able to cope with it.
- Patients report repeated intrusive memories of the critical event. Sometimes they even think that it is important not to forget.
- Patients express thoughts that it no longer matters how they are doing and are even uncertain whether they want the wounds to heal.
- Patients can express suicidal ideation.
- Additional emotions are dysphoria, aggression, and down-heartedness, which can resemble melancholic depressive states with somatic syndromes.
- Patients show a variety of unspecific somatic complaints such as loss of appetite, sleep disturbances, and pain.
- Patients can report phobic symptoms with respect to the place or to persons related to the event.
- Drive is reduced and blocked. Patients experience themselves not so much as drive inhibited but rather as drive unwilling.
- Emotional modulation is not impaired and patients can show normal affect when they are distracted or can even smile when engaged in thoughts of revenge.

Duration: Longer than 3 months.

Impairment: Performance in daily activities and roles is impaired.

As mentioned above, if one wants to describe and classify the different facets of embitterment, this can be done analogous to anxiety. Anxiety, like embitterment, is known by all human beings, both emotions are triggered by situations, are dimensional in intensity, and can become pathologic with increasing intensity. In the same way that anxiety is a pervasive emotion, about half of the normal population report that they harbor feelings of embitterment in relation to recent experiences (Linden et al., 2007). About 5% say that this emotion is so strong that they feel impaired in daily activities, cannot let go, have retreated from daily activities or social contacts, and are haunted by intrusive memories. An interesting question is whether, similar to anxious personalities, there are also embitterment-prone personalities. Easily offended and misanthropic individuals can be prone to embitterment, and it can also occur in the context of other mental disorders. Rotter (2011) presented data that show that patients with personality disorders have increased rates of embitterment. This can be a part of the emotional spectrum of respective personality disorders, but also a consequence of the underlying disorder, as those with personality disorders are prone to be treated unfairly by others, which also results in secondary feelings of embitterment.

Finally, there is also a specific embitterment disorder, the posttraumatic embitterment disorder (PTED) (Linden, 2003; Linden et al., 2007; Linden, Baumann, Lieberei, Lorenz, & Rotter, 2011), which can be seen parallel to the posttraumatic stress disorder, an anxiety disorder. PTED is characterized by embitterment, feelings of humiliation, of having been let down, by help- and hopelessness, aggression against oneself and others, reduction in drive, multiple somatoform symptoms, phobic avoidance of selected places and persons, or reduction from social activities. The diagnostic criteria for PTED are summarized in Table 10.1. (Linden, Baumann, Rotter, & Schippan, 2008).

Embitterment and Culture: Aspiration Level, Injustice, and Violation of Basic Beliefs

PTED is seen in the aftermath of negative life events, which are known to everybody though they are still exceptional. Their common feature is injustice, betrayal and breach of confidence, humiliation, and violation of basic beliefs (i.e., important values in life). Examples are events of injustice (Pirhacova, 1997), enduring unemployment (Zemperl & Frese, 1997), or major negative life events (Baures, 1996). This makes embitterment a culturally sensitive disorder, more so than other mental disorders. What is perceived as injustice, humiliation, and a violation of basic beliefs is dependent on personal values and beliefs that have been learned from the social environment since childhood. Before we understand how culture may impact the prevalence of embitterment, we should first clarify what we mean by injustice and basic beliefs.

"Belief in a just world" is an important part of general psychology. It is the prerequisite for social behavior. There is a large body of research on this psychological dimension (Dalbert, 1999, 2011; Lerner, 1980; Rubin & Peplau, 1975). The belief in a just world gives the security that others will respond to one's own behavior in a similar way so that one can influence others by one's own behavior. That is to say, positive behavior will be rewarded and negative behavior will be punished. This is the basis for mutual trust. This explains why belief in a just world and well-being are correlated with each other.

In case of an injustice, individuals will revolt and retreat from the transgressor. They will initially not change their expectations of justice. Instead, they will try to incorporate their negative experiences into their views of the world by reframing or additional explanations regarding the reasons (Bulman & Wortman, 1977, Lipkus & Siegler, 1993; Strelan, 2007). They will also react with counteraggression against persons, institutions, or even fate (Willebrand, Kildal, Andersson, & Ekselius, 2002). If there is no way out, help- and hopelessness will emerge and aggression turn toward the individual themselves because they did not prevent the negative event from the start. If experiences of injustice can no longer be reconciled with the individual's basic beliefs and values, adaptive reactions will stop and break down, and severe embitterment emerge.

The special feature of injustice is that it is a form of aggression. In modern societies, open aggression, such as beating others, is not accepted. However, individuals can still treat each other with aggression – by inflicting injustice. Deliberate acts of injustice require the power to do so on the part of the perpetrator; this implies the vilification of the victim. Acts of injustice particularly include the aspects that were described earlier as steps to embitterment.

Although people in general hold beliefs in a just world, it still depends on individual factors what is experienced as injustice in a certain situation or by a given person. This is largely dependent on their basic beliefs (Bolby, 1969; Beck, Rush, Shaw, & Emery, 1979; Janoff-Bulman, 1992, Hautzinger, 2008). Cognitive psychotherapy makes a distinction between automatic thoughts, cognitive schemata, and basic beliefs. Cognitive schemata and basic beliefs are, like language, culturally determined and learned in childhood and adolescence. They are needed for coherent behavior throughout an individual's life span (e.g., "keep your goods together/don't be wasteful," which leads to thriftiness in thousands of situations over many years, leading to wealth). They also define large groups of persons (e.g., "belief in Jesus Christ" denotes Christians). Finally, they are passed on from generation to generation and define culture (Jews or Palestinians, Muslims or Christians, French or British).

These values, judgment dispositions, or basic beliefs and schemata are core features of any culture (Schwartz, 1997). Culture is defined by Schwartz (1997) as the summary of all patterns of thinking, feeling, and behavior that are held in common by members of a delimited group of persons, be it ethnic, religious, national, and so forth. Accordingly, they should differ between cultures or other social groups, because only by this can one group be differentiated from the other. To the degree that persons have some experiences in common with other members of their group, they can be part of a social group. But every person also has their very individual life experience, so there will be as many individual cognitive sets as there are persons (Schwartz, 1997).

Therefore, if one wants to predict whether a person will react with embitterment, one has to know their individual basic beliefs. As already mentioned, the content of basic beliefs is culturally determined. Similar to language, we learn basic beliefs. We take them from parents, teachers, and other reference groups in which we are included between the ages of five and twenty. As such views on life differ from culture to culture, the same emotional state can be elicited by different contexts in different social reference groups, while the same event can lead to very different emotional reactions in different cultures. Persons for whom their career is the highest value in life will not have a breakdown when they are left by their spouse. They will just look for another partner who fits in better with their present career. They will, however, react when they are not promoted, especially when they experience this as an act of injustice or deviousness. In contrast, somebody who thinks that family is the most important part of life will not react particularly strongly to being laid off, but more so to the unfaithfulness of a spouse. Similarly, persons will react differently to infidelity depending on their cultural background. In Islamic countries infidelity may be a disaster, while in some African or European countries nobody will care.

It is a well-known fact that negative life events have negative effects on people's lives, not as negative events but depending on the meaning the event has for an individual (i.e., attributions), and also depending on the fit between the event and the individual's capacities to cope with the event (Filipp, 1995; Klauer & Greve, 2005; Lazarus, 1995, 1999; Paykel, 2001, 2003a, 2003b; Schwarzer, 2005; Van der Kolk, Herron & Hostetler, 1994; Van der Kolk, McFarlane, & Weisaeth, 2000; Veenhoven, 1996). Cognitions give meaning to events. If values and preferences are stable over time, this is called "judgment disposition" (Asendorpf, 2007) and seen as a personality trait. Such judgment dispositions do not only refer to an individual's own behavior but also include expectations of others' behavior. They are standards for the evaluation of events and persons. According to Hofstede (1991), they can also be called mental processes. Veenhoven (1996) uses the term cognitive frame of reference. An example for different meanings of the same event in different cultures is premarital virginity. While in modern Western societies a woman who is about to get married at the age of twenty and who is still a virgin may be suspected of having some emotional problem, a non-virgin will be seen as a source of shame for the whole family and not be accepted as a wife in strict Muslim cultures.

In addition to the individual and societal content of basic beliefs there is also a situational aspect. An experience of injustice depends not only on the event as an absolute entity but even more so on its relative evaluation (Biswas-Diener, 2008; Helliwell & Putnam, 2004; Veenhoven, 1991, 1996). Whether an individual thinks that they receive enough salary for their work or are underpaid, for example, depends in part on how much others earn, and on the person's level of aspiration. The aspiration level has been defined as a personal standard for the evaluation of events and state of affairs (Festinger, 1954; Frey, Dauenheimer, Parge, & Haisch, 1993). The evaluation of standards depends on comparisons with others and earlier experiences. According to the theory of social comparison (Festinger, 1954; Frey et al., 1993) aspiration levels are developed in reference to other individuals or social groups that are similar to oneself. Similar to the theory of aspiration psychology, Michalos (1985) developed the Multiple Discrepancies Theory. Individuals are content if reality comes close to (a) what the individual wanted to achieve, (b) what relevant reference they have, (c) what they had in the past, and (d) what they expect from the future (Diener, Suh, Lucas, & Smith, 1999; Michalos, 1985; Veenhoven, 1996).

The individual, societal, cultural, and political role of cognitions, basic beliefs, and aspiration levels explains why this is a very strong psychological factor. It shapes the environment and resists changes in the environment for a long time. People will not easily change their views of the world and their basic beliefs. Thus, it can be understood that there must be intense feelings if basic beliefs are jeopardized by external events or other persons. The defense of basic beliefs creates martyrs or causes wars. The violation of basic beliefs without remedy will cause breakdowns in individuals and societies. One reaction is embitterment, aggression, and rampage against all others, and against one's own self.

Injustice and Basic Beliefs in Societal Change

Another approach to study the relation between embitterment, injustice, and social or individual basic beliefs is to refer to populations that undergo large societal changes. Actually, the studies on postraumatic embitterment disorders started in the wake of German reunification (Linden, 2003). Seventeen million people in Eastern Germany had to adjust to major changes in their lives; that is, in their social status, their working conditions, the legal system, housing, and social relations. Persons with high social standing in the communist system were out of work or driving taxis afterwards. However, individuals who had not been involved in the old system and had expected a new and better life were disappointed during the following years. Many East Germans still felt like second-class citizens 10 years after reunification. This was the time when persons with PTED presented as patients in greater numbers. Similar observations have been reported for the Czech Republic (Balon, 2004). There are further reports of this kind for Turkish immigrants in Western Europe (Hasanoğlu, 2008) who often found themselves disappointed as they were unable to realize the expectations that had led them to leave Turkey, even though they worked hard and spent their lives under dire conditions, and were not respected by their fellow countrymen nor their children. When studying Iranian emigrants (Teherani, 2006) it could be shown that individuals who had been forced to leave their country for political reasons had significantly higher rates of embitterment than those who had left the country in search of a better life elsewhere.

Similarly, there are data that unemployed people in areas with generally high unemployment rates show higher degrees of well-being than those in regions with low unemployment rates (Biswas-Diener, 2008; Clark & Oswald, 1994). In a study with unemployed individuals (Linden, Neumann, & Rotter, 2012; Muschalla & Linden, 2011), 59.8% of the participants indicated that they experienced their unemployment as unjust and unfair, 53.9% reported feelings of embitterment, 69.6% had to think about their unemployment over and over again, and 53.9% said that their unemployment had led to a noticeable and persistent change for the worse in their mental well-being. Significant correlations were found between the sum score of the PTED scale and the item "feelings of injustice in connection to unemployment" with unemployment appraisal, duration of unemployment, and age, while appraisal and duration of unemployment did not correlate with the GHQ-18, which measures unspecific mental symptoms (Linden et al., 2012).

Of special interest in this respect are data from South Africa (Sandau, 2009). Years after the end of apartheid, there are still major differences in social status between black and white citizens with respect to education, occupation, professional status, unemployment, or monthly income (South Africa Statistics, 2003, 2007). When black and white South Africans were compared, black individuals reported significantly higher scores on the PTED scale. However, looking at the rate of embitterment in greater detail showed significant correlations between unemployment and embitterment in white individuals but not in black ones.

Treatment

The aforementioned individual, societal, cultural, and political role of cognitions, basic beliefs, and aspiration levels explain why treatment of embitterment, and especially PTED, is difficult. Patients are reluctant to cooperate with therapists, turn aggressively against everyone, have a negative outlook, are fatalistic and resigning, and feel hopeless, especially as they think that the environment must change, but not they themselves. They often bluntly reject therapeutic help in a demonstrative way ("the world shall see what they did to me").

One approach to treating this problem has been wisdom psychotherapy (Baumann & Linden, 2008; Linden, 2006; Linden et al., 2007; Schippan, Baumann, & Linden, 2004). This is a form of cognitive behavior therapy that aims to enable the patient to come to terms with the negative life event, to let go, and to reconcile themselves with what has happened. A recent controlled clinical study suggests that this treatment can help to ameliorate embitterment (Linden et al., 2011). The overall approach refers to techniques of behavioral description and analysis of the critical event, establishing a working alliance with the patient, exposure treatment, increasing the patient's activities, fostering social contacts, and so forth. Of special importance are reframing techniques. This is where reference is made to modern developments of wisdom psychology (Baltes & Smith, 1990; Böhmig-Krumhaar, Staudinger, & Baltes, 2002; Staudinger & Baltes, 1996; Staudinger, Lopez, & Baltes, 1997; Sternberg, 1998; Mickler & Staudinger 2008, Meeks & Jeste 2009).

Every human being has the capacity for wisdom, similar to assertiveness. Wisdom can, in short, be defined as the capacity to solve unsolvable problems in life. Every life is full of situations in which no clear direction is evident, situations of uncertainty or of contradictory consequences, be it where to go on vacation or whether to marry someone. Like assertiveness, wisdom has several dimensions: (1) change of perspective, (2) empathy, (3) perception and acceptance of emotions, (4) emotional serenity, (5) factual knowledge, (6) procedural knowledge, (7) contextualism, (8) value relativism,

(9) uncertainty acceptance, (10) long-term perspective, (11) distance from oneself, (12) reduction in the level of aspiration (Baumann & Linden, 2008).

Specific psychotherapeutic methods are available that can help to develop and strengthen these capacities in patients. One is the method of unsolvable life problems. Patients are given a little case vignette such as the following:

> Ms. Miller lived with a man for many years and stayed with him and even nursed him for a long time before he died. Afterwards she had to learn that he had given all his money to his former wife and she was left with nothing in poverty.

Patients are then asked to comment on this case from the view of Ms. Miller. Then they are asked to take on the role of the former wife or the deceased partner. They might be asked how other persons would comment this experience: a lawyer who is interested in justice and money, a psychologist who is interested in motives, a grandmother who knows everything about human behavior and life, or a priest who thinks beyond life on earth. The patient can be asked what one might do to make the situation worse or, by contrast, to make the best of it. All this can teach the patient a change of perspective, contextualism, long-term perspective, and so forth.

The goal of this treatment approach is not to solve the problem, nor to say what and who is right or wrong. Instead, the patient learns skills that are needed to solve an unsolvable problem. Change of perspective, empathy, acceptance of one's own emotions, contextualism, value relativism, uncertainty acceptance, or taking a long-term perspective are universal psychological capacities and processes and not culture bound.

Implications for Treatment of Immigrants

As shown earlier, immigrants might be at a particularly heightened risk for embitterment/PTED due to acculturation stress, discrimination, unfulfilled expectations, and higher rates of unemployment (Kogan, 2004) (for an interesting case example, see Hasanoğlu, 2008). Additionally, this group may frequently face unsolvable problems, such as feeling connected with the home culture/dreaming about returning to it on the one hand and being bound to the host culture for political or economic reasons on the other hand. Thus, special attention should be paid to the differentiation between PTSD, depression, and embitterment/PTED in this group. Furthermore, when implementing wisdom psychotherapy in immigrant patients, cultural aspects should be considered. The case vignettes have to be culture embedded. They must be adapted to the cultural background of the patient. Some of the responses to the suggested situations may also be culture bound. Introducing a priest to ask the question of spiritual meaning of the critical event ("what does God want to tell you by loading this burden on your shoulder?") requires knowledge of the patient's religious background, of their *Weltanschauung* and their philosophy of life.

Conclusions

Embitterment is known to all human beings. If it becomes too intense, it can, similar to anxiety, result in a disabling and severe pathological condition such as posttraumatic embitterment disorder.

Modern classification of mental disorders in ICD-10 or DSM is by and large free of etiological assumptions. This is also true for PTED. Diagnosis is cross-sectional and based on the syndrome. This does not mean that etiological knowledge is unimportant for the understanding and treatment of such an illness.

In the diagnosis and treatment of PTED, a dual approach is needed. On the one hand, diagnosis is based on a specific psychopathological profile; that is, prevailing embitterment and intrusions. On the other hand, the understanding and treatment of the disorder must take into account the cultural context, comprising the individual basic beliefs of the patient and the type of event that has violated these basic values in an idiosyncratic way.

In many cases, PTED is seen in the aftermath of experiences of injustice, infidelity, and humiliation. This makes it, more than other mental disorder, a culturally sensitive disorder. What is conceived as unjust depends on personal values and beliefs learned from the social environment in early life. It also depends on an individual's current living conditions and aspiration levels, which are directly linked to processes of social comparison.

Interestingly, the treatment of embitterment and PTED is by and large again independent of the specific cause. It starts by teaching general skills of how to cope with severe and irreversible negative life events such as having been let down, cheated or humiliated. Cultural aspects are used only to the degree that they offer possibilities for the reframing of events and the integration of negative events in an individual's existing framework of basic beliefs and values.

References

Alexander, J. (1960). The psychology of bitterness. *International Journal of Psycho-Analysis, 41*, 514–520.

Asendorpf, J. B. (2007). *Psychologie der Persönlichkeit. Springer-Lehrbuch* [The psychology of personality. Springer textbook] (4th. ed.). Heidelberg, Germany: Springer.

Balon, R. (2004). Reflections on relevance: Psychotherapy and psychosomatics in 2003. *Psychotherapy and Psychosomatics, 73*(1), 5–9.

Baltes, P. B., & Smith, J. (1990). Weisheit und Weisheitsentwicklung. Prolegomena zu einer psychologischen Weisheitstheorie [Wisdom and the development of wisdom. Prolegomena on a psychological theory of wisdom]. *Zeitschrift für Entwicklungspsycholie und Pädagogische Psychologie, 22*, 95–135.

Baumann, K., & Linden, M. (2008). *Weisheitskompetenzen und Weisheitstherapie – Die Bewältigung von Lebensbelastungen und Anpassungsstörungen* [Wisdom competencies and wisdom therapy – Dealing with life problems and adjustment disorders]. Lengerich, Germany: Pabst Science Publishers.

Baures, M. M. (1996). Letting go bitterness and hate. *Journal of Humanistic Psychology, 36*, 75–90.

Beck, A. T., Rush A. J., Shaw B. F., & Emery, G. (1979). *Cognitive therapy of depression*. New York: Guilford.

Biswas-Diener, R. (2008). Material wealth and subjective well-being. In M. Eid & R. J. Larsen (Eds.), *The science of subjective well-being* (pp. 307–322). New York: Guilford.

Böhmig-Krumhaar, S. A., Staudinger, U. M., & Baltes, P. B. (2002). Mehr Toleranz tut Not: Lässt sich wert-relativierendes Wissen und Urteilen mit Hilfe einer wissensaktivierenden Gedächtnistrategie verbessern? [More tolerance is needed: Is it possible to improve value-relativizing knowledge and judgment using a knowledge-activating memory strategy?] *Zeitschrift für Entwicklungspsycholie und Pädagogische Psychologie, 34*, 30–43.

Bolby, J. (1969) *Attachment and loss: Vol. 1, attachment*. New York: Basic Books.

Bulman, R. J., & Wortman, C. B. (1977). Attributions of blame and coping in the "real world": Severe accident victims react to their lot. *Journal of Personality and Social Psychology, 35*, 351–363.

Clark, A. E. & Oswald, A. J. (1994). Unhappiness and unemployment. *The Economic Journal, 104*, 648–659.

Dalbert, C. (1999). The world is more just for me than generally: About the personal belief in a just world scale's validity. *Social Justice Research, 12*, 79–98.

Dalbert, C. (2011) Embitterment – from the perspective of justice psychology. In M. Linden & A. Maercker (Eds.), *Embitterment* (pp. 30–34). Vienna, Austria: Springer.

Diener, E., Suh, E. M., Lucas, R. E., & Smith, H. L. (1999). Subjective well-being: Three decades of progress. *Psychological Bulletin, 125*, 276–302.

Ekman, P. (1997). Expression or communication about emotion. In N. L. Segal, G. E. Weisfeld, & C. C. Weisfeld (Eds.), *Uniting psychology and biology: Integrative perspectives on human development* (vol. 48, pp. 348–392). Washington, DC: American Psychological Association.

Felber, W., Lammel, M., Sutarski, S., & Lau, S. (Eds.). (2010). *Plurale Suizide* [Multiple suicides]. Berlin: MWV Wissenschaftliche Verlagsgesellschaft.

Festinger, L. (1954). A theory of social comparison processes. *Human Relations, 7*(2), 117–140.

Filipp, S.-H. (Eds.). (1995). *Kritische Lebensereignisse* [Critical life events] (3rd ed.). Weinheim: Beltz.

Frey, D., Dauenheimer, D., Parge, O., & Haisch, J. (1993). Theorie sozialer Vergleichsprozesse [Theory of social comparison processes]. In D. Frey & M. Irle (Eds.), *Kognitive Theorien. Theorien der Sozialpsychologie* (2nd ed., pp. 81–122). Bern, Switzerland: Huber.

Hasanoğlu, A. (2008). Suggestion of a new diagnostic category: Posttraumatic embitterment disorder. *Turkish Journal of Psychiatry, 19*(1), 94–100.

Hautzinger, M. (2008). Grundüberzeugungen ändern [Changing basic beliefs]. In M. Linden & M. Hautzinger (Eds.). *Verhaltenstherapiemanual*. Berlin: Springer-Verlag.

Helliwell, J. F., & Putnam, R. D. (2004). The social context of well-being. *Philosophical Transactions of the Royal Society, 359,* 1435–1446.

Hofstede, G. (1991). *Cultures and organizations: Software of the mind.* New York: McGraw-Hill.

Janoff-Bulman, R. (1992). *Shattered assumptions: Toward a new psychology of trauma*. New York: Free Press.

Klauer, T., & Greve, W. (2005). Kritische Lebensereignisse und Gesundheit [Critical life events and health]. In R. Schwarzer (Ed.), *Enzyklopädie der Psychologie – Gesundheitspsychologie* (vol. 1, pp. 237–259). Göttingen, Germany: Hogrefe.

Kogan, I. (2004). Last hired, first fired? The unemployment dynamics of male immigrants in Germany. *European Sociological Review, 20*, 445–461.

Lazarus, R. S. (1991). *Emotion and adaption.* New York: Oxford University Press.

Lazarus, R. S. (1995). Stress und Stressbewältigung – ein Paradigma [Stress and coping with stress – a paradigm]. In S.-H. Filipp (Eds.), *Kritische Lebensereignisse* (3rd ed.) (pp. 198–233). Weinheim: Beltz.

Lazarus, R. S. (1999). *Stress and emotion: A new synthesis*. New York: Springer.

Lerner, M. J. (1980). *The belief in a just world: A fundamental delusion*. New York: Plenum Press.

Linden, M. (2003). The posttraumatic embitterment disorder. *Psychotherapy and Psychosomatics, 72*, 195–202.

Linden, M. (2006). Reaktionen auf belastende Lebensereignisse und Anpassungsstörungen [Reactions to problematic life events and adjustment disorders]. In F. Hohagen & T. Nesseler (Eds.), *Wenn Geist und Seele streiken. Handbuch seelische Gesundheit.* Munich, Germany: Südwest Verlag.

Linden, M., Baumann, K., Lieberei, B., Lorenz, C., & Rotter, M. (2011). Treatment of posttraumatic embitterment disorder with cognitive behaviour therapy based on wisdom psychology and hedonia strategies. *Psychotherapy and Psychosomatics, 80*, 199–205

Linden, M., Baumann, K., Rotter, M., & Schippan, B. (2008). Diagnostic criteria and the standardized diagnostic interview for posttraumatic embitterment disorder (PTED). *International Journal of Psychiatry in Clinical Practice, 12*, 93–96.

Linden, M., & Maercker, A. (Eds). (2011). *Embitterment. Societal, psychological, and clinical perspectives.* Vienna, Austria: Springer.

Linden, M., Neumann, A., & Rotter, M. (in press). Feelings of injustice and reactive embitterment in connection to job loss and unemployment. *Social Psychiatry and Psychiatric Epidemiology.*

Linden, M., Rotter, M., Baumann, K., & Lieberei, B. (2007). *The post-traumatic embitterment disorder (PTED).* Göttingen, Germany: Hogrefe & Huber Publishers.

Lipkus, I. M., & Siegler, I. C. (1993). The belief in a just world and perceptions of discrimination. *Journal of Psychology, 127*, 465–474.

Meeks, T. W., & Jeste, D. V. (2009). Neurobiology of wisdom: A literature overview. *Archives of General Psychiatry, 66*, 355–365.

Merten, J. (2003). *Einführung in die Emotionspsychologie* [An introduction to the psychology of emotions]. Stuttgart, Germany: Kohlhammer.

Michalos, A. C. (1985). Multiple Discrepancies Theory (MDT). *Social Indicators Research, 16*, 347–413.

Mickler, C., & Staudinger, U. M. (2008). Personal wisdom: Validation and age-related differences of a performance measure. *Psychol Aging, 23*, 787–799.

Muschalla B., & Linden, M. (2011). Embitterment and the workplace. In M. Linden & A. Maercker (Eds.). *Embitterment. Societal, psychological, and clinical perspectives.* Vienna, Austria: Springer.

Paykel, E. S. (2001). Stress and affective disorders in humans. *Seminars in Clinical Neuropsychiatry, 6*(1), 4–11.

Paykel, E. S. (2003a). Life events and affective disorders. *Acta Psychiatrica Scandinavica, 108,* 61–66.

Paykel, E. S. (2003b). Life events: Effects and genesis. *Psychological Medicine, 33(7)*, 1145–1148.

Pirhacova, I. (1997). Perceived social injustice and negative affective states. *Studia Psychologica, 39*, 133–136.

Plutchik, R. (1980). *Emotion. A psychoevolutionary synthesis.* New York: Harper & Row.

Plutchik, R. (2001). The nature of emotions. *American Scientist, 89*, 344–350.

Rotter, M. (2011). Embitterment and personality disorder. In M. Linden & A. Maercker (Eds.), *Embitterment. Societal, psychological, and clinical perspectives* (pp. <author: please provide page numbers>). Vienna, Austria: Springer.

Rubin, Z., & Peplau, L. A. (1975). Who believes in a just world? *Journal of Social Issues, 31*, 65–89.

Sandau, E. (2009). *Verbitterungsreaktionen im Kontext sozialer Referenzsysteme* [Embitterment reactions in the context of social reference frameworks]. Diploma thesis, Department of Psychology, Free University, Berlin, Germany.

Scherer, K. R. (2004). Feelings integrate the central representation of appraisal-driven response organization in emotion. In A. S. R. Manstead, N. H. Frijda, & H. Fischer (Eds.), *Feelings and emotions: The Amsterdam symposium* (pp. 136–157) . Cambridge: Cambridge University Press.

Schippan, B., Baumann, K., & Linden, M. (2004). Weisheitstherapie. Kognitive Therapie der Posttraumatischen Verbitterungsstörung [Wisdom therapy. Cognitive therapy of posttraumatic embitterment disorder]. *Verhaltenstherapie, 14*, 284–293.

Schwarzer, R. (Ed.). (2005). *Enzyklopädie der Psychologie: Gesundheitspsychologie* [Encyclopedia of psychology: Health psychology] (vol. 1). Göttingen, Germany: Hogrefe-Verlag.

Schwartz, S. H. (1997). Values and culture. In D. Munro, J. F. Schumaker, & S. C. Carr (Eds.), *Motivation and culture* (pp. 69–84). New York: Routledge.

South Africa Statistics. (2003). *Census 2001: Census in brief.* Retrieved from http://www.statssa.gov.za/census01/html/CInBrief/CIB2001.pdf

South Africa Statistics. (2007). *Stats in brief: 2007*. Retrieved from http://www.statssa.gov.za/Publications/StatsInBrief/StatsInBrief2007.pdf

Staudinger, U. M., & Baltes, P. B. (1996). Weisheit als Gegenstand psychologischer Forschung [Wisdom as a subject of psychological research]. *Psychologische Rundschau, 47*, 57–77.

Staudinger, U. M., Lopez, D., & Baltes, P. B. (1997). The psychometric location of wisdom-related performance: Intelligence, personality, and more? *Personality Social Psychology Bulletin, 23*, 1200–1214.

Sternberg, R. J. (1998). A balance theory of wisdom. *Review of General Psychology, 2*, 347–365.

Strelan, P. (2007). The prosocial, adaptive qualities of just world beliefs: Implications for the relationship between justice and forgiveness. *Personality and Individual Differences, 43*, 881–890.

Teherani, A. (2006). *Lebenszufriedenheit, Gesundheit und Verbitterungserleben: Ein Vergleich iranischer Immigranten und einheimischer Iraner*. [Life satisfaction, health, and embitterment experiences: A comparison of Iranian immigrant and native Iranians]. Diploma thesis, Department of Psychology, University of Potsdam, Germany.

Van der Kolk, B. A., Herron, N., & Hostetler, A. (1994). The history of trauma in psychiatry. *Psychiatric Clinics of North America, 17*, 583–600.

Van der Kolk, B. A., McFarlane, A., & Weisaeth, L. (Eds.). (2000). *Traumatic stress: Grundlagen und Behandlungsansätze. Theorie, Praxis und Forschungen zu posttraumatischem Streß sowie Traumatherapie.* [Traumatic stress: Foundations and treatment approaches. Theory, practical application, and research on posttraumatic stress and trauma therapy]. Paderborn, Germany: Junfermann.

Veenhoven, R. (1991). Is happiness relative? *Social Indicators Research, 24*(1), 1–34.

Veenhoven, R. (1996). Developments in satisfaction-research. *Social Indicators Research, 37*(1), 1–46.

Willebrand, M., Kildal, M., Andersson, G., & Ekselius, L. (2002). Long-term assessment of personality after burn trauma in adults. *Journal of Nervous and Mental Disease, 190*, 53–56.

Zemperl, J., & Frese, M. (1997). Arbeitslose: Selbstverwaltung überwindet die Lethargie [The unemployed: Self-management conquers lethargy]. *Psychologie Heute, 24*, 36–41.

Znoj, H. (2008). *BVI. Berner Verbitterungs Inventar. Manual* [Bern embitterment inventory. Manual]. Bern, Switzerland: Verlag Hans Huber.

Znoj, H. (2011). Embitterment – A larger perspective on a forgotten emotion. In M. Linden & A. Maercker (Eds), *Embitterment. Societal, psychological, and clinical perspectives* (pp. 5–16). Vienna: Springer.

Michael Linden
Charité Research Group Psychosomatic Rehabilitation
FPR, Hs. II, Rm. E01
Hindenburgdamm 39
12200 Berlin
Germany
E-mail: michael.linden@charite.de

Chapter 11

Suicide in Cultural Context

From Etiology to Prevention: The Case of China

Kenneth R. Conner[1] and Liang Zhou[2]

[1]University of Rochester Medical Center, Rochester, NY, USA
[2]School of Public Health, Central South University, Changsha, Hunan, China

Abstract
Suicide is a leading cause of death in China where, uniquely, there are more suicides among women than men. We discuss how the four United Nations (UN) recommendations to prevent suicide are applicable in China. Implementing UN recommendation 1, treat mental disorders, is justified by the pronounced risk for suicide in China conferred by depressive disorders. Although there is solid evidence from the general literature that depression treatment can prevent suicide, the limited infrastructure for depression treatment in China would seem to rule this out as a primary strategy for the foreseeable future, particularly in rural China where the suicide rate is highest and most suicides occur. Implementing UN recommendation 2, limit means, is justified by the widespread use of pesticides in suicide in rural areas and the high case fatality rate associated with these events. There is strong evidence from the general literature that means restriction can reduce suicides, and implementing steps to restrict pesticides in rural China is likely to be the most cost effective strategy. Implementing UN recommendation 3, enhance social support, is justified by some data showing low social support and related variables (e.g., interpersonal stressors) confer suicide risk in China. There are limited data in the general literature concerning the effectiveness of social support interventions to lower suicide risk, and the potential effectiveness of such interventions in China requires study. Implementing UN recommendation 4, change social norms, is justified by some fascinating preliminary data on role conflict conferring risk for suicide among women in China, although research on this topic is in its infancy, and the potential effectiveness in China of interventions focused on changing social norms requires study.

Keywords: suicide, prevention, cultural context, China

Unique Epidemiology of Suicide in China

About 900,000 individuals kill themselves worldwide each year (Nock et al., 2008). The study and prevention of suicide in China is essential because it is the world's most populous country and has a moderately high suicide rate; therefore it contributes substantially (more than 250,000 suicides per year occur in China alone) to the world total (Ji, Kleinmann, & Becker, 2001). The rate of suicide in China has been estimated to be more than 20 per 100,000 per year (Phillips, Li, & Zhang, 2002; Phillips & Yang, 2004). To put this rate in context, it is about double the rate in the US (~11) or Germany (~10), although lower than the rates in some Eastern European countries where the highest rates in the world are generally found.

Suicide in China has a unique epidemiology as it is the only country in the world where there are more suicides among women than men and indeed some have estimated that more than half the world's suicides among women occur in China (Phillips, Li et al., 2002; Phillips & Yang, 2004). Interestingly, the male to female ratio appears to be shrinking and is now fairly close at about 0.9 to 1.0 (Yip & Liu, 2006). Rates of suicide in China peak at two age periods in the life course, between ages 15 to 34 and again after age 70. Most suicides occur in rural areas where the rate of suicide is approximately three times that of urban areas (Ji et al., 2001). Fortunately there appears to be a decrease in the rate of suicide in recent years (Yip, Liu, Hu, & Song, 2005); the reason for the decline is unclear.

Prevention in Cultural Context

Although there remain many unanswered questions about suicide in China, there has been intensive research on suicide in the country over the past 15 years, including completion of two very large, rigorous, controlled postmortem studies (Phillips, Yang et al., 2002; Zhang, Xiao, & Zhou, 2010). These research efforts have led to probably more and better knowledge about suicide in China than in any country in Asia. This gathering knowledge informs suicide prevention efforts that are relevant to China. United Nations (UN) has made four general recommendations for suicide prevention for countries to implement: (1) treat mental disorders, (2) limit means, (3) enhance social support, and (4) change social norms (United Nations, 1996). For the remainder of the chapter the focus is on research on suicide in China that informs implementation of the UN recommendations in a culturally relevant manner. Research on suicide is emphasized, as opposed to nonfatal suicide attempts or suicidal ideation, because generalization of the latter outcomes to suicide deaths is unclear (Nock et al., 2008).

Application of UN Recommendations

Recommendation 1: Treat Mental Disorders

Well-designed controlled studies in China have firmly established that depressive disorders play a key role in suicide. In a large national study depressive disorder was the most prevalent disorder among suicide decedents, affecting 40% of cases (Phillips, Yang et al., 2002). After adjusting for other risk factors, moderate depressive symptoms conferred increased risk for suicide (OR = 6.4, 95% CI [4.2, 10.0]), and high depressive symptoms conferred massive risk for suicide (OR = 41.5, 95% CI [17.2–100.2]). Indeed, high depressive symptoms conferred greater risk for suicide than any of the risk factors studied. Similarly, in a large study in China of individuals ages 15 to 34, depressive disorder was the most prevalent disorder among suicide decedents, affecting 35% of cases (Zhang, Xiao et al., 2010). Moreover, psychiatric diagnosis (including, but not limited to depression) was the most potent risk factor for suicide studied (OR = 10.9, 95% CI [5.8–20.3]). These studies firmly established that depressive disorders are prevalent among suicide decedents in China and confer high risk (Phillips, Yang et al., 2002; Zhang, Xiao et al., 2010). Therefore, the treatment of depression should be a component in the overall strategy for suicide prevention in China, consistent with the UN recommendation. Laypersons in China are generally unlikely to view suicide as the product of depression (Ji et al., 2001), suggesting the need for public education about depression and its consequences.

Although important to address, prevention efforts in China should not be limited to the treatment of depression or other mental disorders. First, some mental disorders that are firmly established risk factors in other countries, for example, alcohol use disorders, have not been shown (as of yet) to confer risk for suicide in China (Phillips, Yang et al., 2002), although this situation may change as rates of drinking and alcohol use disorders increase in China (Zhou et al., 2009; Zhou et al., 2011). Second, the prevalence rate of mental disorders among suicide decedents in China is considerably lower than in Western countries, where up to 90% suicides have a mental disorder (Phillips, 2010). As a result, the population attributable risk (an estimate of the extent to which suicide could be reduced by eliminating a risk factor) associated with mental disorders is almost certainly lower in China than in the West. Third, the infrastructure to treat depression and other mental disorders in China is not well developed, particularly in rural China where most of the suicides occur (Yu, Liu, & Ma, 2010).

Recommendation 2: Limit Means

An international panel of experts concluded that limiting means for suicide (e.g., firearm restrictions) is one of only two proven methods for suicide prevention (Mann et al., 2005). More than half of suicides in China are carried out by ingesting pesticides used for agriculture and to kill rodents (Ji et al., 2001), making such pesticides the most sensible target for means restriction. A large study of Chinese individuals ages 15 to 34 showed that pesticide access increased risk for suicide after rigorous adjustment for other risk factors, with risk being accounted for by insecticide access in particular as opposed to other pesticides (Kong & Zhang, 2010).

Although these (and other) data make it clear that pesticides confer risk to individuals in China, a bolder argument has been made that use of pesticides is *the key* to understanding the high rate of suicide in China in rural areas (Gunnell & Eddleston, 2006; Eddleston & Phillips, 2004). Along these lines, it has been estimated that there is a 7.4% case fatality rate (defined as the percentage of time that enacting a method leads to death) associated with the deliberate ingestion of pesticides in rural parts of Asia (Gunnell & Eddleston, 2006). This high fatality rate is attributable to the high toxicity of pesticides that are routinely used in rural areas along with poor access to medical care in the countryside. In contrast, the case fatality rate for ingestion of substances in Western countries is many times lower, explained by the ingestion of generally far less toxic substances (e.g., over-the-counter medications) together with superior access to emergency medical care. According to the case fatality argument, the high rate of suicide in rural China is *not* attributable to generally elevated suicidality (i.e., high prevalence of suicidal behavior including suicide attempts and suicide) among the population but rather, a pronounced risk to die as the result of an act of suicide (Gunnell & Eddleston, 2006; Eddleston & Phillips, 2004). This case fatality perspective is supported by survey data from rural areas in China that does *not* show high a prevalence of nonfatal suicide attempts in the population (Dai et al., 2011).

Pesticide restrictions can take a variety of forms, including enactment of laws to ban or dilute the most lethal substances and laws or education campaigns to promote safer storage. Conceptually, successful method restriction efforts may make their greatest impact on the reduction of suicides that are unplanned (i.e., impulsive). According to this view, individuals who carry out planned acts of suicide have the time to choose a lethal alternative if their preferred method is blocked (for example, through means restriction). However, means restriction could be lifesaving for individuals who carry out unplanned acts of suicide because these acts tend to occur during short-lived emotional crises that follow acute stressful events, for example, a bad argument with a spouse (Conner, 2004). In support of this argument, reanalysis of a national study of suicide in China showed that individuals carrying out unplanned suicides were especially likely to ingest pesticides stored in the home, suggesting these substances were readily available and ingested hurriedly (Conner et al., 2005). Interestingly, the widespread use of pesticides in suicide in China may go a long way to explain the high prevalence of suicide among young women in rural areas. Worldwide, young women have the highest rate of suicide attempt by ingestion, a pattern that extends to China (Conner et al., 2005), and so a high case fatality rate associated with pesticide ingestion may be expected to increase the rate of suicide among young women in particular. Accordingly, pesticide restrictions in China may be especially beneficial to lowering the suicide rate among young rural women (Eddleston & Phillips, 2004), a testable hypothesis.

Recommendation 3: Enhance Social Support

In a large study in China of individuals ages 15 to 34 (Zhang, Xiao et al., 2010), those with low social support were at high risk for suicide after adjusting for other risk factors (OR = 12.74, 95% CI [7.15–22.68]). Stratified analyses confirmed that high risk applied to females (OR = 10.73, 95% CI [4.84–23.80]) and males (OR = 16.40, 95% CI [6.65–40.41]. In an inventive follow-up analysis, the authors further demonstrated that low social support moderated (increased) the risk for suicide associated with mental disorders. In other words, the combination of mental disorders and low social support appeared to be an especially suicidogenic combination in young Chinese individuals (Zhang, Wieczorak et al., 2010). The results suggest that efforts to reduce suicide risk among young Chinese should include a focus on enhancing social support, consistent with the UN recommendation. Moreover, vulnerable individuals (i.e., those with mental disorders) may especially benefit from these efforts.

The other major controlled postmortem study of suicide in China did not examine social support per se (Phillips, Yang et al., 2002). However, this study showed that acute interpersonal stressful life events as well as strained interpersonal relationships (tapped by a measure of "chronic stress") conferred risk for suicide (Phillips, Li et al., 2002), underscoring the importance of interpersonal stress in suicide in China. Indeed, interpersonal stress (measured in various ways) is among the most well-established risk factors for suicide in the world literature (Van Orden et al., 2010). One potential remedy to strained interpersonal relations is to seek to improve social support, consistent with the UN recommendation. Such efforts may take the shape of broad-based interventions to enhance social support in a community or through more indicated interventions (e.g., extending assistance to couples in conflict). More than 10% of the whole population in China are migrant workers, most of them are young and middle-aged people that move from rural to urban areas. Therefore, rural elderly are left behind. A survey in 2006 showed that 30.9% of rural elderly often felt lonely, higher than 18% among urban elderly (Liang, Li, & Yang, 2006). There is a paucity of data on the impact of such interventions to reduce suicide risk in China (and indeed throughout the world), although there are some encouraging hints in the literature. For example, a successful effort in the US Air Force to lower the suicide rate emphasized enhancing social support, among other foci (Knox, Litts, Talcott, Feig, & Caine, 2003).

Recommendation 4: Change Social Norms

Some of the ground covered thus far pertains in part to the recommendation to change social norms. For example, providing basic education about depression along with efforts to improve awareness of the role of depression in suicide among the Chinese public could be viewed as an effort to change social norms. Similarly, efforts to reduce access to dangerous pesticides may be most successful if they have take into consideration local norms around use and storage and solicit local input in problem-solving.

An inventive study that addressed the issue of social norms more squarely used a large Chinese sample of individuals ages 15 to 34 to test the hypothesis that young Chinese rural women who simultaneously held modern gender values and traditional Confucian gender values would experience conflict that would put them at risk for suicide (Zhang, Wieczorak et al., 2010). The author measured modern values, described as "Communist [gender] egalitarianism," based on agreement with items such as "[women] going to work," "equality for men and women," and "marriage by self-choice." They measured traditional values, described as "Confucian gender discrimination," based on agreement with items such as "women should stay at home and work only at home," "caring for her husband," and "bearing a son." These novel scales showed acceptable internal consistency ($\alpha = 0.69$ for the traditional scale; $\alpha = 0.88$ for the modern scale). Consistent with the authors' hypothesis, females who simultaneously obtained high scores on both scales were at an increased risk for suicide after adjusting for other risk factors. In contrast, men who held conflicting values were at no greater risk.

Broadly consistent with the UN recommendation, the results of the study suggest that efforts to change social norms in rural China concerning gender roles, in particular to relieve young women of the bind to choose between modern and traditional values, may lower risk for suicide in vulnerable women (Zhang, Wieczorak et al., 2010). A very low percentage of Chinese women enter treatment for depression or other behavioral disorders (Yu et al., 2010). However, this can be expected to change as the health care system in China continues to evolve with its increasing wealth, with the potential for treatment providers to therapeutically assist vulnerable women, and their families to navigate competing gender roles and values. A cautionary note is that the degree of suicide risk for women holding conflicting values (OR = 2.91, $p = .023$, confidence interval not given) was considerably smaller than risk among those with low social support or mental disorder (Zhang, Xiao et al., 2010). Moreover, it was a novel finding that requires replication. Therefore, whether or not social norms regarding this conflict per se should be a priority for prevention efforts requires further study.

Conclusion

Empirical evidence has been presented to show that each of the UN's recommendations to lower rates of suicide may be applied in China. In terms of strength of the evidence, there are "good" data to support agendas to improve treatment of mental disorders (in particular depression) and to promote means restriction (in particular pesticides). There is broad empirical support for these two suicide prevention approaches (and indeed, only these two approaches), based on the recommendations of an international panel of experts (Mann et al., 2005). Of the two strategies, means restriction is the more cost effective and practical for widespread implementation in China at the present time (Phillips, 2010). Addressing social support has a "fair" evidence base. An advantage of this focus is that there is the potential for community-based interventions to promote social support broadly (Knox et al., 2003), as well as more targeted interventions for at-risk individuals, for example, those with mental illness or in troubled marriages. Concerning the UN recommendation to change social norms, there is "preliminary" evidence that young women in China experiencing gender role conflict are at increased risk for suicide (Zhang, Xiao et al., 2010), suggesting such conflict may be a target of prevention efforts, although more research is needed. Finally, although the UN recommendations are useful they are not exhaustive and prevention activities that fall outside of these ideas should also be considered. For example, a multisite randomized controlled trial that included a site from China showed that providing patients in the emergency department who have made a suicide attempt with a brief educational intervention followed by a series of brief supportive contacts by telephone decreased the rate of suicide over follow-up (Fleischmann et al., 2008). As suicide attempt is generally the best predictor of eventual suicide (Nock et al., 2008), this type of brief, practical intervention that focuses on attempters presenting to emergency treatment is sensible for use in China and many other countries.

References

Conner, K. R. (2004). A call for research on planned vs. unplanned suicidal behavior. *Suicide and Life-Threatening Behavior, 34*, 89–98.

Conner, K. R., Phillips, M. R., Meldrum, S., Knox, K. L., Zhang, Y., & Yang, G. (2005). Low-planned suicides in China. *Psychological Medicine, 35*, 1197–1204.

Dai, J., Chiu, H. F., Conner, K. R., Chan, S. S. M., Hou, Z. J., Yu, X., & Caine, E. D. (2011). Suicidal ideation and attempts among rural Chinese aged 16–34 years – Socio-demographic correlates in the context of a transforming China. *Journal of Affective Disorders, 130*, 438–446.

Eddleston, M., & Phillips, M. R. (2004). Self poisoning with pesticides. *British Medical Journal, 328*, 42–44.

Fleischmann, A., Bertolote, J., Wasserman, D., De Leo, D., Bolhari, J., Botega, N., … Huong Tran Thi Thanh. (2008). Effectiveness of brief intervention and contact for suicide attempters: A randomized controlled trial in five countries. *Bulletin of the World Health Organization, 86*, 703–709.

Gunnell, D., & Eddleston, M. (2006). Why suicide rates are high in China? *Science, 311*, 1709–1710.

Ji, J., Kleinman, A., & Becker, A. (2001). Suicide in contemporary China: A review of China's distinctive suicide demographics in their sociocultural context. *Harvard Review of Psychiatry, 9*, 1–12.

Knox, K. L., Litts, D. A., Talcott, G. W., Feig, J. C., & Caine, E. D. (2003). Risk of suicide and related adverse outcomes after exposure to a suicide prevention programme in the US Air Force: Cohort study. *British Medical Journal, 327*, 1376.

Kong, Y., & Zhang, J. (2010). Access to farming pesticides and risk for suicide in Chinese rural young people. *Psychiatry Research, 30*, 217–221.

Liang, Q., Li, Y., & Yang, S. (2006). Loneliness and living status among rural elderly. *Chinese Journal of Gerontology, 9*, 1259–1260.

Mann, J. J., Apter, A., Bertolote, J., Beaturais, A., Currier, D., Haas, A., … Hendin, H. (2005). Suicide prevention strategies: A systematic review. *Journal of the American Medical Association, 294*, 2064–2074.

Nock, M. K., Borges, G., Bromet, E. J., Cha, C. B., Kessler, R. C., & Lee, S. (2008). Suicide and suicidal behavior. *Epidemiologic Reviews, 30*, 133–154.

Phillips, M. R. (2010). Rethinking the role of mental illness in suicide. *American Journal of Psychiatry, 167*, 731–733.

Phillips, M. R., Li, X., & Zhang, Y. (2002). Suicide rates in China, 1995–99. *The Lancet, 359*, 835–840.

Phillips, M. R., Yang, G., Zhang, Y., Wang, L., Ji, H., & Zhou, M. (2002). Risk factors for suicide in China: A national case-control psychological autopsy study. *The Lancet, 360,* 1728–1736.

Phillips, M. R., & Yang, G. H. (2004). Suicide and attempted suicide in China, 1990–2002. *Morbidity and Mortality Weekly Report, 53*, 481–484.

United Nations. (1996). *United Nations. Prevention of suicide: Guidelines for the formulation and implementation of national strategies.* New York: United Nations.

Van Orden, K. A., Witte, T. K., Cukrowicz, K. C., Braithwaite, S., Selby, E. A., & Joiner, T. E. (2010). The interpersonal theory of suicide. *Psychological Review, 117*, 575–600.

Yip, P. S., & Liu, K. Y. (2006). The ecological fallacy and the gender ratio of suicide in China. *British Journal of Psychiatry, 189*, 465–466.

Yip, P. S., Liu, K. Y., Hu, J., & Song, X. M. (2005). Suicide rates in China during a decade of rapid social changes. *Social Psychiatry and Psychiatric Epidemiology, 40*, 792–798.

Yu, X., Liu, J., & Ma, H. (2010). Community mental health: A panacea to confront the challenge in China? *Chinese Mental Health Journal, 24*, 885.

Zhang, J., Wieczorek, W., Conwell, Y., Tu, X., Wu, B. Y. W., Xiao, S., & Jia, C. (2010). Characteristics of young rural Chinese suicides: A psychological autopsy study. *Psychological Medicine, 40*, 581–589.

Zhang, J., Xiao, S., & Zhou, L. (2010). Mental disorders and suicide among young rural Chinese: A case-control psychological autopsy study. *American Journal of Psychiatry, 167*, 773–781.

Zhou, L., Conner, K. R., Caine, E. D., Xiao, S., Xu, L., Gong, Y., … Phillips, M. R. (2011). Epidemiology of alcohol use in rural men in two provinces of China. *Journal of Studies on Alcohol and Drugs, 72*, 333–340.

Zhou, L., Conner, K. R., Phillips, M. R., Caine, E. D., Xiao, S., Zhang, R., & Gong, Y. (2009). Epidemiology of alcohol abuse and dependence in rural Chinese men. *Alcoholism: Clinical & Experimental Research, 33*, 1770–1776.

Kenneth R. Conner
University of Rochester Medical Center
300 Crittenden Blvd.
Rochester, NY 14642
USA
E-mail: kenneth_conner@urmc.rochester.edu

Chapter 12

Substance Abuse and Addiction Among Divergent Ethnic Groups

Hans-Jörg Assion[1] and Eckhardt Koch[2]

[1]LWL-Hospital , Dortmund, Germany
[2]Vitos Hospital for Psychiatry and Psychotherapy, Marburg, Germany

Abstract

Substance use disorder (SUD) remains one of the most common and significant problems around the world. Irrespective of the cultural background, addictive behavior is of high prevalence, causing escalating medical and economic costs. The increasing mobility of humans with intense interchange of nations will further contribute to the worldwide growing use of psychotropic drugs. In contrast to the emerging general research on substance use disorders, the scientific database on addictive behavior considering cultural aspects is rather limited. Nationwide data (e.g., for Germany) are still missing. The aim of this contribution is to discuss the prevalence, etiology, and treatment of addictive behavior with special emphasis on ethnical factors. Additionally, some of the relevant studies considering the ethnical background and the impact of acculturation of the patients suffering from SUD will be summarized in this chapter.

Keywords: substance use disorder, migrant, culture, acculturation

Empirical Data: Prevalence of Substance Use Around the World

Alcohol is consumed worldwide, but average alcohol intake per person differs depending on regions of the world. The highest intake of alcohol is found in Europe, America, and the West Pacific, with an intake of 5.5 to 8.5 litres per person per year. For instance, according to a study (Strategy Unit, 2004) conducted in the UK, at present, it is estimated that 4.7 million of the UK population are abstainers; 6.4 million are drinking

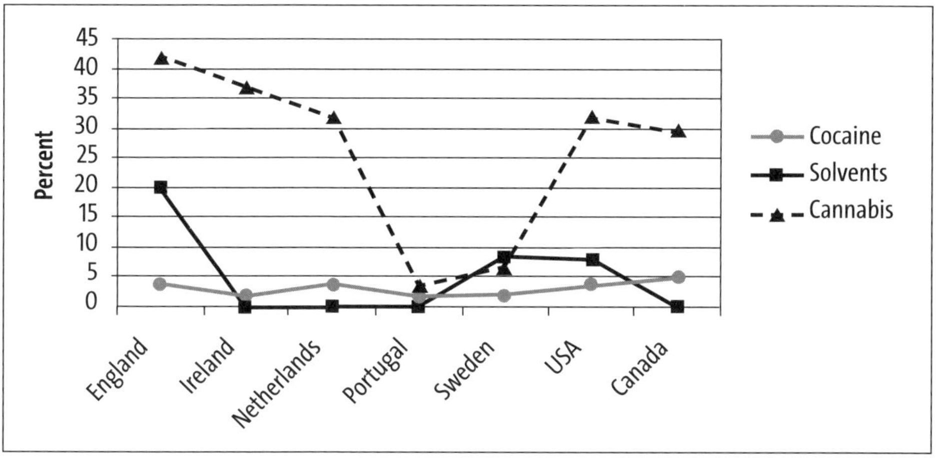

Figure 12.1. Cannabis, cocaine, and solvents consumption in adolescents in various countries (data from European Monitoring Centre for Drugs and Drug Addiction (1999)).

up to 35 units[1] (women) or 50 units (men), while 1.8 million drink at the 35/50 level or over. Moreover, the per capita consumption was found to be 8.6 litres of pure alcohol with an increase of 121% since 1951. Within the period between 1970 and 2000, consumption rate increased five times over. In comparison to other countries, UK consumption is rising, especially in women and young people, although UK adults are not among the heaviest consumers in Europe. British teenagers however, are among the heaviest consumers in Europe (Crome & Bloor, 2008). In contrast, less than one litre of alcohol per person per year is consumed in Africa, Asia, or the Middle East. Not only cultural, but also sociological and economic reasons contribute to these differences in the levels of consumption (European Monitoring Centre for Drugs and Drug Addiction, 1999). Accordingly, Global Burden of Disease study for the year 2000 has demonstrated that alcohol is not among the first 15 causes of disability-adjusted life years (DALYs) lost in the Eastern Mediterranean Region, while in Europe alcohol-related problems rank fourth and in America they rank second (Murray, Lopez, Mathers, & Stein, 2001).

Of further interest is the data pool concerning the consumption of cannabis, cocaine, and solvents in various European and North American countries. At first glance the low intake of cannabis products is obvious and comparably frequent in Portugal and Sweden. The consumption of cannabis products is highest in UK, Ireland, and the Netherlands. The use of solvents is also quite prevalent in UK, but to a lower extent in the US, Sweden, and marginally in the other European countries. A comparably high use of cocaine is found in most of the European and North American countries and Australia.

---

[1] One unit is 8 grams of pure alcohol, equivalent to half a pint of ordinary beer, a small glass of wine (9% strength), or one measure of spirits.

Independent of governmental policy, illegal substances are more or less prevalent in these countries (European Monitoring Centre for Drugs and Drug Addiction, 1999). In contrast, the consumption of illegal drugs in non-Western countries such as Turkey was found to be much lower than many of these European and North American countries (Haasen, Heimann, Penka, & Heinz, 2011).

Substance Use Across Different Psychiatric Disorders Among Ethnic Minority Groups

Remarkably, the lifetime rates of alcoholism vary in view of psychiatric disorders. In general, the percentage is fairly high, with more than one-third of patients with bipolar disorder or schizophrenia to be comorbidly addicted to substances such as alcohol. Correlations between attention deficit hyperactivity disorder (ADHD) and addiction have started to attract more attention. Motivational dysfunctions have been postulated

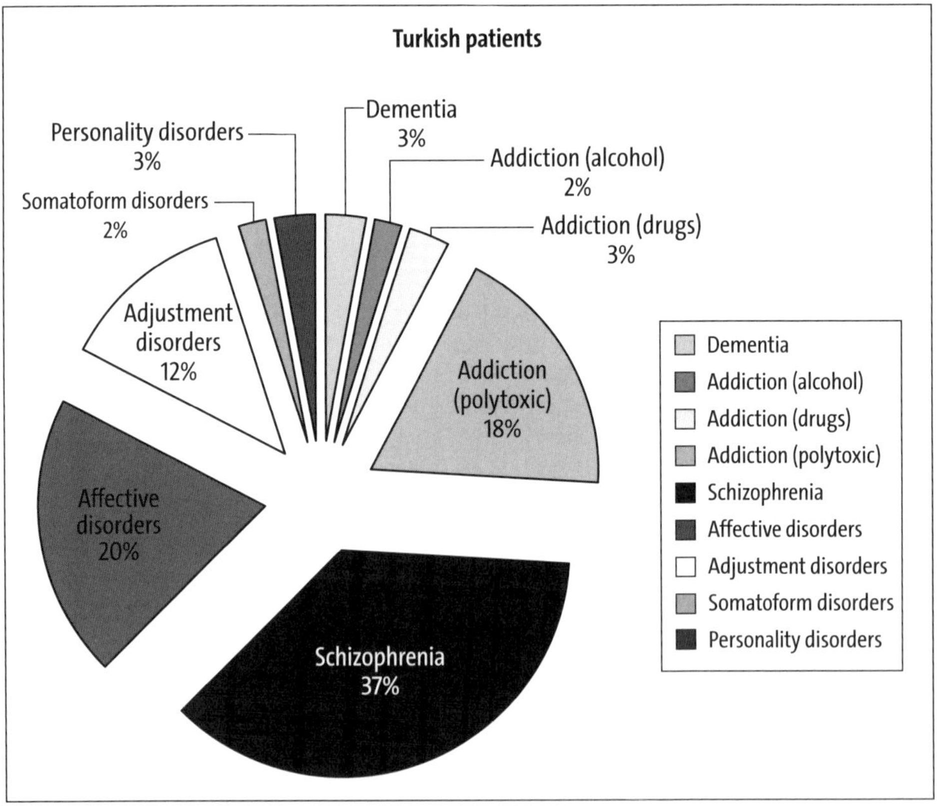

Figure 12.2. Diagnoses in migrants of Turkish origin

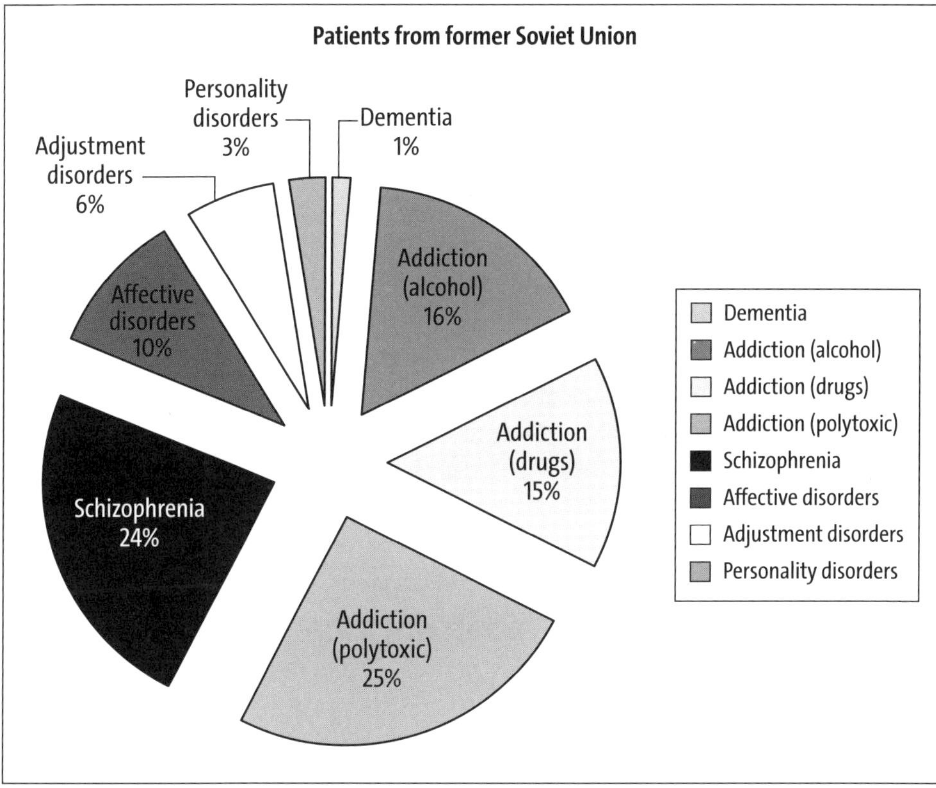

Figure 12.3. Diagnoses in migrants of East European origin

for both disorders. Imaging data suggest that the comorbidity of SUD in adult patients with ADHD could be due to various neuronal dysfunctions in the reward system (Stoy, Wrase, Heinz, & Ströhle, 2006). Pathogenetic relationships between the two disorders indicate a pattern of genetic and neurobiological factors. While the overall prevalence of ADHD in adulthood was estimated between 2– and 6%, SUD was associated with ADHD in about 30 to 50%. For instance, König, Wodarz, Unglaub, and Johann (2007) found out that 35% of the 50 opiate addicts fulfilled the criteria of lifetime ADHD and 19% showed persistent symptoms. Within the same sample, the ADHD (+)-patients were younger at age of onset of substance use, showed lower IQ levels, and were more often judged or imprisoned when compared to ADHD(-)-patients. The authors conclude that ADHD might negatively influence the onset and course of substance use disorder. Despite the strong relationship between adult ADHD and SUD, up to now the literature is missing the data relating to patients with migration.

Likewise, the comorbidity of SUD in patients with depression and anxiety disorders is considerably high as well. Regarding the frequent diagnoses of mood and panic disorders in migrants, this population is likely to suffer from comorbid substance abuse (see also chapters 1 and 14) (Regier et al., 1990). The working group "Migration and Psychiatry" of the Conference of Directors of Psychiatric Hospitals in Germany conducted extensive studies including German psychiatric hospitals and institutions in a survey to get information on diagnoses in migrant populations. These investigations included patients from Turkey and Eastern Europe. Although prevalence rates of depression and anxiety disorders are substantially high among Turkish patients, they were suffering from substance use disorders considerably less often compared to patients from Eastern Europe, with alcohol addiction as the most prevalent subgroup (Koch, Hartkamp, Siefen, & Schouler-Ocak, 2008; Schouler-Ocak et al., 2008) (see Figures 12.2 and 12.3).

Furthermore, according to official data from Bavaria, over the last two decades the rates of addicts committing suicide was significantly increased among Russian settlers. Kornischka, Assion, Ziegenbein, and Agelink (2008) found out in a review of all relevant publications concerning settlers from CiS in Germany until 2008 that depression and addiction were the most common diagnoses, as were functional disorders or somatization (see chapter 8).

Etiology of SUD: Considering General and Culture-Specific Risk Factors for Migrants

The multifactorial etiology of addictive behavior comprises individual, social, cultural, and biological factors, each partially contributing to the onset of substance use disorders. Nevertheless, neurobiology of addiction is currently the main field of research, and genetic risk factors account for presumably 50% of the onset of substance use disorders. Alcohol dependence is cross-culturally inherited, with high concordance rates in twins. A quarter of alcohol addicts are children of alcohol-dependent fathers, and in approximately a third of problem drinkers both parents suffer from alcohol addiction (Clark et al., 1997). A further biological aspect is the variable activity of proteins or enzymes in divergent ethnic groups. For example, the human cytochrome P450 (CYP) enzymes are involved in the biotransformation of drugs and substances in the liver. CYP enzymes exhibit increased or decreased activity in various ethnicities. For this reason tolerance of psychotropic drugs vary on the basis of genetic polymorphisms depending on ethnical origin (Assion & Reinbold, 2011).

Furthermore, it has also been demonstrated that alcoholism is a learned behavior (Kiefer, 2009). An important factor to addiction is the imitation learning from parental patterns. Parents' coping strategies and problem solving are of strong influence to children's behavior (Tuna, 1999). A further sociobiological aspect is the effect of stress as a factor for increased alcohol consumption or substance abuse (Zimmermann, Blomeyer, Laucht, & Mann, 2007). Migrants are likely confronted with risky life events, traumatic experiences, or irksome conditions, and have to cope with language problems, economic difficulties, or social exclusion (Patel, Flisher, & Cohen, 2008). All of these factors elevate the level of stress, and there is evidence for chronic stress to cause impairment of brain function or cell sprouting as probable risk factors to mental problems. It is commonly known that alcohol reduces stress symptoms. The effective amelioration of negative affect facilitates the consumption of alcohol in stressful life events. Abstinent addicts with high stress levels are at higher risk to relapse in order to achieve stress reduction. Szaflarski, Cubbins, and Ying (2011) found out that foreign-born respondents (first-generation migrants) had lower rates of alcohol abuse than the US-born second generation, but some variations were noted by race-ethnicity. The risk of clinical diagnosis due to traumatic events was higher for the foreign-born population.

Regarding personality traits, migrants are supposedly confronted with situations that do not strengthen the narcissistic part of their personality, and instead may lower their self-esteem. A person with low self-esteem or restricted coping strategies will more likely tend to exhibit impulsive or aggressive behavior. Erratic or dissocial behavior is possibly aggravated against the background of given family problems. High levels of arousal or excitability are again a trigger to alcohol or substance abuse. However, it should be made clear that no specific addictive personality exists, although comorbid personality disorders and antisocial traits are frequently seen in alcohol addiction.

Social interaction is an additional piece of the puzzle in the discussion of the etiology of SUD. Consider that, on the one hand, the family situation of migrants is precarious, and on the other hand, there are strong bonds within the family. Substance abuse is related to the style of interaction in families with a migration background (Kimil & Salman, 2010). Interestingly, addiction of an index patient may have stabilizing effects on the familial cohesion, masking emotional, traumatic, or financial conflicts. Family-oriented cultures in particular tend toward cohesion into the nucleus of the family. This helps to avoid the loss of credit in the ethnic group, because addiction has a negative attribution in many cultures. In addition, social support within the family tends to minimize negative consequences of addiction for long periods of time, but in the end a loss of self-control may cause social exclusion. It should be taken into consideration that variable cultural patterns, traditions, conventions, or rules may result in obviously diverse patterns of SUD. Accordingly, it is to assume that quantities, types of ingested psychotropic medications, and the various ways of ingestion vary between cultures. Studies of alcohol consumption among Hispanics in the US show different patterns based on gender, country of origin, and economic status. The literature shows a lower frequency but higher volume of consumption among Mexican American and Puerto Rican males than among non-Hispanic white males. Cuban American males have a pattern of relatively moderate consumption that resembles that of non-Hispanic whites. Women from Mexican American, Cuban American, and Puerto Rican populations have low alcohol consumption rates, which appear to increase with the level of acculturation (Randolph, Stroup-Benham, Black, & Markides, 1998).

An ethnocultural differentiation of migrant addicts is problematic and exclusively based on clinical impressions in routine care, but not a result of systematic research. Consequently, classification in categories must be handled with care and not generalized, being applicable only to selected samples. A rough classification into categories under religious aspects allocates addicts from Africa and Turkey to be Muslim in majority. Islam prohibits the use of alcohol and other drugs. Traditional families found in those cultures are rather attached to a hierarchical parent–child relationship. The coping style employed to manage problems is most likely characterized by repression or sanctioning, and the level of social integration tends to be intermediate or low (Boos-Nünning, Siefen, Kirkcaldy, Otyakmaz, & Surall, 2002) (see chapter 6). In such groups, any use of a proscribed substance contains an element of social deviance for the individual. Norm conflicts can be actuated when ideal norms and behavioral norms differ in a culture. Ideal norms may forbid the use of a substance, whereas the actual behavioral norm, especially for younger generations, may expect substance use as a normative behavior (Westermeyer, 2004, p. 87). So it is not really surprising that young people of Turkish origin look for help within the structures of family and ethnic community and do not know much about advice centers (Penka, Heimann, Heinz, & Schouler-Ocak, 2008).

Table 12.1. Ethnocultural differentiation of addiction in migrants (adapted from Boos-Nünning et al., 2002).

Characteristics of individuals with addiction

Origin	Africa	Turkey, Afghanistan	USSR, ethnic Germans	Southern Europe
Identity	Muslim, mostly male	non-orthodox Muslim	atheist or religious	stable identity
Conflicts in family	repressed	sanctioned	variable	discussed
Parents' relationship	attributed role	attributed role	differentiated role	fixed role
Parents–child relationship	hierarchical	ambivalent, hierarchical	child "carries" family	hierarchical
Social integration	low	partial	broad spectrum	enculturated, integrated
Social class	working class, agricultural laborers	working class, agricultural laborers	working class	working class
Attitude to addiction	sin, transfiguration	sin, transfiguration	variable	devaluation
Attitude to therapy	criticism, refusal	criticism, refusal	formal	criticism, acceptance

Families of addicts from Eastern Europe or Russia tend toward a more variable coping style. Alcohol consumption is common in their countries of origin. The familial role of a child is more prominent in relation to the parents and the families are integrated in part. Settlers tend to practice their religion, while most migrants from Russia are nonbelievers. A population-based study that was recently conducted in Germany, for instance, compared a sample of Turkish and Russian migrants and a sample of native Germans regarding their substance use. The age range of the random sample was 16–65 years of age and 35–41 years on average within the three groups, with each group comprised of about 300 persons. Turkish migrants showed the highest rate of nicotine drug dependency, but the lowest rate of alcohol consumption. Both the Russian and German samples were fairly comparable concerning the rate of individuals exhibiting problematic alcohol intake (Zeef, Salman, Krauth, Walter, & Machleidt, 2011). However, as aforementioned, categorizing is always a simplification or even an oversimplification of reality and the variability of cultural or individual expressions will not fit in a simple concept of behavior, conviction, or traits that will result in stereotypes. Nevertheless, in clinical care it is required to rule out the basic motivation and impulses of migrant addicts as a helpful approach. Knowledge about the common peer group, sociopolitical background, and economic situation is beneficial in treatment of migrant addicts and ought to be taken into therapeutic consideration (Boos-Nünning et al., 2002).

Acculturation and Addiction

Cross-cultural psychology has demonstrated important links between cultural context and individual behavioral development. The long-term psychological consequences of the process of acculturation are highly variable, depending on social and personal variables that reside in the society of origin, the society of settlement, and phenomena that both exist prior to, and arise during, the course of acculturation (Berry, 1997).

There are some international publications that deal with acculturation and treatment of alcohol use disorders. For example, in a field study, 50 Afghan migrants residing in Germany and who currently drink alcohol were investigated. Participants were screened with respect to alcohol use problems and then interviewed concerning patterns of use, mental health, and sociodemographic and cultural variables. A significant correlation was found between acculturation stress and mental distress, as well as between mental distress and severity of alcohol use. These correlations did not differ with respect to whether alcohol had been used prior to migration. The findings support the hypothesis of the effect of acculturation on problematic alcohol use (Haasen, Sinaa, & Reimer, 2008).

Quantity and frequency consumption was somewhat higher among the least acculturated males and moderately acculturated females. Further analyses by generational status indicate heavier consumption patterns among second-generation individuals, especially among the less acculturated. The findings highlight inadequacies of using generational status/nativity measures alone to assess acculturation level. Further, joint effects of acculturation level and generational status suggest the viability of a cultural marginality model of acculturation, though many of the effects of acculturation and generational status are explained by demographic and psychosocial factors (Neff & Hoppe, 1992). For instance, Kulis, Marsiglia, and Hurdle (2003) measured four dimensions of gender identity based on the concepts of "machismo" (masculinity) and "marianismo" (femininity) – aggressive masculinity, assertive masculinity, affective femininity, and submissive femininity. In explaining a variety of indicators of drug use behaviors and antidrug norms, gender alone had limited explanatory power, while gender identity was a better predictor. Aggressive masculinity was generally associated with higher risk of drug use, while the other three gender identity measures had selected protective effects. However, the impact of gender identity was strongly mediated by acculturation. Less acculturated Mexican American students reported lower aggressive masculinity scores than non-Latinos. Less acculturated Mexican American girls reported both the lowest aggressive masculinity scores and the highest submissive femininity scores. More acculturated Mexican American students, along with the less acculturated Mexican American boys, did not appear to be following a polarized approach to gender identity (machismo and marianismo) as was expected. The findings suggest that some aspects of culturally prescribed gender roles can have a protective effect against drug use behaviors and attitudes, possibly for both girls and boys. Another study shows evidence that acculturation is related to lower rates of alcohol use disorders among men and a higher frequency of heavy episodic drinking among women. This suggests that acculturation has different effects on drinking for men and women. This finding needs some attention as literature also indicates that women drink more and may develop more alcohol-related problems as they acculturate. The association between acculturation and alcohol use disorders does not appear to be linear and the effect of acculturation is not uniform on individuals' drinking behavior (Caetano, Ramisetty-Mikler, Wallisch, McGrath, & Spence, 2008).

Clinical Implications

Finally, to address therapeutic issues, basic therapeutic goals in SUD integrate alleviation of withdrawal symptoms, initiation of a recovery process, and awareness of harm reduction. Migrants at risk are in need of multiprofessional care under consideration of cultural and migrational factors. Evidence-based treatment procedures according to updated guideline algorithms should be part of an integrated treatment strategy combining pharmacotherapy and psychosocial support to guarantee the most beneficial results (Assion, Bingöl, Ozguerdal, & Basilowski, 2007). Thus, recovery involves a cultural component along with physical and psychological components (see chapters 1 and 15). A study in Hamburg (Haasen, Toprak, Yagdiran, & Kleinemeier, 2001) focused on psychosocial aspects of addiction among migrants. The family structure was still intact for two thirds of the 51 (43 men and 8 women) addicted migrants (66% were of Turkish origin). The severity of addiction was significantly lower in those with a school diploma, as well as in those with vocational training or with a higher proficiency in German and showed a highly significant relationship with conflicts within the family and the surrounding social environment. A good prognostic indicator seems to be a later age of initiation and an intact family structure, which, however, should lead to a stronger family-therapeutic orientation.

The relationship between higher proficiency in German and a less severe course of addiction can be interpreted as a positive effect of better integration. In a later publication (Haasen et al., 2008) the authors emphasize the need for specific early intervention measures both in general medicine as well as in the field of social counseling for migrants. Among the 50 participants, 36 had consulted either a physician or a counselor in the month previous to the interview. The importance of general practitioners in the early detection of alcohol use disorders is not limited to migrants, but has been claimed as a necessary tool for early intervention for many years.

In a multiethnic society preventive strategies do not fit all groups, so it is necessary to adapt programs and therapeutic approaches to different cultural values (Schouler-Ocak & Haasen, 2008). Self-help groups, for example, are not common in some ethnos and there is a need for special information and modification of the setting (Kofahl, Hollmann, & Möller-Bock, 2009). This is necessary because outpatient consultations and evaluations are increasingly becoming the norm (Assion, Zarouchas, Multamäki, Zolotova, & Schröder, 2007). Whenever possible, a family member or close friend who is committed to the patient's recovery should participate as a collateral resource. If there is any doubt of speaking the language of the host country, a translator from the patient's ethnic background can likewise reassure the patient (Westermeyer, 2004, p. 102). So it is no surprise that for Hispanics who received brief motivational intervention, an ethnic match between patient and provider resulted in a significant reduction in drinking outcomes at 12-month follow-up. In addition, there was a tendency for the ethnic match to be most beneficial to foreign-born Hispanics and less acculturated Hispanics. Ethnic concordance between patient and provider may have impacted the effectiveness of the intervention through several mechanisms, including cultural scripts, ethnic-specific perceptions pertaining to substance abuse, and ethnic-specific preferred channels of communication (Field & Caetano, 2010).

Further, comorbid substance use disorders will likely mask, mimic, or exacerbate symptoms of psychiatric disorders, leading to diagnostic difficulties in migrants. SUD varies within ethnic groups and in dependence from environmental factors. An integrated treatment strategy addressing both migration background and SUD is recommended as a beneficial approach (Czycholl, 1998).

Future Perspectives

The topic of migration and addiction is a widespread field with lots of implications and of large social and medical interest. Up to now there is not enough research, and there are more questions than answers. For example, future research should continue to investigate the role of stress, the specific traumatic events most problematic for immigrant groups, and the interplay of the original and host culture in shaping the patterns of alcohol abuse in the immigrant population. Acculturation needs to be focused on the treatment of alcohol use disorders. This chapter shows at least the necessity to pay attention to cultural aspects when dealing with addiction. We need more studies for the consolidation of the diversity of the previous findings. We need questionnaires and rating scales with cross-cultural assessment and we need guidelines for culturally sensitive treatment and cultural sensitivity in medical institutions (Barth & Czycholl, 2006). Thus far, only a few first steps have been taken.

References

Assion, H. J., Bingöl, H., Ozguerdal, S., & Basilowski, M. (2007). Patients of Turkish origin in an institutional psychiatric outpatient service. *MMW-Fortschritte der Medizin, 149*, 57–58.

Assion, H. J., & Reinbold, H. (2011). Pharmakotherapie bei psychisch kranken Migranten [Pharmacotherapy with mentally ill migrants]. In W. Machleidt & A. Heinz (Eds.), *Praxis der interkulturellen Psychiatrie und Psychotherapie* (pp. 485–488). Munich, Germany: Elsevier.

Assion, H. J., Zarouchas, I., Multamäki, S., Zolotova, J., & Schröder, S. G. (2007). Patients' use of alternative methods parallel to psychiatric therapy: Does the migrational background matter? *Acta Psychiatrica Scandinavica, 116*, 220–225.

Barth, W., & Czycholl, D. (2006). *Sucht. Migration. Hilfe* [Addiction. Migration. Help]. Geesthacht, Germany: Neuland.

Berry, J. W. (1997). Immigration, acculturation and adaptation. *Applied Psychology: An International Review, 46*(1), 5–34.

Boos-Nünning, U., Siefen, R., Kirkcaldy, B., Otyakmaz, B. Ö., & Surall, D. (2002). *Migration und Sucht. Expertise im Auftrag des Bundesministeriums für Gesundheit* [Migration and addiction. Expert opinion for the Federal Ministry of Health]. Baden-Baden, Germany: Nomos.

Caetano, R., Ramisetty-Mikler, S., Wallisch, L. S., McGrath, C., & Spence, R. T. (2008). Acculturation, drinking, and alcohol abuse and dependence among Hispanics in the Texas-Mexico border. *Alcoholism: Clinical and Experimental Research, 32*, 314–321.

Clark, D. B., Moss, H. B., Kirisci, L., Mezzich, A. C., Miles, R., & Ott, P. (1997). Psychopathologa in preadolescent sons of fathers with substance use disorders. *Journal of the American Academy of Child and Adolescent Psychiatry, 36*, 495–502.

Crome, I. B., & Bloor, R. (2008). Alcohol problems. In R. M. Murray, K. S. Kendler, P. McGuffin, S. Wessely, & D. J. Castle (Eds.), *Essential psychiatry* (4th ed., pp. 198–229). Cambridge: Cambridge University Press.

Czycholl, D. (1998). Stationäre Therapie für abhängigeitskranke Migranten. Erfahrungen mit einer Spezialisierung [In-patient treatment for migrants with addiction. Experiences with specialization]. In Deutsche Hauptstelle gegen die Suchtgefahren (Ed.), *Sucht in unserer multikulturellen Gesellschaft.* Freiburg, Germany: Lambertus.

European Monitoring Centre for Drugs and Drug Addiction. (1999). *Annual report on the state of the drug problem in the European Union.* Lisbon, Portugal: Author.

Field, C., & Caetano, R. (2010). The role of ethnic matching between patient and provider on the effectiveness of brief alcohol interventions with Hispanics. *Alcoholism: Clinical and Experimental Research, 34*(2), 262–271.

Haasen, C., Heimann, H., Penka, S., & Heinz, A. (2011). Abhängigkeit und Sucht [Dependence and addiction]. In W. Machleidt & A. Heinz (Eds.), *Praxis der interkulturellen Psychiatrie und Psychotherapie.* Munich, Germany: Elsevier.

Haasen, C., Sinaa, M., & Reimer, J. (2008). Alcohol use disorders among Afghan migrants in Germany. *Substance Abuse, 29*(3), 65–70.

Haasen, C., Toprak, M. A., Yagdiran, O., & Kleinemeier, E. (2001). Psychosoziale Aspekte der Sucht bei Migranten [Psychosocial aspects of addiction in migrants]. *Suchttherapie, 2*, 161–166.

Kiefer, F. (2009). Complete suppression of craving in alcohol-dependent individuals. Is it possible? *CNS Drugs, 23*, 361–367.

Kimil, A., & Salman, R. (2010). Migration und Sucht [Migration and addition]. In T. Hegemann & R. Salman (Eds.), *Handbuch Transkulturelle Psychiatrie* (pp. 368–382). Bonn, Germany: Psychiatrie Verlag.

Koch, E., Hartkamp, N., Siefen, R. G., & Schouler-Ocak, M. (2008). German pilot study of psychiatric inpatients with histories of migration. *Nervenarzt, 79*, 328–339.

Kofahl, C., Hollmann, J., & Möller-Bock, B. (2009). Gesundheitsbezogene Selbsthilfe bei Menschen mit Migrationshintergrund [Health-related self-help in individuals with a migration background]. *Bundesgesundheitsblatt - Gesundheitsforschung – Gesundheitsschutz, 52*, 55–63.

König, S., Wodarz, N., Unglaub, W., & Johann, M. (2007). Aufmerksamkeitsdefizit/Hyperaktivitätssyndrom (ADHS) bei erwachsenen Drogenabhängigen [ADHD in adults with drug dependence]. *Psychiatrische Praxis, 34*(1), 71–72.

Kornischka, J., Assion, H. J., Ziegenbein, M., & Agelink, M. W. (2008). Psychosoziale Belastungsfaktoren und psychische Erkrankung bei Spätaussiedlern [Psychosocial stress factors and mental illness in ethnic German migrants]. *Psychiatrische Praxis, 35*, 60–66.

Kulis, S., Marsiglia, F. F., & Hurdle, D. (2003). Gender identity, ethnicity, acculturation, and drug use: Exploring differences among adolescents in the southwest. *American Journal of Community Psychology, 31*(2), 167–188.

Murray, C. J. L., Lopez, A. D., Mathers, C. D., & Stein, C. (2001). *The global burden of disease 2000 project: Aims, methods and data sources.* Geneva: World Health Organization. Retrieved from http://www3.who.int/whosis/discussion_papers/pdf/paper36.pdf

Neff, J. A., & Hoppe, S. K. (1992). Acculturation and drinking patterns among U.S. Anglos, blacks, and Mexican Americans. *Alcohol and Alcoholism, 27*(3), 293–308.

Patel., V., Flisher, A. J., & Cohen, A. (2008). Social and cultural determinants of mental health. In R. M. Murray, K. S. Kendler, P. McGuffin, S. Wessely, & D. J. Castle (Eds.), *Essential psychiatry* (4th ed., pp. 419–433). Cambridge, UK: Cambridge University Press.

Penka, S., Heimann, H., Heinz, A., & Schouler-Ocak, M. (2008). Explanatory models of addictive behaviour among native German, Russian-German, and Turkish youth. *European Psychiatry, 23*(1), 36–42.

Randolph, W. M., Stroup-Benham, C., Black, S. A., & Markides, K. S. (1998). Alcohol use among Cuban-Americans, Mexican-Americans, and Puerto Ricans. *Alcohol Health & Research World, 22*(4), 265–269.

Regier, D. A., Farmer, M. E., Rae, D. S., Locke, B. Z., Keith, S. J., Judd, L. L., & Goodwin, F. K. (1990). Comorbidity of mental disorders with alcohol and other drug abuse. Results from the epidemiologic catchment area (ECA) study. *JAMA, 264*, 2511–2518.

Schouler-Ocak, M., Bretz, H. J., Penka, S., Koch, E., Hauth, I., Rapp, M. A., … Heinz, A. (2008). Patients of immigrant origin in inpatient psychiatric facilities. A representative national survey by the psychiatry and migration working group of the German federal conference of psychiatric hospital directors. *European Psychiatry, 23*(1), 21–27.

Schouler-Ocak, M., & Haasen, C. (2008). Sucht und Migration [Addiction and migration]. *Sucht, 54*, 268–270.

Stoy, M., Wrase, J., Heinz, A., & Ströhle, A. (2006). ADHS und Sucht – Untersuchungen mit bildgebenden Verfahren [ADHD and addiction – studies using imaging techniques]. *Sucht, 52*, 386–394.

Strategy Unit. (2004). *Alcohol harm reduction strategy for England.* London: Prime Minister's Strategy Unit.

Szaflarski, M., Cubbins, L. A., & Ying, J. (2011). Epidemiology of alcohol abuse among US immigrant populations. *Journal of Immigrant and Minority Health, 13*(4), 647–658.

Tuna, S. (1999). Entwicklungskrisen und migrationsbedingte Belastungen als Suchgefährdungspotentiale jugendlicher Migranten [Developmental crises and migration stressors as factors of addiction risk in juvenile migrants] as . In R. Salman, S. Tuna, & A. Lessing (Eds.), *Handbuch interkulturelle Suchthilfe. Modelle, Konzepte und Ansätze der Prävention, Beratung und Therapie.* Gießen, Germany: Psychosozial-Verlag.

Westermeyer, J. (2004). Culture and addiction psychiatry. In W. S. Tseng & J. Streltzer (Eds.), *Cultural competence in clinical psychiatry* (pp. 85–106). Washington, DC: American Psychiatric Publishing.

Zeef, A., Salman, R., Krauth, C., Walter, U., & Machleidt, W. (2011). Prävention bei Migranten am Beispiel der Sucht [Prevention in migrants: The example of addiction]. In W. Machleidt & A. Heinz (Eds.), *Praxis der interkulturellen Psychiatrie und Psychotherapie.* Munich, Germany: Elsevier.

Zimmermann, U., Blomeyer, D., Laucht, M., & Mann, K. F. (2007). How gene-stress-behavior interactions can promote adolescent alcohol use: The roles of predrinking allostatic load and childhood behavior disorders. *Pharmacology Biochemistry and Behavior, 86*, 246–262.

Hans-Jörg Assion
LWL-Hospital Dortmund
Marsbruchstraße 179
44287 Dortmund
Germany
E-mail: Hans-joerg.assion@wkp-lwl.org

Chapter 13

Possible Misclassification of Psychotic Symptoms Among Moroccan Immigrants in The Netherlands

Tekleh Zandi

UGGZ-Centraal Institute for Mental Health Care Amersfoort, The Netherlands

Abstract

Various studies in European countries have reported increased incidence rates of psychotic disorders among immigrant groups compared to the native population. Unexpectedly, there are no studies in the literature that evaluate the possibility of different sources of bias related to the cross-cultural validity of the diagnostic instruments. The current study examined whether the incidence rates of psychotic disorders (including schizophrenia) among Moroccan immigrant patients remain increased when a culture-sensitive diagnostic interview is used. We compared the first contact incidence rates of schizophrenia by using a standard and a culturally sensitive version of a diagnostic interview. First contact incidence of schizophrenia among Moroccans was no longer significantly higher than Dutch patients when a culture-sensitive diagnostic procedure was applied.

Keywords: immigrant, psychosis, standardized, diagnosis, schizophrenia, cultural formulation

Introduction

Ever-increasing cultural diversity in Western societies and the culture-specific psychopathological conditions imported by ethnically diverse immigrant groups have caused engendered diagnostic issues to become more complicated. The dilemma of the cultural differences that may influence the manifestations and definitions of various psychiatric disorders has been a matter of discussion for some decades, as is the need to maintain uniform methods and criteria in cross-cultural studies (Kleinman, 1997). Yet there is a trend in international publications to ignore the possibility of misdiagnosis, reporting extremely deviated rates of incidence of different psychopathologies among immigrants. Kleinman questioned the validity of applying diagnostic concepts to different ethnic groups in Western societies and has introduced the term "categorical fallacy" to describe the misclassification that may result when culturally sanctioned idioms of expressing distress are interpreted as diagnosable pathological phenomena (Kleinman, 1980, 1987) (see chapter 7).

Over the last decades, there has been an increasing interest within transcultural psychiatry on the high incidence of psychotic disorders among several immigrant groups. Apart from two published reviews of the literature on the incidence of psychotic disorders among immigrants (Fearron et al., 2006; Hutchinson & Haasen, 2004), two meta-analyses have collected the results of English-language publications in European countries more systematically (Cantor-Graae & Selten, 2005; Bourque, Van der Ven, & Malla, 2011). Different epidemiological studies in the UK consistently reported increased incidence rates of schizophrenia among ethnic minority groups compared to the native population (Harrison et al., 1997; Wessely, Castle, Der, Murray, 1991; Van Os, Castle, Takei, & Murray, 1996; Bhugra & Cochrane, 2001). For instance, the reported relative risk (RR) to develop schizophrenia for the first generation of Caribbean immigrants in the UK ranges from 0.6 (Thomas, Stone, Osborn, Thomas, & Fisher, 1993) to 8.9 (Harrison, Owens, Holton, Neilson, & Boot, 1988). The RR among first-generation West-Africans in the UK was 26.1 (Rwegellera, 1997). Furthermore, in the Netherlands, particularly high rates have been reported among Surinamese and Moroccans (Selten, Veen, & Feller, 2001). According to the study, RR for Moroccan and Surinamese was found to be 4.5 and 3.2, respectively, and for Turkish immigrants this rate was 0.8 (see chapter 1).

Several authors have postulated that cross-cultural biases may have influenced admission rates and diagnostic evaluations among immigrants and thus may have led to an overestimation of the incidence rates among ethnic minorities (Mckenzie, 1999; Littlewood & Lipsedge, 1981; Sashidharan, 1993; Strakowski et al., 1996). Unfortunately, very few studies have been conducted to assess the potential impact of a cultural formulation on diagnostic decisions.

Examinations of two areas of pathology (i.e., hallucinations and dissociative symptoms considering patients' sociocultural contexts) are said to be pivotal in the accurate diagnosis of schizophrenia among culturally divergent patients. In some cultures, such as Moroccan, hearing voices and seeing images or faces of relatives is quite common and not necessarily pathological. Hearing voices may actually be a key presenting symptom of emotional problems, which sometimes is perceived to be related to supernatural events (Al-Issa, 2000; Alsughayir, 1996). Hearing voices, especially if experienced as originating from inside the head, can be a normal experience of thought (Van Gemert, 1998). Thus, the differentiation between traditional, nonpathological idioms of distress and religious experiences and true positive symptoms of psychosis can be very crucial in diagnostic procedures (Rack, 1983; Zarrouk, 1975; Al-Jadiri, 1996; Mezzich et al., 1999).

The second area of possible misinterpretation is that of dissociative experiences. For instance, in Morocco, as in some other areas in Africa, the Middle East, and Asia, people can enter a state of trance or dissociation during religious ceremonies. Many people have either had such an experience themselves or have observed other people in such states. In these regions, sensations of floating above or outside of the body are not necessarily a medical condition, but a religious phenomenon or a culturally appropriate idiom of distress (Van Duijl, Cardena, & De Jong, 2005). In such a state a person experiences that his or her mind and body is taken over by an external force such as a spirit. In many parts of the world witchcraft and possession are idioms of distress and are culturally sanctioned ways of accounting for misfortune and are socially accepted. A "possessed" person may perform actions that are totally out of character. They are sometimes misdiagnosed as schizophrenia and treated as such (Dein, 1997).

These two areas of possible false positive symptoms can be the source of misclassification in epidemiological studies. The American Psychiatric Association recommends using a "cultural formulation" as an aid to assist the proper interpretation of symptoms against the patient's cultural background (APA, 1994). Unfortunately, very few studies have been conducted to assess the potential impact of a cultural formulation on diagnostic decisions.

To address this issue, we designed an incidence study with the aim of examining whether incidence rates of first contact schizophrenic disorders among Moroccan immigrants in the Netherlands remained higher compared to native Dutch population when a culturally sensitive diagnostic interview was used (Zandi et al., 2008). For this purpose we compared the risk of schizophrenia and other psychotic disorders among Moroccans and native Dutch, with a standardized diagnostic assessment and one based on a culturally sensitive adapted version of the same instrument based on cultural formulation. To our knowledge this is the first study to assess the impact of a systematic application of the principles of cultural formulation in the context of a standardized diagnostic interview.

Sample and Study Design

Our study took place in the city of Utrecht, the Netherlands; every patient aged 15 to 54 years who was referred to the mental health services in Utrecht with a suspected psychotic disorder for the first time during two years was screened for eligibility. Within the 2–year study period, a total of 145 patients were registered after having contacted the mental health services with a suspected psychosis (55% native Dutch). Patients with a clear substance-induced psychosis were excluded. Finally, 102 patients (65 males and 37 females) were eligible for the study: 48 native Dutch (52% male), 29 Moroccan (68% male), and 25 with other ethnicities. All native Dutch and Moroccan immigrants are included in this study. All registered Moroccan patients with a suspected psychosis were born in Morocco, and all were considered first generation.

All included patients were interviewed two times: (1) with the standard Dutch version of the Comprehensive Assessment of Symptoms and History (CASH) (Andreasen,

Flaum, & Arndt, 1992); (2) with a modified, culturally sensitive version of the CASH (CASH-CS) (Zandi et al., 2008). The two versions of the instrument were administered in random order within an interval of three weeks.

The Cross-Cultural Adaption of the Standard Diagnostic Interview

The CASH is a semistructured diagnostic interview designed to provide a comprehensive description of phenomenology for patients suffering from a broad range of psychotic disorders, including mood disorders and substance abuse disorders. We modified this diagnostic interview with the purpose of arriving at a culturally sensitive, unbiased interpretation of psychotic symptoms, taking into account the cultural background of Moroccan immigrants, which can determine the content of illness and the way that it is expressed.

The adapted culturally sensitive instrument, which we call CASH-Cultural Supplement (CASH-CS), was developed to differentiate between true positive symptoms of psychosis and other cultural idioms of distress among Moroccan patients (please see the appendix in Zandi et al. 2008).

As a first step in the development of CASH-CS, a number of focus group sessions were held in which each of the CASH items was reviewed for comprehensibility and appropriateness of formulation for use among patients of Moroccan descent. The members of these groups were trained psychiatrists, psychologists, and a translator, all with extensive experience in working with Moroccan patients. Some of them were themselves of Moroccan origin.

One focus of attention was how to differentiate between nonpathological idioms of distress (described in the introduction to this chapter), and true positive symptoms of psychosis. The second area of misinterpretation of symptoms is the presence or absence of depressive symptoms. There is no word for depression in Berber, the most commonly spoken language by Moroccan immigrants in the Netherlands, and admitting to such feelings is a taboo in this culture. A third area was that of dissociative phenomena, which is also discussed in our introduction. For each of these areas we formulated ways to introduce the item, words that could be used to describe the item, and appropriate translations to make sure all items were easy to understand. In addition, guidelines were formulated to make sure the patient would feel fully at ease to freely discuss his or her experiences, without breach of taboos of feeling shame (Zandi et al., 2008).

For both standard CASH and CASH-CS, the medical files of the subjects were screened and if necessary the rater contacted the physician. The culturally sensitive interviews also included an interview with a key informant and the patient to elicit additional cultural background information. A consensus on DSM-IV diagnosis was made based on this information.

Results

Table 13.1 gives an overview of the population at risk and relative risks of all cases where referred to the central reporting office with suspected signs of psychosis during the observation period.

The overall first contact rate for a *suspected psychotic disorder* was 3.0 (95% CI 2.3–3.7) per 10,000 population. This rate was significantly different for native Dutch and Moroccan immigrants: 2.0 (95% CI 1.5–2.7) and 11.9 (95% CI 8.0–17.1) per 10,000 population, respectively. The age- and gender-adjusted RR for Moroccans was 5.6 (95% CI 3.5–9.0).

According to the results obtained from CASH (see Table 13.2), all Moroccan and 84% of native Dutch participants with a possible psychotic disorder were diagnosed with one of the psychotic disorders; 65% of the Moroccan and 51% of the native Dutch participants with a possible psychotic disorder were diagnosed as having schizophrenia.

However, according to data based on CASH-CS, 58% of Moroccan and 86% of Dutch native participants with a possible psychotic disorder were diagnosed to have one of the psychotic disorders, and 15% of the Moroccan patients and 59% of the native Dutch participants with a possible psychotic disorder received a diagnosis of schizophrenia, according to the CASH-CS.

Table 13.1. Adjusted rate ratios for a suspected psychosis for Moroccan immigrants in Utrecht, April 1, 2002 to April 1, 2004.

Sample (*N* = 77)		Person – years at risk, 15–54 years	First contact cases suspected psychosis	Incidence rate[1] (95% CI) suspected psychosis	RR_{adj} (95% CI) suspected psychosis
Moroccan	all	24,334	29	11.9 (8.0–17.1)	5.6 (3.5–9.0)*
	male	12,794	20	15.6 (9.5–24.1)	6.5 (3.6–11.8)**
	female	11,540	9	7.8 (3.6–14.8)	4.4 (2.0–9.6)**
Dutch	all	236,338	48	2.0 (1.5–2.7)	reference
	male	114,930	25	2.2 (1.4–3.2)	reference
	female	121,408	23	1.9 (1.2–2.8)	reference

Notes: [1]Incidence rates are per 10,000; *age- and sex-adjusted; **age-adjusted.

Table 13.2. Comparison of incidence rate, age- and sex-adjusted relative risk ratio, and frequency of psychotic disorders and nonpsychotic disorders according to CASH and CASH-CS

	Study participants (*N* = 63)	All psychotic disorders[1]			Schizophrenic disorders[2]			Nonpsychotic disorders[3]		
		cases (m/f)	incidence rate[4] (95% CI)	RR_{adj} (95%CI)	cases (m/f)	incidence rate (95% CI)	RR_{adj} (95%CI)	cases (m/f)	incidence rate (95% CI)	RR_{adj} (95%CI)
CASH	total	35/22	2.2 (1.7–2.8)		23/13	1.4 (1.0–1.9)		3/3	0. 2 (0.08–0.5)	
	Moroccan	19/7	10.7 (7.0–15.7)	7.9 (4.7–13.5)	14/3	7.0 (4.1–11.2)	7.8 (4.0–15.2)	0/0	0 (0–1.5)	cannot be estimated
	Natives	16/15	1.3 (0.9–1.9)		9/10	0.8 (0.5–1.3)		3/3	0.3 (0.09–0.6)	
CASH-CS	total	28/19	1.8 (1.4–2.4)		15/11	1.0 (0.7–1.5)		10/6	0.6 (0.4–1.0)	
	Moroccan	11/4	6.2 (3.5–15.7)	4.2 (2.3–7.9)	4/0	1.6 (0.4–4.2)	1.5 (0.5–4.3)	8/3	4.5 (2.3–8.1)	23 (8.0–68)
	Natives	17/15	1.4 (0.9–1.9)		11/11	0.9 (0.6–1.4)		2/3	0.2 (0.07–0.5)	

Notes: m/f = male/female; [1] Includes DSM-IV categories schizophrenia, schizophreniform disorder, schizoaffective disorder, delusion disorder, brief psychotic disorder, and psychotic disorder not otherwise specified, and major depressive or bipolar disorder with psychotic features; [2] Includes DSM-IV categories schizophrenia, schizophreniform disorder, and schizoaffective disorder; [3] Includes mood disorders without psychotic features, factitious disorders, and dissociative disorders; [4] Incidence rates are per 10,000 and RRs are adjusted for age and sex.

Discussion

The aim of this study was to investigate whether first contact incidence of schizophrenia and other nonaffective psychotic disorders among Moroccan immigrants would remain higher than among the native Dutch if a culturally sensitive instrument was used instead of a standard diagnostic interview.

In our incidence study the RR 95% CI for broadly defined psychosis, including affective psychosis, was substantially attenuated when a culturally sensitive diagnostic procedure was applied but remained statistically significant (7.9–4.2), while the RR for schizophrenia became nonsignificant (7.8–1.5) (Zandi et al., 2010). Based on the CASH-CS, 42% of the Moroccan patients with a suspected psychotic disorder were found not to be psychotic at all. For the native Dutch patients this occurred only in 14% of cases. The main differences between the outcomes based on the two versions of the CASH resulted from high percentage of Moroccan patients who were reclassified from schizophrenia to nonpsychotic disorders (29%, or affective psychosis 47%).

In our earlier study (Zandi et al., 2008) we presented that the observed differences in agreement among CASH, CASH-CS, and clinical diagnoses were mainly attributable to different scores for positive symptoms and the hierarchy of affective symptoms. In view of the results it looks like additional information by considering the cultural beliefs could appropriately guide psychiatrists in The Netherlands to distinguish the typical idioms of distress among Moroccan patients from psychotic symptoms and to more correctly identify mood symptoms.

It is important to mention that during the observation period no second-generation Moroccan immigrants contacted the central reporting office in Utrecht. This was independent of the type of interview used. Thus, we did not replicate the extremely high relative risks reported in The Hague (Selten et al., 2001; Veling et al., 2006). This cannot be explained by the number for the second-generation Moroccans in Utrecht: the number of person–years at risk for the study period for this group in Utrecht was almost twice as much as for the same period in The Hague. The main reason why we reclassified many patients as nonpsychotic on the basis of the culturally sensitive version of the standardized instrument for the diagnosis was that with this instrument the presence of hallucinatory and delusion-like symptoms among immigrant patients is not automatically interpreted as perception disturbance or thought disorder indicative of psychosis. Likewise, in another study of our research group conducted with Moroccan patients in Casablanca, Morocco (Zandi et al., 2008), hearing voices (mostly animals, a deceased parent, or a voice just calling his name), seeing a strange, dark man, or feeling insects (mostly ants) in the whole body were the most commonly reported symptoms in all patients, regardless of diagnosis. These results might imply that hallucinations and delusions are taken to be indicative of schizophrenia, which is not necessarily the case for patients from other cultural backgrounds (Cochrane & Bal, 1987). Moreover, in the aforecited study of our research team, we showed that diagnoses based on the culturally sensitive version of the CASH displayed much better concordance with diagnoses made by local Moroccan psychiatrists than the standard version of CASH, with substantially lower numbers of schizophrenia cases according to CASH-CS and local clinicians.

The other source of difference between CASH and CASH-CS might stem from the poor recognition of mood symptoms in the Moroccan population with the standard version of the instrument. In the current study, we observed that most of Moroccan patients with putative acute psychotic symptoms had been suffering from mood symptoms for quite a while before asking professional help, usually in combination with one or more of these "psychosis-like" cultural expressions of distress. The reason for this might be that psychotic symptoms as a reaction to distress may be more characteristic in some cultures, while the European equivalent would be different symptoms of depression (Cochrane & Bal, 1987).

A limitation of the current study, or at least a deviation from the study we partly replicated (Selten et al., 2001), is that the background information obtained by key informants was not available for the diagnosis based on the standard CASH. This difference in availability of information, therefore, may explain why we found even higher RRs with the standard CASH than The Hague study (Selten et al., 2001). We think that the method used by them, which was also used in the AESOP (Aetiology and Ethnicity in Schizophrenia and Other Psychoses) incidence study (Fearon et al., 2006) takes away some of the ethnic bias at the level of diagnostic decision making. It cannot preclude misinterpretation of culturally appropriate expressions of distress as signs of psychosis at the time of the interview when symptom ratings are assigned. This may, therefore, still lead to overdiagnosis of schizophrenia in ethnic minorities. However, one could argue that in our study clinicians who used the adapted version of the CASH may have been reluctant to diagnose schizophrenia among Moroccans (Zandi et al., 2008; Selten & Hoek, 2008). In the absence of a gold standard to ascertain which of the two diagnostic procedures renders the most "truthful" results, we have to rely on the results of a follow-up study investigating the possible differences between the two diagnostic procedures in terms of the stability of the diagnoses and the course and outcome of the disorders over an extended period of time (predictive validity). In a 30-month follow-up of the patients in this study, we showed that the prognosis for patients with a schizophrenia diagnosis according to the CASH was significantly better for Moroccan compared to native Dutch patients, whereas the outcome for nonschizophrenic patients according to the CASH was similar for Moroccan and native Dutch patients. In contrast, the prognosis for patients with schizophrenia according to the CASH-CS was very similar in Moroccan and native Dutch patients, whereas the outcome in nonschizophrenic patients according to the CASH-CS was significantly better in Moroccan compared to native Dutch patients (Zandi et al., submitted). These findings indicate that the diagnoses according to the culturally sensitive CASH-CS had better predictive validity than those according to the standard CASH. We therefore feel that the absence of a significant difference between Moroccans and native Dutch patients in the treated incidence of schizophrenia according to a culturally sensitive diagnostic procedure is a valid observation and not the result of some reluctance of the interviewers to apply the diagnosis of schizophrenia to Moroccan patients.

Our study raises the question whether, if not schizophrenia, perhaps the incidence of affective psychosis is increased. However, our incidence study does not warrant a final conclusion on this issue since it was at measuring the incidence of cases where psychotic symptoms are the main presenting feature. The study was not developed to find patients with a primary mood disorder. In fact, cases with a clear affective (nonpsychotic) disorder were excluded from the study. The high numbers of affective psychosis and nonpsychotic disorders among Moroccan patients detected by CASH-CS in this sample is probably a result of a failure to detect affective symptoms at the screening level.

Conclusion

Our study demonstrates the vital importance of knowledge about the cultural background of the patient and the use of the principles of cultural formulation for a valid evaluation of symptoms in ethnic and culturally different populations (Vega, Scribney, Miskimen, Escobar, & Aguilar-Gaxiola, 2006; Arnold et al., 2004; Littlewood & Lipsedge, 1981; Karno, Burnam, Escobar, Hough, & Eaton, 1983). In the current study a culture-sensitive approach resulted in a substantial attenuation of the relationship between immigrant status, and as a consequence the elevated rate of schizophrenia became statistically nonsignificant. However, given the limited sample size, no final conclusion can be drawn about the presence or absence of a difference in incidence rates between native Dutch and Moroccan immigrant patients within the society at large. On the other hand, similar attenuations might have occurred in other immigrant studies that failed to (adequately) adjust for possible cultural bias in the diagnostic process. Misinterpretation of symptoms may have serious consequences on the prescription of potentially beneficial medicine and on the prognosis of this particular patient group. We therefore would like to encourage the use of cultural formulation as a central element in the assessment of the symptoms of psychotic and affective disorders among immigrants with ethnically diverse origins (see chapter 7). Misdiagnosis in psychiatry, particularly in cross-cultural psychiatry, is a complex problem and not only knowledge in different fields is needed to analyze the possible bias but also the link between culture and behavior should take the debate forward.

References

Al-Jadiri, A. (1996). *Hallucinations in chronic schizophrenia*. Paper presented at the VII Pan-Arab Congress of Psychiatry, Kaslik, Lebanon.

Al-Issa, I. (Ed.). (2000). *Al Junun: Mental Illness in the Islamic World*. Madison, CT: International Universities Press.

Alsughayir, Ma. (1996). Public view of the evil eye and its role in psychiatry. A study in Saudi society. *The Arab Journal of Psychiatry,* 7, 152–160.

American Psychological Association. (1994). *Diagnostic and statistical manual of mental disorders* (4th ed.). Washington, DC: APA.

Andreasen, N., Flaum, M., & Arndt, S. (1992). The Comprehensive Assessment of Symptoms and History (CASH): An instrument for assessing psychopathology and diagnosis. *Archives of General Psychiatry, 49*, 615–623.

Arnold, L. M., Keck, P. E., Jr., Collins, J., Wilson, R., Fleck, D. E., Corey, K. B., ... Strakowski, S. M. (2004). Ethnicity and first-rank symptoms in patients with psychosis. *Schizophrenia Research, 67*, 207–212.

Bhugra, D., & Cochrane, R. (Eds.). (2001). *Psychiatry in multicultural Britain*. London: Gaskell.

Bourque, F., Van der Ven, E., & Malla, A. (2011). A meta-analysis of the risk for psychotic disorders among first- and second-generation immigrants. *Psychologic Medicine, 41*, 897–910.

Cantor-Graae, E., & Selten, J. P. (2005). Schizophrenia and migration: A meta-analysis and review. *American Journal of Psychiatry, 162*, 12–24.

Cochrane, R., & Bal, S. S. (1987). Migration and schizophrenia: An examination of five hypotheses. *Social Psychiatry, 22(4)*, 181–191.

Dein, S. (1997). ABC of mental health. Mental health in a multiethnic society. *British Medical Journal, 315*, 473–476.

Fearon, P., Kirkbride, J. B., Morgan, C., Dazzan, P., Morgan, K., Lloyd, T., ... Murray, R. M. (2006). On behalf of the AESOP study group. Incidence of schizophrenia and other psychoses in ethnic minority groups: Results from the MRC AESOP study. *Psychological Medicine, 36*, 1541–1550.

Harrison, G., Glazebrook, C., Brewin, J., Cantwell, R., Dalkin, T., Fox, R., . . . Medley, I. (1997). Increased incidence of psychotic disorders in migrants from the Caribbean to the United Kingdom. *Psychological Medicine, 27*, 799–808.

Harrison, G., Owens, D., Holton, A., Neilson, D., & Boot, D. (1988). A prospective study of severe mental disorder in Afro-Caribbean patients. *Psychological Medicine, 18*, 643–657.

Hutchinson, G., & Haasen, C. (2004). Migration and schizophrenia. The challenges for European psychiatry and implications for the future. *Social Psychiatry and Psychiatric Epidemiology, 39*(5), 350–357. doi: 10.1007/s00127-004-0766-0

Karno, M., Burnam, A., Escobar, J. I., Hough, R. L., & Eaton, W. W. (1983). Development of the Spanish-language version of the National Institute of Mental Health Diagnostic Interview Schedule. *Archives of General Psychiatry, 40*, 1183–1188.

Kleinman, A. (1980). *Patients and healers in the context of culture*. Berkeley, CA: University of California Press.

Kleinman, A. (1987). Anthropology and psychiatry: The role of culture in cross-culture research on illness. *British Journal of Psychiatry, 151*, 447–454.

Kleinman, A. (1997). Triumph or pyrrhic victory? The inclusion of culture in DSM-IV. *Harvard Review of Psychiatry, 4*(6), 343–344.

Littlewood, R., & Lipsedge, M. (1981). Some social and phenomenological characteristics of psychotic immigrants. *Psychological Medicine, 11*(a), 289–302.

Mckenzie, K. (1999) Moving the misdiagnosis debate forward. *International Review of Psychiatry,* II, 153–161.

Mezzich, J. E., Kirmayer, L. J., Kleinman, A., Fabrega, H., Jr., Parron, D. L., Good, B. J., ... Manson, S. M. (1999). The place of culture in DSM-IV. *The Journal of Nervous and Mental Disease, 187*, 457–464.

Rack, P. (1983). *Race, culture and mental disorder*. London: Tavistock.

Rwegellera, G. G. C. (1997). Psychiatric morbidity among West Africans and West Indians living in London. *Psychological Medicine, 7*, 317–329.

Sashidharan, S. P. (1993). Afro-Caribbeans and schizophrenia: The ethnic vulnerability hypothesis re-examined. *International Review of Psychiatry, 5*, 129–144.

Selten, J. P., & Hoek, H. (2008). Does misdiagnosis explain the schizophrenia epidemic among immigrants from developing countries to Western Europe? *Social Psychiatry Psychiatric Epidemiology, 43*, 937–939. doi: 10.1007/s00127-008-0390-5

Selten, J. P., Veen, N., & Feller, W. (2001). Incidence of psychotic disorders in immigrant groups to the Netherlands. *British Journal of Psychiatry, 178*, 367–372.

Strakowski, S. M., Flaum, M., Amador, X., Bracha, H. S., Pandurangi, A. K., Robinson, D., & Tohen, M. (1996). Racial differences in the diagnosis of psychosis. *Schizophrenia Research, 21*, 117–124.

Thomas, C. S., Stone, K., Osborn, M., Thomas, P. F., & Fisher, M. (1993). Psychiatric morbidity and compulsory admission among UK-born Europeans, Afro-Caribbeans and Asians in central Manchester. *British Journal of Psychiatry, 163*, 91–99.

Van Duijl, M., Cardena, E., & De Jong, J. T. (2005). The validity of DSM-IV dissociative disorders categories in south-west Uganda. *Transcultural psychiatry, 42*, 219–241.

Van Gemert, F. (1998). *Ieder voor zich. Kansen, cultuur en criminaliteit van Marokkaanse jongens* [Each for himself. Opportunities, culture, and criminal behavior in Moroccon youths]. Amsterdam: Het Spinhuis.

Van Os, J., Castle, D. J., Takei, N., & Murray, R. M. (1996). Psychotic illness in ethnic minorities: Clarification from the 1991 census. *Psychological Medicine, 26*, 203–208.

Vega, W. A., Sribney, W. M., Miskimen, T. M., Escobar, J. I., & Aguilar-Gaxiola, S. (2006). Putative psychotic symptoms in the Mexican American population: Prevalence and co-occurrence with psychiatric disorders. *Journal of Nervous & Mental Disease, 194*, 471–477.

Veling, W., Selten, J. P., Veen, N., Laan, W., Blom, J. D., & Hoek, H. W. (2006). Incidence of schizophrenia among ethnic minorities in the Netherlands: A four-year first-contact study. *Schizophrenia Research, 86*, 189–193. doi:10.1016/j.schres.2006.06.01

Wessely, S., Castle, D. J., Der, G., & Murray, R. (1991) Schizophrenia and Afro-Caribbeans. A case-control study. *British Journal of Psychiatry, 159*, 795–801.

Zandi, T., Havenaar, J. M., Limburg-Okken, A. G., van Es, H., Sidali, S., Kadri, N., … Kahn, R. S. (2008). The need for culture sensitive diagnostic procedures: A study among psychotic patients in Morocco. *Social Psychiatry Psychiatric Epidemiology, 43*, 244–250.

Zandi, T., Havenaar, J. M., Smits, M., Limburg-Okken, A. G., van Es, H., Cahn, W., … van den Brink, W. (2010). First contact incidence of psychotic disorders among native Dutch and Moroccan immigrants in the Netherlands: Influence of diagnostic bias. *Schizophrenia Research, 119*, 27–33. doi:10.1016/j.schres.2010.02.1059

Zarrouk, E. T. A. (1975). The frequency of visual hallucinations in schizophrenic patients in Saudi Arabia. *British Journal of Psychiatry, 127*, 553–555.

Tekleh Zandi

Tekleh Zandi
UGGZ-Centraal
Institute for Mental Health Care
Amersfoort
The Netherlands
E-mail: t.zandi@ggzcentraal.nl

V. Treatment

Taking Culture Into Account

Chapter 14

Mental Illness Models and Help-Seeking Behaviors Among Turkish Immigrant Patients in Europe

Nazli Balkir

Department of Clinical Psychology and Psychotherapy, Institute of Psychology,
University of Heidelberg, Germany

Abstract

Although Turkish immigrants in Europe are identified as a vulnerable group with respect to higher prevalence rates of mental disorders, numerous studies constantly report that they fall outside the existing mental health care services. In order to provide insights into the underutilization of mental health care services, premature treatment termination, and low treatment adherence among this patient group, an examination of their help-seeking behavior is essential. Therefore, this chapter examines the antecedents of help-seeking behavior among Turkish patients suffering from psychiatric disorders, considering their social and cultural context. Despite modernizing and acculturative influences, studies have demonstrated that culture is a major determinant of Turkish patients' symptom recognition and of how they interpret, make sense, and react to distress, all of which determines the choice of and adherence to treatment. A better understanding of cultural determinants of help-seeking pathways may provide practical solutions for (but not limited to) Turkish immigrant patients' differential utilization of mental health care services and therefore compensate the existing treatment gap. The clinical implications of the findings are discussed.

Keywords: Turkish, immigrants, somatic, symptoms, causal attribution, help seeking, mental health care

Introduction

The demographic profile of the European population is currently far from being homogenous. Migration is a key force in this demographic diversity of the European population, involving 56 million international migrants (Carta, Bernal, Hardoy, & Haro-Abad, 2005). Turkish immigrants form the largest immigrant group in Western Europe, numbering nearly 4 million. The largest number of Turkish immigrant workers is found in Germany, followed by France, The Netherlands, Austria, Belgium, Switzerland, the UK, Sweden, Denmark, Italy, and Norway (Manco, 2004).

Immigrants tend to bring their own values and practices with them as they settle in a new country, and these may be very different from those of the host culture. The adaptation to their new environment creates difficulties that immigrants have to cope with when they integrate new styles and norms of interpersonal relationships, social habits and rules, organization of community services, and so forth, to start a new life in a different culture (Rios, 2008). The psychological effect derived from an adaptive situation of this kind, known as acculturative stress, is added to the difficulties that usually characterize immigration (e.g., loss and bereavement). According to a recent report, the risk of distress in immigrants as compared to natives was found to be 1.0 in Belgium, 1.2 in The Netherlands, 1.4 in Spain, 4.3 in Germany, and 4.7 in France (The State of the Mental Health in Europe, 2004, cited in Carta et al., 2005). Furthermore, several studies indicated that immigration and its related acculturation stress are associated with a higher risk for mental disorders, such as anxiety and depression (e.g., Bhugra, 2003). This might be especially true for Turkish immigrants, as they are the largest but also one of the least integrated groups in Europe (German Federal Office for Statistics, 2008). The strong clash of values places them at a particularly high risk of social isolation and psychological distress compared to immigrants from other parts of Europe and the native population. In support of this, an epidemiological study in Belgium by Levecque, Lodewyckx, and Vranken (2007) demonstrated that immigrants originating from Turkey and Morocco reported significantly higher levels of depression and anxiety in comparison with other European immigrant groups and Belgian natives. Comparably, a recent study conducted in Germany indicated that Turkish patients in general practice showed an increased number of psychological symptoms and a higher rate of mental disorders compared to German patients. Notably, the study also indicated higher rates of mental disorders among Turkish women immigrants (55%) compared to their male counterparts (35%). Most prevalent were anxiety and depressive disorders (Tydecks, Temur-Erman, Schoular-Ocak, & Fydrich, 2009). Likewise, a recent study carried out with a sample of Turkish immigrants in The Netherlands found a higher prevalence rate of minor psychiatric disorders[1] (33.4% in general, 36.1% in females, 27.9% in males) than is normally found in community-based samples. This increased prevalence of depression in female immigrants can be attributed to sex differences in biological and/or psychosocial functioning (Bengi-Arslan, Verhulst, & Crijnen, 2002) (see chapter 1).

In order to minimize the difficulties, compensation of the treatment gap (i.e., the absolute difference between the prevalence of the disorder and the treated proportion of the individuals affected) is essential (Kohn, Saxena, Levav, & Saraceno, 2004).

[1] Minor psychiatric disorders (MPD) are understood as symptoms such as depression, anxiety, fatigue, irritability, insomnia, and memory and concentration deficits (see Harding et al., 1980).

However, despite higher prevalence rates of mental disorders, Turkish immigrants are less likely to seek professional care and exhibit higher drop-out rates and lower rates of treatment compliance than the native population. For instance, studies conducted in Germany provide evidence for lower rates of admission to mental health care services in immigrants compared to the native population (Haasen, Lambert, Yagdiran, & Krausz, 1997). Moreover, language barriers were found to be associated with more frequent involuntary hospital admissions and less speedy release from hospital after regular treatment for Turkish patients (Künzler, Garcia-Brand, Schmauss, & Messer, 2004). A study on service utilization in female immigrants in Amsterdam found that Surinamese, Antillean, Turkish, and Moroccan women made considerably less use of mental health care services than native-born women. It was discovered that immigrant women instead consulted social work facilities and crisis intervention centers for women nearly 1.5 times more often than mental health care services (Ten Have & Bijl, 1999). A similar situation was found in Switzerland. For instance, Lay, Lauber, and Rossler (2005) demonstrated that female Turkish inpatients had higher rates of compulsory admission, were more unlikely to be readmitted, and spent significantly shorter time in hospital compared to female Swiss inpatients. To summarize, these results demonstrate a significant underutilization of mental health services and delayed treatment among (Turkish) immigrants. Thus, a broader understanding of the factors associated with their lower rates of service utilization is necessary.

Numerous studies report service underutilization among Turkish immigrants in Europe, however, it is still not sufficiently understood why many Turkish immigrants are reluctant to use the mental health care system, or what they experience before their encounter with it and during their exposure to it. This is largely because most research on service use in Turkish immigrants has failed to consider the social and cultural context in which help seeking is initiated (McKinlay, 1972). It has been demonstrated that people from all cultures seek help for their suffering based on the meaning their culture ascribes to the suffering (White & Marsella, 1982). A better understanding of cultural determinants of help-seeking pathways might therefore provide insights into ethnic group differences in mental health care utilization.

Cultural Determinants of Help-Seeking Behavior

In this chapter, *help seeking* refers to attempts to maximize well-being or to minimize illness (Saint Arnault, 2009). A comprehensive understanding of help-seeking pathways requires an enlarged scope of the research agenda, beginning with the time when a problem is first recognized. Once a problem is recognized, labeled, and interpreted, the decisions regarding help seeking and the selection of a help provider take place. A large amount of empirical psychological and anthropological literature clearly documents that cultural models determine the perceptual, explanatory, and behavioral options for understanding and responding to illness (e.g., Mechanic, 1972; Fabrega, 1974; Chrisman & Kleinman, 1983). Culture therefore has an extensive influence on all stages of the help-seeking pathway, including recognition (i.e., what to attend to or ignore?), labeling (i.e., what does it mean?), and interpretation of the problem (i.e., what is the cause? how serious is it?), and therefore the choice of treatment provider(s) (i.e., what can be done, who can heal it?) (e.g., Cauce et al., 2002; Bhui et al., 2003; Briones et al., 1990).

Recognition and Labeling: Somatic Symptoms in Turkish Patients

Kirmayer and Sartorious (2007) pointed out that analyses of sensations and symptoms are the pivotal units in understanding illness experience. In their comprehensive work, Hinton and Hinton (2002) denoted that cultural models guide processes of sensation amplification that alter the perception and awareness of arousal sensations. Likewise, Zola (1966, 1973) provided empirical evidence that culture has a significant effect on the recognition of symptoms, which in turn affects health communication. Some cultures are said to have a deep awareness of physiological shifts. Conversely, others are portrayed as paying less attention to bodily sensations but having a more extensive emotional awareness (Saint Arnault, 2009). There is, for instance, a precise separation between physical and emotional experience in Western European languages. In the Turkish language, however, emotional perceptions are figuratively expressed through representations of physical sensations (Nickel et al., 2006) (see chapter 8). Whether physical or emotional, the alterations in an individual's sense of well-being are then said to be cognitively differentiated into the categories of normal or abnormal. A number of psychological and anthropological studies have documented that culture has a profound impact on categorizations of states as normal or abnormal. At this point, normality is assessed through comparisons with the average health status of an individual's reference group. If an abnormal physical or emotional condition is prevalent in the reference group, then an individual is less likely to attribute great significance to it. This categorization regarding normality is what Angel and Thoits (1987) called "first-order categorizations." They argued that the lack of predictive power of most of the large-scale surveys investigating help-seeking behavior among culturally diverse patients is mainly due to the influence of culture on this pre-symptom, which has cumulative effects on the entire help-seeking behavior. There is a lack of empirical studies on the early stages of the illness modeling process in this particular patient population.

Once the physical or emotional change is noticed and referred to as abnormal, second-order categorizations are made in order to determine whether this abnormal state is indicative of an illness (i.e., symptom). Sequentially, a further evaluation is made according to whether the underlying disorder is physical or psychological in nature (Angel & Thoits, 1987). There is some evidence that the organization of symptoms into consistent categories is considerably influenced by folk knowledge. Members of traditional cultures such as the Turkish one may differentiate little between psychological and physical symptoms and therefore experience them in a holistic fashion. Given that emotions also have a physical effect on bodily functions, both physical and emotional symptoms may be viewed as a physical disorder. Individuals with a more "scientific" orientations differentiate between mental and physical types of disorders to a greater degree (Angel & Thoits, 1987; Saint Arnault, 2009). The traditional Turkish, who experience as a physical illness what modern Western medicine recognizes as depression, are a prime example. There is considerable evidence demonstrating a high prevalence of somatic symptoms among this patient group living in Germany (Diefenbacher & Heim, 1994), in the Netherlands (Limburg-Okken 1989), and in Denmark (Mirdal, 1985). Likewise, Schmelling-Kludas, Frfschlin, and Boll-Klatt (2003) reported that the most prevalent psychiatric disorder diagnosed in this population is some type of somatoform disorder (over 60%), which can be interpreted as related to a culturally-patterned perceptual focus on the body rather than a difference in levels of distress (Nickel et al., 2006). In light of the aforementioned facts, Turkish immigrants with their traditional Eastern cultural background might label such psychological distress as somatic illness and present distress as physical illness in medical settings (Karasz, 2005). Given that this particular population hardly relates bodily symptoms to psychoemotional factors, it may be that these patients rarely view psychiatric treatment as an acceptable or valuable tool for recovery. Thus, help seeking among Turkish immigrants is usually organized around the presentation of bodily complaints rather than explicit mention of emotional disturbance or family conflict, and they seek a physical cure in primary care settings. Thus, an overexpression of somatic symptoms should alert physicians to considering the possible existence of minor psychiatric disorders in order to improve patient care (Bengi-Arslan et al., 2002).

Interpretations of Illness: Causal Attributions as a Cultural Product

Further categorizations in the construction of illness meaning involve additional dimensions, such as cause, seriousness, prognosis, and responsibility, in terms of which patients undertake further evaluations of their disorder and thus decide upon an appropriate source for help (Angel & Thoits, 1987). A similar perspective, the explanatory model (EM) introduced by the medical anthropologist Arthur Kleinman (1978), has also directed attention to eliciting the cognitive aspects of patients' understanding of their illness in order to unravel their help-seeking behaviors and responses to clinical interventions.

The EM is the patient's understanding of the cause, severity, and prognosis of an illness, of the expected treatment, and of how the illness affects their life (Kleinman, 1980). In essence, it is the meaning of the illness for the patient affected by it. It has been stated that patients' explanatory models of illness are, to a large extent, culturally determined. These explanations, in turn, are said to set up expectations that influence the ways in which individuals attend to their bodies and the sorts of symptoms they recognize and report to others (Groleau, Young, & Kirmayer, 2006) (see chapter 15).

Causal attributions are suggested to be a pivotal cognitive process in the construction of illness Ems (Kirmayer, Young, and Robbins, 1994). Given that the EMs are said to be coherent with general cultural beliefs about sickness and health care as well as historical and sociopolitical constructs, several anthropological studies have differentiated between Western and non-Western causal beliefs (i.e., causal attributions) about mental distress (Marsella & White, 1982). It has been stated that social and supernatural etiologies are associated with more traditional societies of non-Western cultures whereas natural or patient-centered explanations of distress are more commonly found in Western industrialized societies (Landrine & Klonoff, 1992). For instance, among Europeans, the causes of psychological illness are more likely to be located within the individual, whereas many non-Western and minority cultures cite supra-individual or social relationships as causal (Marsella & White, 1982). Moreover, with the advantage of a medical and social science history that encompasses hundreds of years, a medical agenda is commonly adopted by Western societies to understand and interpret the experience of mental illness. Such an understanding of psychopathology does not exist in traditional Eastern societies. Furthermore, Littlewood and Lipsedge (1997) underlined the historical importance of religion in traditional cultures and its significance for the understanding of mental illness. In support of the aforementioned arguments, a study conducted in rural areas of Turkey revealed that lay beliefs concerning causes of mental illnesses are strongly religious in nature and involve possession by jinns, spiritual entities whose existence is accepted by Islam, sorcery, or the evil eye rather than organic causes (Öztürk & Vamik, 1971). Similarly, a study conducted with Turkish immigrants in Australia revealed two dimensions of causal beliefs distinctly interpretable as natural and supernatural. The findings showed that while beliefs in natural causes (e.g., stress, infections, and organ damage) are more common, beliefs in supernatural causes (e.g., fate, sorcery, mysticism-breaking taboos, disrespect of religious and cultural practices) persist despite modernizing and acculturating influences (Minas, Klimides, & Tuncer, 2007). Additionally, in a study of Turkish psychiatric outpatients in Turkey, Karanci (1986) found that these patients mainly attribute the cause of their disorder to interpersonal conflicts, conflicts within the current family, conflicts in the family of origin, fate and marital problems, personal characteristics, blame on others, and a lack of willpower. In a similar study of psychiatric outpatients in Turkey, a total of seven different dimensions for causal beliefs were revealed, namely conflict with the current family and family of origin, personal characteristics and behaviors, problems with work, interpersonal conflicts, and bad luck. The highest values were obtained for conflict within the current family (Karanci, 1993). By contrast, Townsend (1975) demonstrated in a cross-cultural study that German patients regarded mental illness as biologically determined whereas American patients believed mental illness to be a behavioral phenomenon.

Notably, the findings also suggest that patients' beliefs regarding the cause of their illness play an important role in the organization of effective healing strategies (Hall & Tucker, 1985). It has likewise been suggested that the beliefs people hold regarding their illness have an impact on the decision to seek medical care, adherence to treatment, and adjustment to prognosis (Sensky, 1997). Thus, psychiatric patients who attribute their illness to supernatural agents, witchcraft, and possession by evil spirits are likely to seek help for their problems from traditional healers (Razali, Hasanah, Aminah, & Subramaniam, 1998), whereas, as demonstrated by Foulks, Persons, and Merkel (1986), patients who endorse more medical beliefs about the causes of their illness are more likely to seek help from medical sources and exhibit higher levels of treatment compliance than patients who hold more nonmedical beliefs.

Given that most of the Turkish immigrants in Europe came from rural areas of Turkey, had relatively little education and a strong commitment to Islamic religious practices as well as the extended family, and had (and still have) to deal with an urban and individualistic Western society (Al-Issa & Tousignant, 1997), it may be argued that the underutilization of mental health care services, premature treatment termination, and low treatment adherence among Turkish immigrant patients may be attributed to suh cultural variations in the EM of mental illness. Although there is considerable evidence demonstrating culturally diverse causal attributions among Turkish patients, their link to patients' choice of treatment providers has so far been little investigated.

To address this issue, our research team aimed to explore the ethnic differences in causal beliefs about major depression and whether ethnicity or discrepant causal beliefs are most relevant for decisions regarding an appropriate source of help (Balkir, Arens, & Barnow, 2012). To this aim, a qualitative study design was used based on an EM of illness. Thirty-nine female Turkish immigrant and 27 female German depressive inpatients were interviewed with a semistructured interview protocol regarding their beliefs concerning the factors responsible for their illness (causal beliefs) and the appropriate source of help. A content analysis procedure was employed through focus group discussions to identify and code specific categories within the data. Causal beliefs involved three main domains composed of social (interpersonal versus noninterpersonal), psychological (personality, psychological trauma, etc.), and biological (genetic/neurological, biomedical attributions) factors. Ethnicity was not a significant predictor for adopting social factors as causes. However, Germans, as compared to Turkish patients, were more likely to address psychological and biomedical factors responsible for their health conditions. With regard to treatment, they were far more likely to recommend professional treatment (e.g., psychotherapy, medication, psychoeducation, alternative therapies such as relaxation or occupational therapy) as the most valuable tool for recovery. On the other hand, Turkish patients were more likely than Germans to recommend nonprofessional sources of help (e.g., social support, self initiation) (see Table 14.1). Further, it was revealed that causal beliefs (attribution to psychological and biological factors) mediate the relationship between ethnicity and preference for professional treatment resources (see Figure 14.1). These results indicate that the difference between Turkish and German depressive patients concerning the preference for seeking professional help could be explained by the differences in their beliefs concerning the causes of depression (predominance of psychological and biological attributions in German patients).

Table 14.1. Causal beliefs and treatment preferences among Turkish immigrant and German patients

	Turkish patients (n = 39)	German patients (n = 27)	F/χ^2	p-value
Age (mean)	43.68	43.26	.04	$p > .05$
	2.26	1.49	14.28	$p < .0001$
Causal attributions (%)				
Social	**%68.4**	**%47.8**	**2.55**	**$p > .05$**
Interpersonal (Family & marital conflicts)	%63.2	%8.7	17.38	$p < .0001$
Non-interpersonal (severe working conditions, life burden)	%13.2	%47.8	8.9	$p < .001$
Psychological	**%15.1**	**%60.9**	**13.21**	**$p < .0001$**
Personality	%15.8	%17.4	0.3	$p > .05$
Psychological trauma	%0	%43.5	19.76	$p < .0001$
Biological	**%21.1**	**%60.9**	**9.85**	**$p < .001$**
Genetic/neurological	%2.6	%60.9	26.21	$p < .0001$
Biomedical	%18.4	%26.1	.50	$p > .05$
Treatment preferences (%)				
Professional	**%26.3**	**%91.3**	**24.21**	**$p < .0001$**
Psychotherapy	%13.2	%73.9	22.94	$p < .0001$
Psycho-education	%2.6	%13	2.54	$p > .05$
Medication	%15.8	%43.5	5.68	$p < .05$
Alternative therapies (relaxation or occupational therapy)	%10.5	%17.4	.59	$p > .05$
Non-professional	**%76.3**	**%26.1**	**14.78**	**$p < .0001$**
Social satisfaction	%64.9	%13	15.39	$p < .0001$
Self initiation	%29.7	%17.4	1.15	$p > .05$

Our findings clearly document the gap between popular Turkish lay beliefs about the cause of mental distress, which are said to rely mainly on familial or social conflicts, and the culture of Western medicine, in which mental distress is mainly seen as a result of malfunctioning in or maladaptation of biological and/or psychological processes in addition to social problems. Thus, the Turkish patient group rarely sees professional treatment (e.g., psychotherapy, psychotropic drugs, psychoeducation) as a valuable tool for recovery. Instead, the road to recovery is seen to lie in regaining social harmony within the family and the social environment. Similar empirical

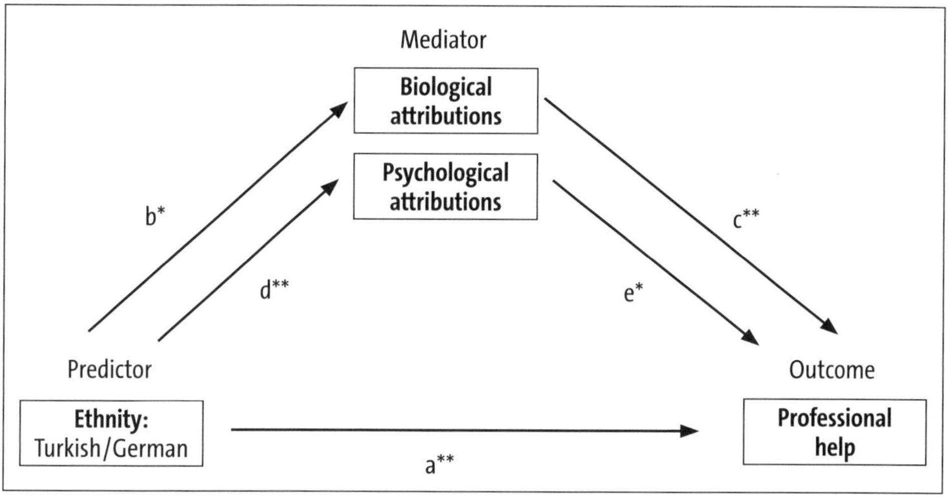

Figure 14.1. Determinants of patients' preference to seek professional help: Ethnicity or discrepant causal beliefs?

Notes: a = (β = 3.61, W = 8.45), $p < .01$; b= (β = 1.99, W = 5.12), $p < .05$; c = (β = 2.94, W = 8.52), $p < .01$; d = (β = 2.04, W = 7 .43), $p < .01$; e = (β = 2.44, W = 6.67), $p < .05$.

evidence supporting this argument is provided by another recent comparative study (Calliess et al., 2007), which illustrated that, overall, the Turkish population reported a less positive attitude toward psychotherapy in comparison to the German population. Turkish immigrants with a less traditional cultural background reported a more positive attitude toward psychotherapy when compared to Turkish immigrants of a more traditional cultural background. Not surprisingly, another study reported that female Turkish immigrants in Amsterdam consulted social work facilities and crisis intervention centers for women nearly 1.5 times more than mental health care services (Ten Have & Bijl, 1999). Although religion, prayer, and spirituality were shown by previous studies to be the key aspects of beliefs about the nature of mental illness and coping styles of the patients in rural areas of Turkey, our research did not reveal any religious aspect of causal beliefs or treatment preferences (Sunter, Guz, Ozkan, & Peksen, 2006; Öztürk & Vamik, 1971). As Kirmayer and Sartorius (2007) also noted, the aforementioned results suggest that these patients are not only seeking mitigation of symptoms but also individually and socially meaningful explanations and psychosocial or spiritual treatment for their illness.

Given that mental illness is perceived to be a result of a disruption in social relationships or in the spiritual realm in most Turkish patients, they usually prefer informal solutions for their mental health problems, such as seeking support from friends or family, rather than from mental health professionals. They may implement religious practices such as praying or work out problems on their own and delay the decision to seek professional assistance until problems have got severe. When Turkish patients finally decide to seek help, they usually prefer contacting nonprofessional sources such as religious healers (Sunter et al., 2006; Röder, 1988), social work facilities, or crisis intervention centers for women (Ten Have & Bijl, 1999). Additionally, it is well-documented that drop-out and premature treatment termination after initial contact with mental health professionals are also common among these patients (Haasen et. al., 1998; Künzler et al., 2004). These findings may suggest that patients sought nonprofessional treatment when they evaluated professional treatment as ineffective. Literature has pointed to the need for culturally competent providers who are able to recognize and share the patient's illness model and present interventions that fit patient expectations (Good & Delvecchio-Good, 1981; Kleinman, 1978; Lin and Lin, 1978; White and Marsella, 1982). It has also been suggested that matching problem conceptualization between service provider and client is crucial to increasing service utilization by minority clients (Zane, Sue, Castro, & George, 1982). Furthermore, empirical evidence suggests that patients are most satisfied when their psychiatrist shares their model of understanding distress and treatment (Callan & Littlewood, 1998). Thus, Turkish patients who have difficulties in initiating and maintaining contact with mental health providers may be more likely to stay in treatment if they encounter such culturally congruent aspects of the care process.

Social Context: Stigma and Emotional Display Rules in Turkish Culture

Alternatively, illness evaluation may also be related to its social significance. For instance, Turkish culture's condemnation of expressing emotional complaints to people who are not members of the family or the close social environment may also influence culture-specific styles of expressing distress (somatic symptoms). Thus, patients may decide that seeking help for emotional problems is simply not a socially appropriate behavior. Moreover, the underreporting of psychological symptoms and somatic presentation may also be related to limited opportunities for the expression of psychosocial distress available to members of traditional collectivistic societies (Arens, Balkir, & Barnow, 2012). Indeed, in a study conducted with somatisizing Turkish inpatients in Germany it was shown that expressions of their emotional distress ranged from open use of culturally traditional expressions to complete avoidance, in which cross norms contributed to emotional suppression (Nickel et al., 2006). A study in Sweden showed that first-generation Turkish immigrants with somatization avoided discussing illness and healing within the family or social contexts in order to avoid causing concern (Bäärnhielm and Ekblad, 2000). By contrast, so-called individualistic and autonomous cultures less frequently use suppression to regulate emotions because of the higher acceptance of psychological problems in these cultures (Haga, Kraft, & Corby, 2009; Butler, Lee, & Gross, 2007; Matsumoto, Yoo, & Fontaine, 2008, Arens et al., 2012). When trust is established with the physician, patients in such cultures may acknowledge significant psychoemotional problems such as marital and family problems (see Figure 14.2 for an overview of the help-seeking process).

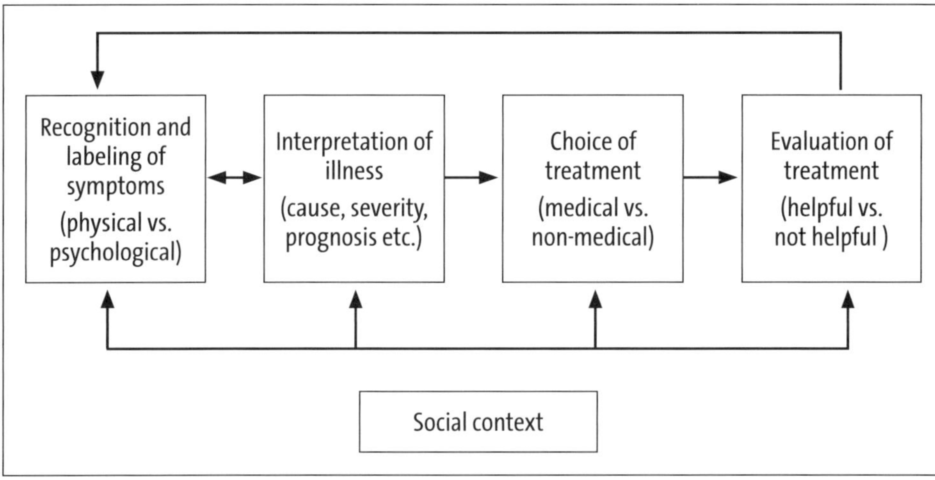

Figure 14.2. Determinants of help-seeking

Conclusions and Clinical Implications

Despite modernizing and acculturating influences, culture is a major determinant of Turkish patients' symptom recognition and of how they evaluate and react to distress, all of which impacts the choice of and adherence to treatment. These findings have several implications for clinical practice.

First, the overexpression of somatic symptoms in Turkish patients may lead to underrecognition and delayed treatment of psychiatric disorders. For various reasons, Turkish patients do not usually report affective symptoms in primary care settings. Physicians therefore often employ diagnostic tests and medical treatments to examine patients' physical complaints (Lipowski, 1990) while psychological diagnosis is often neglected. In order to avoid this, explicitly asking such patients about possible psychological symptoms might be useful. Moreover, eliciting patients' mood symptoms with a culture-sensitive terminology would help to minimize the social and moral stigma attached to mental disorders (Yeung & Kam, 2005).

Second, collectivistic values often held by these patients point toward the importance of addressing person–society conflicts in addition to intra-psychic conflicts and the involvement of family members in the therapy process in order to increase treatment adherence and promote positive treatment outcomes. This highlights the importance of psychosocial treatment in Turkish immigrant patients. Treatment solely relying on medication, without ameliorating personal, familial, or social conflicts, will in many cases probably not lead to the desired outcome.

Third, treatment provideers' openness to multiple explanatory models, including biomedical, psychological, religious, and traditional ones, has been shown to be cricial to enhancing communication with minority patients (Kirmayer & Robbins, 1996). This may involve recognition that while clinicians provide psychological treatment, patients may maintain that what they believe/practice is also effective for their treatment. That is to say, in order to keep these patients in treatment it may be helpful to remain open not only to alternative explanatory models but also to the use of traditional forms of treatment (De Jong, 1994; Razali et al., 1998) (see chapter 15). Finally, increasing communication between primary care settings and mental health care services may facilitate the recognition and treatment of psychiatric disorders, especially in culturally diverse patient groups.

References

Al-Issa, I., & Tousignant, M. (1997). *Ethnicity, Immigration, and Psychopathology.* New York: Plenum Press.

Angel, R. J., & Thoits, P. (1987). The impact of culture on the cognitive structure of illness. *Culture, Medicine, and Psychiatry, 11*, 23–52.

Arens, E. A., Balkir, N., & Barnow, S. (2012). *Ethnic variations in emotion regulation: Do cultural differences end where psychopathology begins?* Manuscript submitted for publication.

Bäärnhielm, S., & Ekblad, S. (2000). Turkish migrant women encountering health care in Stockholm: A qualitative study of somatization and illness meaning. *Culture, Medicine and Psychiatry, 24*, 431–452.

Balkir, N., Arens, E. A., & Barnow, S. (2012). *Determinants of help-seeking among Turkish immigrant and German depressive inpatients. Cultural origin or illness model?* Manuscript in preparation.

Bengi-Arslan, L., Verhulst, F. C., & Crijnen A. A. (2002). Prevalence and determinants of minor psychiatric disorder in Turkish immigrants living in The Netherlands. *Social Psychiatry Psychiatric Epidemiology*, *37*, 118–124.

Bhugra, D. (2003). Migration and depression. *Acta Psychiatrica Scandinavica Supplementum, 418*, 67–73.

Bhui, K., Stansfeld, S., Hull, S., Priebe, S., Mole, F., & Feder, G. (2003). Ethnic variations in pathways to and use of specialist mental health services in the UK. Systematic review. *British Journal of Psychiatry, 182,* 105–116.

Briones, D. F., Heller, P. L., Chalfant, H. P., Roberts, A. E., Aquirre-Hauchbaum, S. F., & Farr, W. F. Jr. (1990). Socioeconomic status, ethnicity, psychological distress, and readiness to utilize a mental health facility. *American Journal of Psychiatry, 147,* 1333–1340.

Butler, E. A., Lee, T. L., & Gross, J. J. (2007). Emotion regulation and culture: Are the social consequences of emotion suppression culture-specific. *Emotion, 7*, 30–48.

Callan, A., & Littlewood, R. (1998). Patient satisfaction: Ethnic origin or explanatory model? *International Journal of Social Psychiatry, 44*, 1–11.

Calliess, I. T., Schmid-Ott, G., Akquel, G., Jaeger, B., & Ziegenbein, M. (2007). Einstellung zu Psychotherapie bei jungen türkischen Migranten in Deutschland [Attitudes towards psychotherapy of young second-generation Turkish immigrants living in Germany]. *Psychiatrische Praxis, 34*, 343–348.

Carta, M. G., Bernal, M., Hardoy, M. C., & Haro-Abad, J. M. (2005). Report on the Mental Health in Europe Working Group (2005): Migration and mental health in Europe (the state of the mental health in Europe working group: Appendix 1). *Clinical Practice and Epidemiology in Mental Health*, 1–13.

Cauce, A. M., Domenech Rodríguez, M., Paradise, M., Shea, J. M., Cochran, B., Srebnik, D., & Baydar, N. (2002). Cultural and contextual influences in mental health help seeking: A focus on ethnic minority youth. *Journal of Consulting and Clinical Psychology, 70,* 44–55.

Chrisman, N. J., & Kleinman, A. (1983). Popular health care, social networks, and cultural meanings: The orientation of medical anthropology. In D. Mechanic (Ed.), *Handbook of health, health care, and the health professions* (pp. 569–590). New York: Free Press.

De Jong, J. T. V. M. (1994). Ambulatory mental health care for migrants in The Netherlands. *Curare, 17,* 5–34.

Diefenbacher, A., & Heim, G. (1994). Somatic symptoms in Turkish and German depressed patients. *Psychosomatic Medicine, 56,* 551–556.

Fabrega, H. Jr. (1974). *Disease and social behavior: An interdisciplinary perspective.* Cambridge, MA: MIT Press.

Foulks, E. F., Persons, J. B., & Merkel, R. L. (1986). The effect of patients' beliefs about their illnesses and compliance in psychotherapy. *American Journal of Psychiatry, 143,* 340–344.

German Federal Office for Statistics. (2008, March 11). Leichter Anstieg der Bevölkerung mit Migrationshintergrund [Small increase in population proportion with a migration background]. [Press release]. Berlin: author.

Good, B. J., & Delvecchio-Good, M. J. (1981). The meaning of symptoms: A cultural hermeneutics model for clinical practice. In L. Eisenberg & A. Kleinman (Eds), *The relevance of social science for medicine* (pp. 165–196). Boston, MA: Reidel.

Groleau, D., Young, A., & Kirmayer, L. J. (2006). The McGill illness narrative interview (MINI): An interview schedule to elicit meanings and modes of reasoning related to illness experience. *Transcultural Psychiatry, 43,* 671– 691.

Haasen, C., Lambert, M., Yagdiran, O., & Krausz, M. (1997). Psychiatric disorders among migrants in Germany: Prevalence in a psychiatric clinic and implications on services and research. *European Psychiatry, 12,* 305–310.

Haga, S. M., Kraft, P., & Corby, E.-K. (2009). Emotion regulation: Antecedents and well-being outcomes of cognitive reappraisal and expressive suppression in cross-cultural samples. *Journal of Happiness Studies, 10,* 271–291.

Hall, L. E., & Tucker, C. M. (1985). Relationships between ethnicity, conceptions of mental distress and attitudes associated with seeking psychological help. *Psychological Reports, 57,* 907–916.

Harding, T. W., De Arango, M. V., Baltazar J., et al. (1980). Mental disorders in primary health care: A study of their frequency and diagnosis in four developing countries. *Psychological Medicine, 10,* 231–241.

Hinton, D., & Hinton, S. (2002). Panic disorder, somatization, and the new cross-cultural psychiatry: The seven bodies of a medical anthropology of panic. *Culture, Medicine & Psychiatry, 26,* 155–178.

Karanci, A. N. (1986). Causal attributions for psychological illness among Turkish psychiatric inpatients and their relationship with hope. *International Journal of Social Psychiatry, 32,* 3–13.

Karanci, A. N. (1993). Causal attributions for illness among Turkish psychiatric out-patients and differences between diagnostic groups. *Social Psychiatry and Psychiatric Epidemiology, 28,* 292–295.

Karasz, A. (2005). Cultural differences in conceptual models of depression. *Social Science & Medicine, 60,* 1625–1635.

Kirmayer, L. J., & Robbins, J. M. (1996). Patients who somatisize in primary care: A longitudinal study of cognitive and social characteristics. *Psychological Medicine, 26,* 937–951.

Kirmayer, L. J., & Sartorius, N. (2007). Cultural models and somatic syndromes. *Psychosomatic Medicine, 69*(9), 832–840.

Kirmayer, L. J., Young, A., & Robbins, J. M. (1994). Symptom attribution in cultural perspective. *Canadian Journal of Psychiatry, 39,* 584–595.

Kleinman, A. (1978). Concepts and a model for the comparison of medical systems as cultural systems. *Social Science and Medicine, 12*(2B), 85–93.

Kleinman, A. (1980). *Patients and healers in the context of culture*. Berkeley, CA: University of California Press.

Kohn, R., Saxena, S., Levav, I., & Saraceno, B. (2004). The treatment gap in mental health care. *Bulletin of World Health Organization, 82*, 858–866.

Künzler, N., Garcia-Brand, E., Schmauss, M., & Messer, T. (2004). Deutschkenntnisse psychiatrischer Patienten anderer Kulturen: Einfluss auf Freiwilligkeit und Dauer der stationären Behandlung [German language skills among foreign psychiatric patients: Influence on voluntariness and duration of hospital treatment]. *Psychiatrische Praxis, 31*(Suppl.1), 21–23.

Landrine, H., & Klonoff, E. A. (1992). Culture and health-related schema. *Health Psychology, 11*, 267– 276.

Lay, B., Lauber, C., & Rossler, W. (2005). Are immigrants at a disadvantage in psychiatric inpatient care? *Acta Psychiatrica Scandinavica, 111*, 358–366.

Levecque, K., Lodewyckx, I., & Vranken, J. (2007). Depression and generalized anxiety in the general population in Belgium: A comparison between native and immigrant groups. *Journal of Affective Disorders*, *97*, 229–239.

Limburg-Okken, A. (1989). Migranten in de psychiatrie [Immigrants and psychiatry]. *Van Loghum Slaterus*, Deventer 31.

Lin, T., & Lin, M. (1978). Service delivery issues in Asian-North American communities. *The American Journal of Psychiatry*, *135*, 454–456.

Lipowski, Z. J. (1990). Somatization and depression. *Psychosomatics, 31*(1), 13–21.

Littlewood, R., & Lipsedge, M. (1997). *Aliens and Alienists. Ethnic Minorities and Psychiatry* (3rd ed.). London: Routledge.

Manco, U. 2004. Turks in Western Europe. Retrieved from www.flwi.ugent.be/cie/umanco/umanco3.htm

Marsella, A. J., & White, G. M. (1982). *Cultural conceptions of mental health and therapy.* Boston, MA: Reidel.

Matsumoto, D., Yoo, S.H., & Fontaine, J. (2008). Mapping expressive differences around the world: The relationship between emotional display rules and individualism versus collectivism. *Journal of Cross-Cultural Psychology*, *39*(1), 55–74.

McKinlay, J. B. (1972). Some Approaches and Problems in the Study of the Use of Services – an Overview. *Journal of Health and Social Behavior, 13*, 115–152.

Mechanic, D. (1972). Social psychologic factors affecting the presentation of bodily complaints. *New England Journal of Medicine, 286,* 1132–1139.

Minas H., Klimidis S., & Tuncer, C. (2007). Illness causal beliefs in Turkish immigrants. *BMC Psychiatry, 7*, 34–44.

Mirdal, G. M. (1985). The condition of "tightness": The somatic complaints of Turkish migrant women. *Acta Psychiatrica Scandinavica, 71*(3), 287–296.

Nickel, M., Cangoez, B., Bachler, E., Mühlbacher, M., Lojewski, N., Müller-Rabe, N., … Nickel, C. (2006). Bioenergetic exercises in inpatient treatment of Turkish immigrants with chronic somatoform disorders: A randomized, controlled study. *Journal of Psychosomatic Research, 61*, 507–513.

Öztürk, O. M., & Vamık, V. D. (1971). The Theory and Practice of Psychiatry in Turkey. *American Journal of Psychotherapy, 25*, 240–271.

Razali, S. M., Hasanah, C. I., Aminah, K., & Subramaniam, M. (1998). Religious-sociocultural psychotherapy in patients with anxiety and depression. *Australian and New Zealand Journal of Psychiatry, 32*, 867–872.

Rios, P. D. (2008). Migration and Psychopathology. *Annuary of Clinical and Health Psychology, 4*, 15–25.

Röder, F. (1988). Die Bedeutung türkischer Heiler (Hodschas) für die allgemeinärztliche Praxis [The importance of Turkish healers for general medical practice]. *Deutsches Ärzteblatt, 85*, 119–120. Saint Arnault, D. M. (2009). Cultural determinants of help seeking: A theoretical model for research and practice. *Theory for Research and Practice. Research and Theory for Nursing Practice, 23*, 259–278.

Schmeling-Kludas, C., Fröschlin R., & Boll-Klatt, A. (2003). Stationäre psychosomatische Rehabilitation für türkische Migranten: Was ist realisierbar, was ist erreichbar? [Inpatient psychosomatic rehabilitation for Turkish immigrants: What is realistic, what can be accomplished?]. *Rehabilitation, 42*, 363–370.

Sensky, T. (1997) Causal attribution in physical illness. *Journal of Psychosomatic Research, 43*, 565–573.

Sunter, A. T., Guz, H., Ozkan A., & Peksen, Y. (2006) The search for non-medical treatment by patients with psychiatric disorders. *Journal of Religion and Health, 45*, 396–404.

Ten Have, M. L., & Bijl, R. V. (1999). Inequalities in mental health care and social services utilisation by immigrant women. *The European Journal of Public Health, 9*(1), 45–51.

Townsend, J. M. (1975). Cultural conceptions, mental disorders and social roles: A comparison of Germany and America. *American Sociological Review, 40*, 239–252.

Tydecks, S., Temur-Erman, S., Schouler-Ocak, M., & Fydrich, T. (2009). Psychische Störungen, psychische Belastungen und soziale Unterstützung bei türkischen Migranten in zwei Berliner Allgemeinarztpraxen [Mental disturbances, mental stress, and social support in Turkish migrants seen in two general medical practice offices in Berlin]. *Zeitschrift für Medizinische Psychologie, 18*, 101–107.

White, G.M., & Marsella, A. J. (1982). Introduction: Cultural Conceptions in Mental Health Research and Practice. In A. J. Marsella & G. M. White (Eds.), *Cultural Conceptions of Mental Health and Therapy* (pp. 3–38). Dordrecht, The Netherlands: Reidel.

Yeung A. S., & Kam, R. (2005). Illness beliefs of depressed Asian Americans in primary care. In A. M. Georgiopoulos & J. F. Rosenbaum (Eds.), *Perspectives in cross-cultural psychology* (pp. 21–36). Philadelphia, PA: Lippincott Williams & Wilkins.

Zola, I. K. 1966. Culture and symptoms: An analysis of patients' presenting complaints. *American Sociological Review, 31*, 615–630.

Zola, I. K. 1973. Pathways to the doctor: From person to patient. *Social Science & Medicine, 7*, 677–689.

Zane, N., Sue, S., Castro, F. G., & George, W. (1982). Service system models for ethnic minorities. In L. Snowden (Ed.), *Reaching the underserved: Mental health of neglected populations* (pp. 229–258). Beverly Hills, CA: Sage.

Nazli Balkir
Department of Clinical Psychology and Psychotherapy
Institute of Psychology
University of Heidelberg
Hauptstraße 47–51
69117 Heidelberg
Germany
E-mail: nazli.balkir@psychologie.uni-heidelberg.de
nazlibalkir@gmail.com

Chapter 15

Training for Overcoming Health Disparities in Mental Health Care

Interpretative-Relational Cultural Competence

Adil Qureshi[1] and Francisco José Eiroa-Orosa[2]

[1]Vall d'Hebron University Hospital, Barcelona, Spain
[2]Autonomous University of Barcelona, Spain

Abstract

Cultural and racial diversity is increasingly becoming a reality in many countries worldwide, to the extent that nearly every mental health professional will treat patients from other countries, cultures, and/or races. Research from both the US and Europe indicates that immigrants and racial minority patients receive a lower quality of care, which may in part be related to a lack of professional competence. Few professional training programs provide trainees with comprehensive preparation for work with racial or cultural diversity. Cultural competence training represents an approach to reducing health disparities framed by culture, diversity, and difference. This article presents an interpretive-relational approach to cultural competence conceptualized as a process of self-introspection rather than knowledge gathering. Disparities are understood to stem from both cultural and racial difference, and to that end, the basic concepts of culture and race are defined and their relationship to health disparities explored. Cultural competence training, it is argued, must strive to provide trainees with the tools necessary to overcome the principle barriers to the provision of quality mental health care, and can do so by focusing on the knowledge, skills, and attitudes necessary for this process. Because of cultural differences in the way in which mental distress is experienced, expressed, and explained, and because of cultural variation in the expectations of both course and treatment, clinicians must develop a knowledge base about these underlying mechanisms. As racial prejudice contributes significantly to health disparities, it is essential that training is provided that effectively works to reduce the negative impact of racial prejudice rather than a narrative focused on its suppression.

Keywords: cultural competence, training, transcultural psychiatry, racial prejudice

Introduction

In the face of cultural and racial diversity that is increasingly the reality in mental health care in much of the world, "cultural competency training" (or some derivative thereof) has become one of the most highly recommended means of addressing the challenges that said diversity presupposes (Bhui, Warfa, Edonya, McKenzie, & Bhugra, 2007; Qureshi, Collazos, Ramos, & Casas, 2008). The need for cultural competency training in psychiatry is very simply a function of the barriers to quality mental health care for ethnic minority and migrant patients. Large-scale research reports carried out in the UK (Department of Health, 2003; Healthcare Commission, 2005) and the US (Institute of Medicine, 2002) and diverse studies in Europe (Lindert, Schouler-Ocak, Heinz, & Priebe, 2008) demonstrate that health disparities are present in the mental health care system (see chapter 1). That is to say, access to mental health services, entry into them, diagnosis, treatment, and adherence are all of a poorer quality for ethnic minority patients and those with a migration background than for the "mainstream" white population.

Research on cultural competence in mental health care is relatively scant (Bhui, et al., 2007; Vega, 2005) due, it would appear, to methodological challenges that pertain to the isolation of the "ingredients" that actually impact treatment outcome (Brach & Fraser, 2000). Two studies indicate that clients who rate their psychotherapists as more culturally competent are more satisfied with the therapy received (Constantine, Kindaichi, Arorash, Donnelly, & Jung, 2002; Fuertes & Brobst, 2002), although in these studies no objective measure for therapist cultural competence was used. Without specific reference to cultural competence, various studies of some form of cultural adaptation in psychotherapy indicate that treatment that is responsive to cultural difference, in the broadest sense, can be more effective than treatment as usual (Bernal, Jiménez-Chafey, & Domenech Rodríguez, 2009). There is no shortage of research indicating that responsiveness and sensitivity to difference enhances treatment, which provides the basis for some of what is presented here. At the same time, almost every competency model is predicated on inferences as to what constitutes cultural competence rather than any clear empirical evidence (Qureshi et al., 2008).

What remains certain, with or without a formalized research base, is that clinicians need to be trained to work with racial and cultural diversity, although as will be suggested below, "all mental health interactions are intercultural." That is to say, it will be argued that the competencies discussed in this chapter are applicable to everyday work as we propose that cultural competence should be conceptualized as a process of self-introspection rather than knowledge gathering. We also contend that the most important barrier to effective care is a poor or compromised therapeutic relationship (Lindert et al., 2008; Qureshi & Collazos, 2011), such that cultural competence training is in the service of developing the capacity to build a solid working alliance with all patients, regardless of cultural or racial background. The same fundamental issues are at play in the work with all patients, even if the disparities diminish as cultural and racial differences between client and clinician diminish. All mental health care is "multicultural," because all people are "cultural," and culture is perhaps best understood subjectively. Each individual has been socialized into a micro-culture, and as such the good clinician is always attending to and able to respond to the particularities of each individual patient, taking context into account; general clinical competence, then, implicitly demands cultural competence.

Some 30 years after Sue et al. published their groundbreaking position paper entitled "Cross-cultural counselling competencies" (1982), there exist a wide array of cultural competence models as well as local training approaches, only some of which have been formally incorporated into the accreditation of professional training programs, as is the case in American psychology under the auspices of the American Psychological Association (Committee on Accreditation, 2005). The recommendations made in this chapter are a response to the continental European context in which cultural competence remains a relatively recent concept and, although recognized as an important component of professional competence, is not, to the authors' knowledge, required for accreditation nor professional licensing. To that end, the discussion of this chapter, although applicable in any sort of training context, is developed with a view to postgraduate, continuing education training.

In the perspective of cultural competence adopted in this chapter, the basic issues of interest in cultural competence training are (1) that there is considerable variation in how a person experiences, expresses, and explains distress as well as in their expectations of treatment, and that (2) clinicians need to be mindful that their preconceptions and prejudices may interfere with their capacity to engage with and "see" the patient. These are applicable in all clinical encounters.

A Note on Terminology

A central yet perhaps underaddressed component of cultural competence is terminological and conceptual; how key terms and concepts are understood largely circumscribes how cultural competence training will be carried out. To that end, in the interests of developing solid training programs, it may be worth exploring some terminological and conceptual conundrums that haunt the field of transcultural psychiatry. The parameters delineating the population of interest itself are rather underspecified, as are the specific variables or factors of relevance. Culture, ethnicity, immigration, race, poverty, minority status, and social exclusion amongst others are germane to transcultural psychiatry and may influence mental health and its treatment, however the specific and differential nature of this influence is explicated, and some, such as race, are hotly contested (Omi & Winat, 1993). Even the specific name of the field is contested (e.g., transcultural or cultural psychiatry; cross-cultural versus cultural psychology; multicultural counseling, etc.), and indeed replete with disagreements as to whether they constitute distinct but overlapping fields of study or rather are like a rose by any other name. Furthermore, the different options listed all focus on culture, which raises the question about race, further confounding the issue.

The concept of health disparities at least as developed in much of the literature, differentiates between two population groupings, one of which is identified as subject to systematic disadvantage in mental health care; "haves" and "have-nots". In the UK and North America, the haves are typically considered to be some variation on "whites" or European Americans whereas the have-nots are generally "ethnic minorities," "people of color," or "Black minority ethnic." On the continent, the haves are the "autochthonous" population and the have-nots are seen to be immigrants. Notwithstanding this differentiation, there are multiple factors related to health disparities that are not reducible to simple and neat categories. Poverty, poor housing, underemployment, irregular immigration status, traumatic experiences, lower education, and other characteristics associated with marginalization are often coincident with immigration or ethnic minority status, but are by no means inherently related. Most categories used in transcultural psychiatry are problematic, replete with both stricter denotations and broader, more enigmatic connotations. For example, in much of Europe, the term "immigrant" implicitly includes poverty and political instability; "culture" on the other hand, tends to be exoticized and essentiallized as the dominion of the "ethnic other" (as if the European mental health professional's culture were in effect the default, and invisible at that). Furthermore, much of the study of culture and mental health implicitly assumes both homogenous and discrete groups. Publications abound that characterize groups according to various dimensions or put them into certain categories ("Counseling Asian Americans" or a recent publication in *Science*, "Differences between tight and loose cultures: A 33–nation study," Gelfand et al., 2011). It is apparently assumed that individuals can be unproblematically identified as a member of a specific "cultural" or "ethnic" group on the one hand, and, on the other hand, that group membership is in some capacity meaningful in that it confers on a given individual certain characteristics. This would be an example of a "totalizing typology" which implicitly confers explanatory power on the group category in question. Such an approach runs the risk of treating group membership as a psychological characteristic on the one hand, and, on the other, assuming that group boundaries are discrete and unproblematic. In this day and age of globalization, neoliberalism, and worldwide migration, the very notion of discrete and homogenous groups is increasingly untenable (Bhugra & Mastrogianni, 2004); in addition, the ever increasing number of "mixed marriages" means that there are more and more people of mixed race and ethnicity, who are clearly not easy to categorize.

For the purposes of this chapter, two broad, contested, and decidedly imperfect constructs will be used in the discussion of cultural competence, namely culture and race. "Culture" itself would appear to be a more palatable construct, in which health disparities are broadly understood to be a function of "cultural differences" in terms of experience, expression, explanation, and expectations related to mental health and its care. "Race", considerably less palatable, is nonetheless increasingly identified as the more basic crucible of disparities, which is related not to any "inner" difference on the part of the patient but rather to differential treatment on the part of society, institutions, and clinicians.

Clarification of these two constructs is central to cultural competence, not simply for conceptual elegance but also because both the specific conceptions themselves and the differential manner of engagement with the two in and of itself will have an impact on how training proceeds and how one will enact cultural competence. To that extent, prior to entering into the relevant competencies, it may be useful to define the two constructs.

Culture

Culture is a highly complex construct, to the extent that anthropologists have extensively debated its meaning, use, and relevance to the extent that some have even called for its abandonment (Brightman, 1995). Given psychology's and psychiatry's penchant for the "scientific method," culture has often been quantified, however, with no consensus as to what sort of variable it might "really" be. For the purposes of cultural competency training, the culture construct is central, and its conceptualization will inevitably impact many aspects of how clinicians view the very complex and fuzzy relationship between culture, the person, and psychopathology. Because of the relative importance of meaning in clinical communication, the following definition of culture is provided:

> A context of more or less known symbols and meanings that persons dynamically create and recreate for themselves in the process of social interaction. Culture is thus the orientation of a people's way of feeling, thinking, and being in the world – their unself-conscious medium of experience, interpretation, and action. As a context, culture is that through which all human experience and action – including emotions – must be interpreted. This view of culture attempts to take into consideration the quality of cultures as something emergent, contested, and temporal, thereby allowing theoretical breathing space for individual and gender variability and avoiding notions of culture as static, homogenous, and necessarily shared or even coherent. (Jenkins, 1996, p. 74)

From this perspective, culture is about how we experience and make sense of the world. At the same time culture is not to be reified, or frozen, or even unified. To that end, the very notion of "knowing" a culture becomes a highly dubious if not counter-conceptual project, precisely because culture is much more a socially given idiographic process, context, or condition than any sort of knowable entity. Culture is of interest for clinicians in the context of one's encounter and interaction with as well as interpretation and sense-making of the world.

Race

Race is a decidedly contested construct, largely because of its historical association with biology and behavior. Few would argue that race is a "real" construct at all, however, there is no agreement as to whether it should stand as a category in the human sciences. With concern about its use to disempower or disadvantage, it is often argued that the construct should be abandoned, yet at the same time, doing so renders it complicated to address racism, as Smedley & Smedley (2005) argue in an article aptly entitled, "Race as biology is fiction, racism as a social problem is real." Because of the very strong indications that racism is a central part of health disparities, replacing it with "ethnicity" appears to serve to divert attention from the issue at hand. To that end, the following definition thematizes the dialectical and political nature of the race construct:

> Race is a dynamic set of historically derived and institutionalized ideas and practices that (1) sorts people into ethnic groups according to perceived physical and behavioural human characteristics; (2) associates differential value, power, and privilege with these characteristics and establishes a social status ranking among the different groups; and (3) emerges (a) when groups are perceived to pose a threat (political, economic, or cultural) to each other's world view or way or life; and/or (b) to justify the denigration and exploitation (past, current, or future) of, and prejudice toward, other groups. (Markus, 2008, p. 654)

Race, then, for our purposes, is strictly a sociopolitical construct, however, a social construct the very existence of which is predicated on power, on control of, and access to resources. To that end, "races" and their delineation are always political.

Background on Cultural Competence Training

The need for cultural competence derives from the existence of health disparities; patients would receive higher quality treatment were specialists to have better competencies. Over the past 30 or so years, a variety of approaches have been taken that have oscillated between a more "race-based" approach and a "culturalist" approach (Carter, 1995; Carter & Qureshi, 1995). Gregg and Saha (2006) make the very powerful point that disparities are due to both, however, it may be that the "race" paradigm is generally eschewed in favor of the culturalist perspective as a means of avoiding the rather more uncomfortable issues related to racism (Helms, 1994; Smith, Constantine, Graham, & Dize, 2008).

The culturalist approach holds that health disparities are largely due to differences in how psychopathology is both expressed and explained. Patients from "other" cultures are misdiagnosed and misunderstood because their manner of living mental distress is distinct from that standard to Western-trained practitioners and to "psychiatry" as a Western phenomenon. The most important manner, then, of reducing disparities from this perspective is by educating clinicians about the ways in which culture influences the experience, expression, and explanation of mental distress along with the expectations regarding treatment, prognosis, and the course of illness. Traditionally, this has often meant focusing on the "cultural characteristics" of the primary patient groups in the region. The race-based approach holds that health disparities are largely due to individual and institutional racism. Patients from "other" races and cultures are misdiagnosed and misunderstood not because of any characteristic proper to the patient but rather due to the prejudiced gaze of the clinician, or, indeed, the sorts of services available. Disparity reduction, then, is not about learning about the culture or race of the patient but rather through a process of introspection and self-awareness, with the goal of reducing the negative impact of racialist thought and behavior.

Cultural Competence Training in a Nutshell

Multicultural counseling competency models, like most competence models, consist of the three domains of (a) knowledge or cognitive competence, (b) skills or procedural competence, and (c) attitudes and beliefs or attitudinal competence. Applied to the two health disparity domains identified, "knowledge" is particularly germane to the culturalist perspective, which demands attention to cultural aspects of experience, expression, and expectations, whereas attitudes are particularly applicable to the race-based approach, which demands attention to racial prejudice. Skills are applicable to both the culturalist and race-based approaches. Cultural knowledge, as Sue and Zane (1987) pointed out, is distal from the clinical encounter, and thus must be effectively applied in order to have any therapeutic value. Identification and modification of racial prejudice

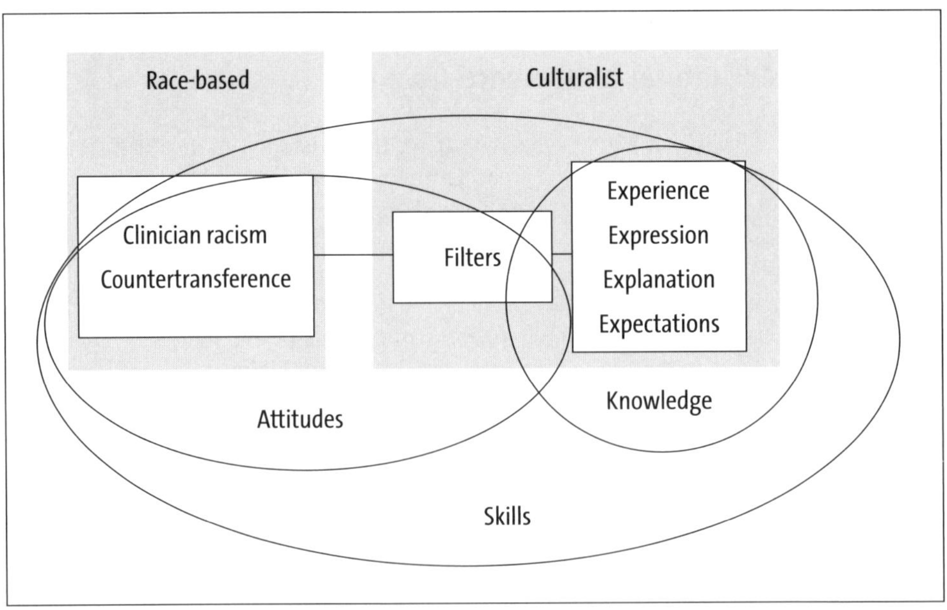

Figure 15.1. Model of cultural competence

and ethnic countertransference is a very demanding and complex process, and requires considerable skill for its realization.

As seen in Figure 15.1, these three domains consist of both culturalist and race-based concepts that are organized on a nonexclusive fashion. Culture includes what we can call the four "exes," all concepts related to subjective experience. Attitudes are more relationally based. Skills involve application of attitudes and knowledge in the clinical context.

An Interpretive Relational Approach

Engagement with a patient in the mental health context is both an interpretive and relational experience. On the one hand, the clinician seeks to make clinical sense of what the patient presents, and on the other, it is through the interaction – the relationship – with the patient that the clinical process advances.

Interpretation and Hermeneutics

Humans are interpretive creatures; we are always already in the process of trying to make sense of our world, implicitly, automatically, and unconsciously, a perspective common to both the cognitive sciences (Banaji, Blair, & Glaser, 1997; von Hecker, 1997) and hermeneutic philosophy (Gadamer, 1960/1997; Weinsheimer, 1985). We approach any new experience, any stimuli, and automatically organize it into a "whole"; we automatically make sense of it.

If asked what they see depicted in Figure 15.2, most people will say they see a square (even if they are aware that there are four 3/4 circles). This is automatic, and

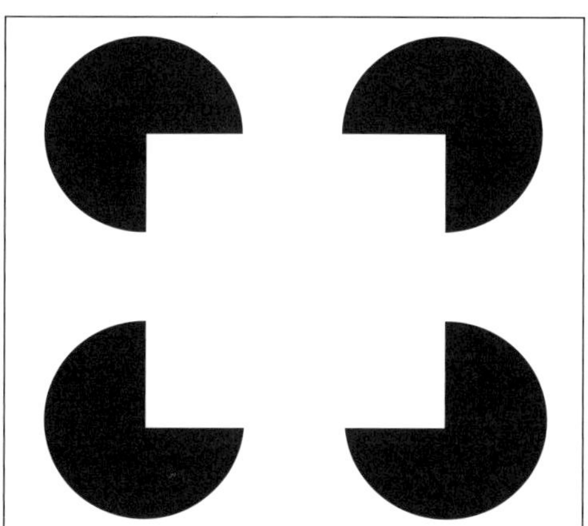

Figure 15.2. What do you see?

it is impossible *not* to see the square that "does not really exist." What this means, then, is that rather than seeing things "as they really are" we see them in accordance with our perceptual devices, on the basis of what is already known, consistent with previous experience. In contrast with his "grand-mentor" Husserl, who maintained that the knowledge of "essences" would only be possible by "bracketing" all previous assumptions (Husserl, 1913), Gadamer (1960) observed that in the human sciences there exists a "prejudice against prejudice," inviting scientists to be aware of their prejudices through analyzing the context in which they work. Rorty (1987) held that we are all of us "ethnocentric," that is, we see and experience the world from our own particular perspective. Research in the area of the "social" brain shows that social interaction (which, by definition, is cultural) influences synaptogenesis and synaptic pruning (Dawson, Ashman, & Carver, 2000) to the extent, for example, that by one year of age the capacity for hearing language sounds is largely determined (Kuhl, 2010) (see chapter 2).

Relational/Dialogical Perspective

In recent years, something of a "relational revolution" has been taking place in the human sciences, in which the self is understood as fundamentally relational or intersubjective, as opposed to the Cartesian notion of a bounded, in effect "separate" individual (Mitchell, 2000; Orange, Atwood, & Stolorow, 2001; Suchman, 2006; Yonteff, 2002), a perspective that is lent support in the neurosciences in the study of the social brain and mirror neurons (Cozolino, 2006).

A relational perspective holds that in effect, as expressed by the African proverb, "I am because we are, and since we are, therefore I am" (Hord & Lee, 1995); human beings are, in effect, a function of their relationships. The idea is that humans are always already in relationships starting from our entry into the world (and some would argue that it is also the case during gestation). The perspective holds that it is not simply internal drives or programming, but rather our relational dynamics and history that in turn impact our being at every level and result in us being who and how we are. As relational creatures, we are not simply onion-like layered selves that have a particular form (though it may be hidden over); how we are at any given moment in time is in part influenced by the specific interaction in which we engage. Hubert Hermans, in his model of the dialogical self (Hermans, Kempen, & Van Loon, 1992), defines the self as extending beyond the skin, to the extent that it includes significant and influential others; i.e., that which I see and experience is, in effect, part of my self.

For mental health care, one of the strong implications of this approach is that, as relational beings, we impact and affect each other. The notion of "mutuality" holds that clinician and patient, in their mutual interaction, have an effect on each other (Aron, 1992; Qureshi, 2005). To that end, a patient's enactments in a clinical encounter will in part be related to the nature of the interaction with the clinician. The clinical process, therefore, requires that the clinician attend not only to the patient's symptom presentation, personal and cultural history, and the like, but also to their own impact on the patient.

As can be seen, the interpretive-relational approach shifts the vision of our clinical work to how we engage with the other, and to that extent cultural competence training will be focalized around the development of the therapeutic relationship. Personal experience as trainers as well as some anecdotal evidence indicates that the biggest barriers to cultural competence may indeed be both personal and contextual. Chun (2010), for example, in her discussion of developing cultural competence training for surgeons, notes that she was surprised by the considerable resistance among trainees that she encountered as she attempted to establish a cultural competency training initiative. It would appear that many people overtly assert that they do not perceive such training as valuable. She also observed that people resisted the self-exploration aspect of the training, apparently related to the fear that they might be labeled as a racist. It would appear that a politically correct context in which there is strong social pressure to exhibit a specific discourse concerning diversity may serve to impede effective training, or even its delivery.

Racism

Research from a variety of fronts indicates that one of the most devastating sources of health disparities is racism (Dovidio et al., 2008; Institute of Medicine, 2002; Kenneth, Klap, Koike, & Sherbourne, 2001; Miranda, McGuire, Williams, & Wang, 2008; Simpson, Krishnan, Kunik, & Ruiz, 2007). Patients receive differential treatment due to their perceived group membership; and in that respect, immigrants and ethnic minorities receive a poorer quality of care. The disparity shows up as poorer access, a lower likelihood of receiving needed care, when treated, reception of poorer quality of care, and elevated rates of involuntary hospitalization and use of restraints (Redmond, Galea, & Delva, 2009; US Department of Health and Human Services, 2001; Whaley, 1998).

That health disparities in mental health care are in part due to racism may appear counterintuitive given that mental health professionals are overwhelmingly liberal in political orientation (Redding, 2001), and as such profess a decidedly antiracist sentiment. At the same time, there is a growing body of research indicating that even the best intentioned among us are prone to respond differently to people of different races and backgrounds, showing a preference for people "like themselves" and greater discomfort faced with those whose appearance is distinct (Dovidio, Gaertner, Kawakami, & Hodson, 2002; Dovidio, Kawakami, & Gaertner, 2002; Greenwald, Poehlman, Uhlmann, & Banaji, 2009; Nail, Harton, & Decker, 2003).

Research in the area of aversive racism (Dovidio, 2001; Dovidio, Gaertner et al., 2002) and implicit attitudes (Banaji, et al., 1997; Greenwald, et al., 2009) differentiate between behavior that is under explicit or conscious control and that which is not. A pencil-and-paper instrument that assesses racism is under conscious control, as is any verbalized expression of attitudes. In the mental health profession in particular and in most Western democracies in general, overt expressions of racism are considered to be both personally and socially repugnant. At the same time, and despite the best of intentions, most people express an own-group preference and discomfort and differential treatment of people from racial groups "different" from their own. In effect, our cognitive and emotional processes are impacted by our own histories of socialization in cultures, which denigrate immigrants and ethnic minorities in contradistinction to majority group members, who are depicted as capable and meritorious. The various tests of unconscious racism developed over the past decade or so utilize reaction time, skin conductance, and other physiological indicators that are beyond conscious control (e.g., the Implicit Association Test, accessible online at the Project Implicit website, http://projectimplicit.net). A growing body of research, although still small, nevertheless strongly indicates that despite our liberal bent, mental health professionals are as prone to implicit racism as anyone else (Boysen, 2009; Penner et al., 2010; van Ryn & Fu, 2003).

Two related and useful concepts are those of "racial microaggressions" and racial or ethnocultural countertransference. The former concerns behaviors or statements made, in general, by majority group members that are experienced by a person from a minority as offensive or hurtful, whereas for the perpetrator the behavior is viewed as benign (Harris, 2008; Sue, Capodilupo, & Holder, 2008; Sue et al., 2007). In the mental health context researchers have begun to chronicle the ways in which clinicians unwittingly "aggress" against their ethnic minority patients (Constantine, 2007; Sue et al., 2007). Included are comments such as "you are a credit to your race," minimization of the patient's experience of racism, a "color-blind" response to the patient ("I do not notice a person's race, rather who they are as a person"). To that end, a growing body of research associates a color-blind stance on the therapist's part with lower levels of perceived empathy (Burkard & Knox, 2004) and cultural competence (Beutler, 1981).

Countertransference has a psychoanalytic conceptual basis, however, as applied to racial and cultural difference, it simply refers to any clinician reactions that are not related to the patient him- or herself. Given that racial difference is rife with uncomfortable associations, particularly for liberal clinicians, it is posited that we compensate for the discomfort provoked by race-related material by transferring onto the patient a response that is less threatening (Altman, 1999; Comas-Diaz & Jacobsen, 1991; Gorkin, 1996; Holmes, 2001). What this means is that we lose sight of the patient and respond to our projections, even though these may be overtly benign, for example, responding to the patient's culture with considerable interest ("oh, I just love [fill in the blank] culture, it is so interesting").

What all of this means is that our attitudes have a tremendous impact on our clinical work with immigrant and ethnic minority patients, to the extent that the American Psychological Association in its *Guidelines on Multicultural Education, Training, Research, Practice, and Organizational Change for Psychologists*, states:

> Psychologists are encouraged to recognize that, as cultural beings, they may hold attitudes and beliefs that can detrimentally influence their

> perceptions of and interactions with individuals who are ethnically and racially different from themselves. (American Psychological Association, 2003)

Addressing race and prejudice in training is complicated, in large part because of the very strong societal taboo that exists concerning race and racism. It is not only the case that we are prejudiced, but also that we live in a society in which discussion of "race" is highly controversial, to the extent that many people insist that race does not exist and must not be discussed. From the perspective of training in cultural competence, semantics are important to the extent that they hinder or help in the exploration of and attention to racist and other beliefs.

Cultural Competence Training and Race

One of the pitfalls of antiracism training has been that it has adopted a moral-ideological perspective, in which trainees are told that they are racists and must adopt a nonracist approach (Bennett & Keating, 2009). The impact of such an approach more often than not is to provoke a highly defensive reaction and a rift between the trainee and trainer; the former feels attacked whereas the latter acts as a crusader.

The research reviewed, combined with the interpretive or hermeneutic approach (Christopher, 2001), demonstrates that having prejudices is not "bad," but rather simply part of the human condition. That is to say, training is not about adopting a certain moral stance but rather striving toward maximizing clinical competence. To that end it is recommended that trainers adopt a collaborative, nonjudgmental, and supportive stance, providing trainees with a forum in which to express and explore frustrations, difficulties, and fears associated with race and culture.

Effectively addressing such issues in the training context demands the creation of a nonthreatening environment in which trainees feel safe to express their "true" feelings. This, in turn, demands that the trainers themselves have engaged in and indeed are engaging in a similar process. One approach is that of the "lab," a sort of group process in which trainees are invited to explore their feelings and reactions related to "diversity" (Carter, 2003). A process orientation means that participants are encouraged to explore and process their feelings and thoughts with an eye to understanding how they interfere with clinical work.

Cultural Filters: Attitudes and Humility; Knowledge

From the hermeneutic perspective, we see and experience the world on the basis of what we already know, through our interpretive filters. Although much of biomedicine has long staked a claim to "objectivity" and "evidence-based" practices, this stance is increasingly questioned (Haraway, 1988; Howard, 1991). If indeed it is the case, as argued here, that experience is culturally circumscribed, then it follows that our interaction with the world is always "from our point of view"; that a "bird's-eye" view is simply the perspective of a bird (and not how things *really are*). Following this line, then, comes the central notion that our experience of and interaction with the world is very much a function of what could be termed our cultural filters, sometimes called worldviews, cultural values, psychological constructs, value orientations, or narratives (Frankl, 1977; Kelly, 1955; Kirmayer, 2007; Koltko-Rivera, 2004).

Taken from this perspective, the Western-trained psychiatrist or psychologist will "see" the immigrant patient both from their perspective as a "Westerner" and as a psychiatrist or psychologist. Similarly, Nancy Andreasen (2007) recently lamented that psychiatrists are trained to "see" mental disorders on the basis of the DSM checklist rather than "see" the patient phenomenologically, or as a whole person; our training and the overall perspective taken therein circumscribes how we "see" the patient.

Thus from the very outset, it becomes essential that trainees are willing to accept their "situatedness," their ethnocentrism, that they see things from a particular perspective, which may constitute the truth in a particular professional context, but not the Truth as it "really is." Indeed, it is worth noting that the quest for the Truth and the assumption that the Truth can be accessed by way of the correct application of the best practice, are themselves cultural values.

The need for perspectivality is all the more pronounced given the "play" of culture. Knowledge, in the cultural competence model presented here, is primarily related to the how, or at least possible "hows," rather than any concrete "whats." Thus specific "knowledge" about a given culture *may* be useful, however, only if deployed in a culturally competent manner. Knowing about the general impact on different facets of life as related to mental health and its care can provide a useful framework through which one can make sense of things. It is worth noting that as clinicians we can be aware that culture impacts experience, expression, and explanation of mental illness and distress *in general*, but we cannot know "how" or even "what" only knowing a person's cultural membership. It makes no sense to say that "Nigerians experience anxiety in such and so a way," or that "Germans express social stress in such and so a way." What we can say is that a given individual's experience is culturally circumscribed, something that I need to take into consideration as I attempt to diagnose and treat this patient.

Experience

In a rather provocative statement, metaphor commentators Lakoff and Johnson (1980) argue that we never experience "the things themselves," but rather do so culturally:

> [...] *every* experience takes place within a vast background of cultural presuppositions [...] Cultural assumptions, values, and attitudes are not a conceptual overlay, which we may or may not place upon experience as we choose. It would be more correct to say that all experience is cultural

> through and through, that we experience our "world" in such a way that our culture is already present in the very experience itself (p.57).

Second-order cybernetics from Heinz von Foerster (1981) could be useful to understand this concept. According to this author, "a brain is required to write a theory of a brain." In other words, whether we realize it or not, when we analyze others we implicitly analyze ourselves.

The current perspective on the interrelationship between nature and nurture, on the cultural or social brain provides further weight to this perspective. By now it would appear that we know that our experience impacts our biology, just as our biology impacts our experience. What this means is that experience itself is cultural, or to put it another way, there is no such thing as pure experience, and our experience is just that – our experience (see chapter 2).

Expression

How we express ourselves, our emotion, our distress, even our psychopathology is in large part related to cultural norms (Furst, 2002; Katz et al., 1988). It has been reasonably well established that "idioms of distress" are culturally circumscribed (see chapter 8). Once again, this is not to say that there is, for example, a "Spanish way of expressing fear," but rather that what we consider normative for the expression of emotion or distress is exactly that, normative within a particular group. In psychiatry we are alert for "flat affect," "anhedonia," "emotional lability" and a discrepancy between affect and speech content. All of these involve cultural norms, that is, what may be "flat affect" for the emotionally volatile Spaniard may be normative emotional expression for the even-keeled and stoic Swede, if we may succumb to stereotypes for illustrative purposes.

Not only the intensity of expression but also the content of expression is culturally circumscribed. In the West, where the Cartesian mind-body dualism is the norm, psychological expression of distress is pretty much standard. In many parts of the world, however, there is no such dualism, and distress is simply distress, with no clear division between somatic and psychic (Kirmayer & Groleau, 2001).

What constitutes a symptom and how that symptom is related to a given mental disorder also comes into play. In the DSM-IV an appendix includes "Culture bound syndromes" such as *ataque de nervios, koro*. These, along with, some would argue, disorders such as anorexia nervosa or borderline personality, comprise culture-specific symptom–pathology matches and constellations that are not universal (Mezzich et al., 1999) (see chapter 7).

Clearly, there is no way to ascertain a priori how anyone will express their distress, and making sense of said expression is not necessarily all that easy, particularly in the face of cultural difference. No recipe book is available; however, the culturally competent clinician will interpret the expression of distress taking into consideration the possible cultural variation therein.

Explanation

As experience and expression of emotion and distress varies cross-culturally, it follows that the explanations that are given for why distress is experienced do as well (Bhui & Bhugra, 2002; Dinh & Groleau, 2008). How a patient explains what is happening to them will in large part depend on their worldview. Although there are clear cross-cultural tendencies, one need not travel far – perhaps down the hall – to find different explanatory models (see chapters 8 and 14). Indeed, in Western mental health we see biological, psychological, social, and systems explanations with greater or lesser degrees of convergence. That is to say, once again it is not that culture *x* uses a supernatural explanation for mental distress whereas culture *y* uses a social one, rather, it is a question of tendencies that show specific patterns (McCabe & Priebe, 2004).

This would appear to be all the more pronounced across cultures, such that the source of the problem is viewed very differently. Given the variation in cultural values, and given the modernist paradigm (in which psychiatry is soundly situated), it follows that many patients hold divergently different views on the source, cause, and even nature of their distress.

Perhaps the most relevant here for training are two related issues. One is that a person who says that he or she is ill due to the position of the planets, a hex, or having been near things that lurk in the dark, the evil eye, and so on is not necessarily crazy, simple minded, gullible, or any such thing, but rather may well be accounting for mental distress in a culturally normative way.

The second is that what constitutes a symptom in the DSM-IV may not in another culture. That is to say, the combination of a supernatural-based explanation and expression may appear to be symptomatic of mental illness, whereas it is simply a culturally normative expression and explanation of a nonpathological life situation.

Expectations

What people expect about their interaction with the mental health professional, the nature of the treatment, and the course of the "problem" can vary considerably, and largely as a function of cultural difference. The very notion of a weekly office visit in which the patient talks about their personal problems with a stranger is itself specific to a particular cultural context.

There is an increased attention to both patient- and relationship-centered care (Suchman, 2006), in which the therapeutic relationship is viewed as collateral and constituted by patient and clinician collaboration, although consistent with the antihierarchical and power differential values endemic in many contemporary therapeutic approaches. This tendency runs decidedly against the grain for many from more hierarchical and authoritarian cultures, for example, to the extent that patients have been known to insist on referring to the psychologist as "doctor," eschewing the use of first names, and questioning the utility of talking, of a focus on insight, exploration of emotions, experience, and the like (Sue, Ivey, & Pederson, 1996). Many patients specifically expect that their psychologist or psychiatrist will provide them with advice and concrete suggestions – after all, they are the experts – as to how they can reduce their distress and live more effective lives.

Expectations about the course of the distress, which are often intimately related to the explanation or understanding of the basis of the distress, can also vary. From a medical perspective, in which illness is a function of some sort of internal biological or psychological dysfunction, the presence of symptomatology at any given moment is not necessarily indicative of an absence of the disease entity; remission does not equal cured. From a supernatural perspective, this is not necessarily the case; absence of symptoms in a given moment most likely indicates an absence of possession, hex, and so forth. What this means, then, is that a patient whose expectation and understanding of distress diverges from that of Western biomedicine may discontinue treatment not because they "lack insight" or are "resistant," but rather because of cultural difference.

Training Issues in the Context of the Cultural Context of Experience, Expression, Explanation, and Expectations

The central premise concerning the four exes is that culture fundamentally circumscribes how a person experiences and makes sense of his or her distress. A postmodern or relativist perspective would train clinicians to understand that a supernatural explanatory model is as valid as a psychiatric one. Although this may make heuristic sense, in our daily clinical work we are not shamans or mystics but Western-trained mental health professionals, meaning that we operate from a fundamentally distinct epistemic paradigm. The challenge, then, is to adopt what Rorty (1986) calls a "benign" ethnocentric attitude. To that end, trainees must learn to appreciate the broad variety of possible ways of experiencing, expressing, and explaining mental distress without opening their minds so much, that, as Rorty laments, their "brains fall out" (p. 526).

The central challenge is one of self-awareness, of excavating one's epistemic filter such that one has a sense of "where one is coming from," while at the same time having the capacity to differentiate between psychopathology and culturally normative behavior. There is no easy way out of this conundrum, precisely because what is normal for one person may be downright strange for another. This does not mean, however, that the strange is simply "cultural" – such a stance of extreme relativism can result in severe underdiagnosis. Yet at the same time, there is a very clear risk of overdiagnosis if cultural variation is not taken into consideration.

Cultural Competency Training, Political Correctness, and Stress

In much of the European context, most clinicians' first contact with cultural competence training may well be postgraduate, once they are working in the field. Given the nature of mental health budgets, this all too often also means that they are working under considerable stress, with a high patient load. When a high patient load is combined with patients coming from other countries and cultures, this can exponentially increment the resultant stress and lead to burn-out.

All too often, the training context is one in which the trainers are implicitly or explicitly proffering the message that they are "less racist," more "culturally on the ball," and so forth, than the trainees. The trainer often comes across as holier-than-thou, spews forth politically correct cant to such an extent and with such fervor that what trainees end up learning is to abide by the cant, by the politically correct narrative. Although this may be vaguely coherent from an institutional demand for compliance with state mandates, it is at best ineffective and at worst counterproductive. The danger of such an approach is that it creates a distance between trainer and trainee, in which the latter is being told (a) that they are "bad" for having racist thoughts or feelings, and that (b) prejudices must be eliminated completely. Evidently, such an approach is rarely effective. It may change the explicit behavior, however, the implicit attitudes do not change. What may come up here is that trainers are no more free from prejudice than anyone else. To that end, trainers must always adopt a dose of cultural humility (Tervalon & Murray-Garcia, 1998) and recognize that no-one is prejudice-free, that we always respond from our subjective perspective, and that simply spouting the right words only operates at the explicit level and the real change is represented by implicit behavior change, not just external. This is all to underscore the importance of the creation of an open, safe, comfortable, and collaborative learning environment.

Participants need to feel safe, feel that it is acceptable for them to express their thoughts and feelings. If the message is that political correctness rather than sincerity is what gets valued, then there is little hope of much progress. Getting beyond the prejudice against prejudice is essential; what is important is recognition and acceptance that all of us experience and interpret the world through our own (prejudiced) filters, and as such the key first step is acknowledgment of this. Therefore, the issue is not that we "should not be prejudiced" but rather that we need to be open to how we engage with the world and actively strive to recognize and reduce the play of prejudice in our intercultural encounters.

Conclusions

The main job of the trainer is to create a safe, open space in which dialogue can flow freely, in which participants do not feel judged and are not afraid to express feelings and opinions that may run counter to those that are socially normative. Our experience as trainers shows that even the most politically committed clinician is at least somewhat ambivalent about these issues, and sharing this ambivalence with colleagues who are committed to providing their patients with a high quality of care is liberating. The discourse then shifts from one of "I shouldn't feel like this" to "OK, given that I sometimes feel like this, what can I, as a clinician, do to improve the services I provide?"

Cultural competence, as discussed in this chapter, is more concerned with how the clinician interacts with patients than with what they know about patients' cultures. It is argued that effective clinical care, particularly when working with patients from diverse backgrounds, demands self-awareness and as such self-exploration. Exploration and interrogation of prejudices allows clinicians greater freedom by which they can become aware of and therefore alter those prejudices that impede effective clinical care. Cultural competence is not an endpoint but rather a process; not something to be achieved, but rather, in the spirit of cultural humility, an orienting paradigm that allows us to be more effective clinicians.

References

Altman, N. (1999). Psychoanalytic perspective on clinical work in the inner city. In H. Kaley, M. N. Eagle, et al., *Psychoanalytic therapy as health care: Effectiveness and economics in the 21st century* (pp. 257–271). Hillsdale, NJ: Analytic Press, Inc.

American Psychological Association. (2003). Guidelines on multicultural education, training, research, practice and organizational change for psychologists. *American Psychologist, 58*(5), 377–402.

Andreasen, N. C. (2007). DSM and the death of phenomenology in America: An example of unintended consequences. *Schizophr Bull, 33*(1), 108–112.

Aron, L. (1992). Interpretation as expression of the analyst's subjectivity. *Psychoanalytic Dialogues: The International Journal of Relational Perspectives, 2*(4), 475–507.

Banaji, M. R., Blair, I. V., & Glaser, J. (1997). Environments and unsconscious processes. In R. S. Wyer (Ed.), *The automaticity of everyday life: Advances in social cognition* (vol. 10, pp. 63–74). Mahwah, NJ: Erlbaum.

Bennett, J., & Keating, F. (2009). Training to redress racial disadvantage in mental health care: Race equality or cultural competence? *Journal of Public Mental Health, 8*(2), 40–46.

Bernal, G., Jiménez-Chafey, M. I., & Domenech Rodríguez, M. M. (2009). Cultural adaptation of treatments: A resource for considering culture in evidence-based practice. *Professional Psychology: Research and Practice, 40*(4), 361-368.

Beutler, L. E. (1981). Convergence in counseling and psychotherapy: A current look. *Clinical Psychology Review, 1*(1), 79–101.

Bhugra, D., & Mastrogianni, A. (2004). Globalisation and mental disorders. *British Journal of Psychiatry, 184*, 10–20.

Bhui, K., & Bhugra, D. (2002). Explanatory models for mental distress: Implications for clinical practice. *British Journal of Psychiatry, 181*, 6–7.

Bhui, K., Warfa, N., Edonya, P., McKenzie, K., & Bhugra, D. (2007). Cultural competence in mental health care: A review of model evaluations. *BMC Health Services Research, 7*, 15.

Boysen, G. A. (2009). A review of experimental studies of explicit and implicit bias among counselors. *Journal of Multicultural Counseling and Development, 37*, 240–249.

Brach, C., & Fraserirector, I. (2000). Can cultural competency reduce racial and ethnic health disparities? A review and conceptual model. *Medical Care Research and Review, 57*(4 suppl), 181–217.

Brightman, R. (1995). Forget culture: Replacement, transcendence, relexification. *Cultural Anthropology, 10*, 509–546.

Burkard, A., & Knox, S. (2004). Effect of therapist color-blindness on empathy and attributions in cross-cultural counseling. *Journal of Counseling Psychology, 51*, 387–397.

Carter, R. T. (1995). *The influence of race and racial identity in psychotherapy: Toward a racially inclusive model*. New York: Wiley.

Carter, R. T. (2003). Becoming racially and culturally competent: The racial-cultural counseling laboratory. *Journal of Multicultural Counseling and Development, 31*(1), 20–30.

Carter, R. T., & Qureshi, A. (1995). A typology of philosophical assumptions in multicultural counseling and training. In J. G. Ponterotto, J. M. Casas, L. A. Suzuki, & C. M. Alexander (Eds.), *Handbook of multicultural counseling.* (pp. 239–262). Thousand Oaks, CA: Sage.

Comas-Diaz, L., & Jacobsen, F. M. (1991). Ethnocultural transference and countertransference in the therapeutic dyad. *American Journal of Orthopsychiatry, 61*, 392–402.

Committee on Accreditation. (2005). *Guidelines and principles for addreditation of programs in professional psychology*. Washington, DC: American Psychological Association.

Constantine, M. G. (2007). Racial microaggressions against African American clients in cross-racial counseling relationships. *Journal of Counseling Psychology, 54*(1), 1–16.

Constantine, M. G., Kindaichi, M., Arorash, T. J., Donnelly, P. C., & Jung, K.-S. K. (2002). Clients' perceptions of multicultural counseling competence: Current status and future directions. *Counseling Psychologist, 30*, 407–416.

Cozolino, L. (2006). *The neuroscience of human relationships: Attachment and the developing social brain*. New York: Norton.

Christopher, J. C. (2001). Culture and psychotherapy: Toward a hermeneutic approach. *Psychotherapy: Theory, Research, Practice, Training, 38*(2), 115–128.

Chun, M. B. J. (2010). Pitfalls to avoid when introducing a cultural competency training initiative. *Medical Education, 44*, 613–620.

Dawson, G., Ashman, S. B., & Carver, L. J. (2000). The role of early experience in shaping behavioral and brain development and its implications for social policy. *Development and Psychopathology, 12*, 695–712.

Department of Health. (2003). *Inside outside: Improving mental health services for black and minority ethnic communities in England*. London: author.

Dinh, N. M., & Groleau, D. (2008). Traumatic amputation: A case of Laotian indignation and injustice. *Cult Med Psychiatry, 32*, 440–457.

Dovidio, J. F. (2001). On the nature of contemporary prejudice: The third wave. *Journal of Social Issues, 57*(4), 829–849.

Dovidio, J. F., Gaertner, S. L., Kawakami, K., & Hodson, G. (2002). Why can't we just get along? Interpersonal biases and interracial distrust. *Cultural Diversity and Ethnic Minority Psychology, 8*(2), 88–102.

Dovidio, J. F., Kawakami, K., & Gaertner, S. L. (2002). Implicit and explicit prejudice and interracial interaction. *Journal of Personality and Social Psychology, 82*(1), 62–68.

Dovidio, J. F., Penner, L. A., Albrecht, T. L., Norton, W. E., Gaertner, S. L., & Shelton, J. N. (2008). Disparities and distrust: The implications of psychological processes for understanding racial disparities in health and health care. *Social Science & Medicine, 67*, 478–486.

Drummond, J. J. (1988). Modernism and postmodernism: Bernstein or Husserl? [Feature]. *The Review of Metaphysics, 42*, 275–300.

Frankl, V. E. (1977). *...trotzdem Ja zum Leben sagen: Ein Psychologe erlebt das Konzentrationslager* [... affirming life in spite of all: A psychologist's experience of the concentration camp]. Munich, Germany: Kösel.

Fuertes, J. N., & Brobst, K. (2002). Clients' ratings of counselor multicultural competency. *Cultural Diversity and Ethnic Minority Psychology, 8*, 214–223.

Furst, L. R. (2002). *Idioms of distress: Psychosomatic disorders in medical and imaginative literature*. Albany, NY: State University of New York Press.

Gadamer, H. G. (1960). *Wahrheit und Methode. Grundzüge einer philosophischen Hermeneutik* [Truth and method: Outlines of philosophical hermeneutics]. Tübingen, Germany: J. C. B. Mohr.

Gadamer, H. G. (1997). *Truth and method* (J. Weinsheimer & D. G. Marshall, Trans., 2nd ed.). New York: Crossroad. (Original work published 1960)

Gelfand, M. J., Raver, J. L., Nishii, L., Leslie, L. M., Lun, J., Lim, B. C., … Yamaguchi, S. (2011). Differences between tight and loose cultures: A 33–nation study. *Science, 332*(6033), 1100–1104.

Gorkin, M. (1996). Countertransference in cross-cultural psychotherapy. In R. M. P. Foster, M. Moskowitz, & R. A. Javiev (Eds.), *Reaching across boundaries of culture and class: Widening the scope of psychotherapy* (pp. 159–176). Northvale, NJ: J. Aronson.

Greenwald, A. G., Poehlman, T. A., Uhlmann, E. L., & Banaji, M. R. (2009). Understanding and using the implicit association test: III. Meta-analysis of predictive validity. *Journal of Personality and Social Psychology, 97*(1), 17–41.

Gregg, J., & Saha, S. (2006). Losing culture on the way to competence: The use and misuse of culture in medical education. *Academic Medicine, 81*, 542–547.

Haraway, D. (1988). Situated knowledges: The science question in feminism and the privilege of partial perspective. *Feminist Studies, 14*, 575–599.

Harris, R. S. (2008). Racial microaggression? How do you know? *American Psychologist, 63*, 275–276; discussion 277–279.

Healthcare Commission. (2005). *Count me in: Results of a national census of inpatients in mental health hospitals and facilities in England and Wales*. London: Healthcare Commission, Mental Health Act Commission & Care Services Improvement Partnership/National Institue for Mental Health in England.

Helms, J. E. (1994). How multiculturalism obscures fracial factors in the psychotherapy process. *Journal of Counseling Psychology, 41*, 162–165.

Hermans, H. J., Kempen, H. J., & Van Loon, R. J. (1992). The dialogical self: Beyond individualism and rationalism. *American Psychologist, 47*(1), 23–33.

Holmes, D. E. (2001). Race and countertransference: Two "blind spots" in psychoanalytic perception. In D. E. Scharff (Ed.), *The psychoanalytic century: Freud's legacy for the future* (pp. 251–268). New Westminster, BC: The Other Press.

Hord, F. L., & Lee, J. S. (1995). *I am because we are: Readings in black philosophy*. Boston, MA: University of Massachusetts Press.

Howard, G. S. (1991). Culture tales. A narrative approach to thinking, cross-cultural psychology, and psychotherapy. *Am Psychol, 46*, 187–197.

Husserl, E. (1913). Ideen zu einer reinen Phänomenologie und phänomenologischen Philosophie. Erstes Buch: Allgemeine Einführung in die reine Phänomenologie [Thoughts on pure phenomenology and phenomenological philosophy. Volume one: General introduction to pure phenomenology] . *Jahrbuch für Philosophie und phänomenologische Forschung, 1*, 1–323.

Institute of Medicine. (2002). *Unequal treatment: Confronting racial and ethnic disparities in healthcare*. Washington, DC: National Academies Press.

Jenkins, J. H. (1996). Culture, emotion, and psychiatric disorder. In C. F. Sargent & M. Thomas (Eds.), *Medical anthropology: Contemporary theory and method* (pp. 71–87). Westport, CT: Praeger.

Katz, M. M., Marsella, A., Dube, K. C., Olatawura, M., Takahashi, R., Nakane, Y., … Jablensky, A. (1988). On the expression of psychosis in different cultures: Schizophrenia in an Indian and Nigerian community. *Culture, Medicine and Psychiatry, 12*, 331–355.

Kelly, G. A. (1955). *The psychology of personal constructs*. New York: Norton.

Kenneth, K., Klap, R., Koike, A., & Sherbourne, C. D. (2001). Ethnic disparities in unmet need for alcoholism, drug abuse, and mental health. *American Journal of Psychiatry, 158*, 2027–2032.

Kirmayer, L. J. (2007). Psychotherapy and the cultural concept of the person. *Transcultural Psychiatry, 44*, 232–257.

Kirmayer, L. J., & Groleau, D. (2001). Affective disorders in cultural context. *The Psychiatry Clinics of North America, 24*, 465–478.

Koltko-Rivera, M. E. (2004). The psychology of worldviews. *Review of General Psychology, 8*(1), 3–58.

Kuhl, P. K. (2010). Brain mechanisms in early language acquisition. *Neuron, 67*, 713–727.
Lakoff, G., & Johnson, M. (1980). *Metaphors we live by*. Chicago, IL: University of Chicago Press.
Lindert, J., Schouler-Ocak, M., Heinz, A., & Priebe, S. (2008). Mental health, health care utilisation of migrants in Europe. *European Psychiatry, 23*(Suppl 1), 14–20.
Markus, H. R. (2008). Pride, prejudice, and ambivalence: Toward a unified theory of race and ethnicity. *American Psychologist, 63*, 651–670.
McCabe, R., & Priebe, S. (2004). Explanatory models of illness in schizophrenia: Comparison of four ethnic groups. *The British Journal of Psychiatry, 185*(1), 25–30.
Mezzich, J. E., Kirmayer, L. J., Kleinman, A., Fabrega, H. J., Parron, D. L., Good, B. J., ... Manson, S. M. (1999). The place of culture in DSM-IV. *The Journal of Nervous and Mental Disease, 187*, 457–464.
Miranda, J., McGuire, T. G., Williams, D. R., & Wang, P. (2008). Mental health in the context of health disparities. *American Journal of Psychiatry, 165*, 1102–1108.
Mitchell, S. A. (2000). *Relationality: From attachment to intersubjectivity*. Hillsdale, NJ: Analytic Press.
Nail, P. R., Harton, H. C., & Decker, B. P. (2003). Political orientation and modern versus aversive racism: Tests of Dovidio and Gaertner's (1998) integrated model. *Journal of Personality and Social Psychology, 84*, 754–770.
Omi, M., & Winat, H. (1993). On the theoretical status of the concept of race. In C. McCarthy & W. Crichlow (Eds.), *Race, identity, and representation in education*. New York: Routledge.
Orange, D. M., Atwood, G. E., & Stolorow, R. D. (2001). *Working intersubjectively: Contextualism in psychoanalytic practice*. Hillsdale, NJ: Analytic Press.
Penner, L. A., Dovidio, J. F., West, T. V., Gaertner, S. L., Albrecht, T. L., Dailey, R. K., & Markova, T. (2010). Aversive racism and medical interactions with black patients: A field study. *Journal of Experimental Social Psychology, 46*, 436–440.
Project Implicit. (2011). *Project Implicit*. Retrieved from https://implicit.harvard.edu/implicit/
Qureshi, A. (2005). Dialogical relationship and cultural imagination: A hermeneutic approach to intercultural psychotherapy. *Am J Psychother, 59*(2), 119–135.
Qureshi, A., & Collazos, F. (2011). The intercultural and interracial therapeutic relationship: Challenges and recommendations. *International Review of Psychiatry, 23*(1), 10–19.
Qureshi, A., Collazos, F., Ramos, M., & Casas, M. (2008). Cultural competency training in psychiatry. *Eur Psychiatry, 23 Suppl 1*, 49–58.
Redding, R. E. (2001). Sociopolitical diversity in psychology: The case for pluralism. *American Psychologist, 56*(3), 205–215.
Redmond, M. L., Galea, S., & Delva, J. (2009). Examining racial/ethnic minority treatment experiences with specialty behavioral health service providers. *Community Mental Health Journal, 45*(2), 85–96.
Rorty, R. (1986). On ethnocentrism: A reply to Clifford Geertz. *Michigan Quarterly Review, 25*, 525–534.
Rorty, R. (1987). Science as solidarity. In J. S. Nelson, A. Megill, & D. N. McCloskey (Eds.), *The rhetoric of the human sciences: Language and argument in scholarship and public affairs* (pp. 38–52). Madison, WI: University of Wisconsin Press.
Simpson, S., Krishnan, L., Kunik, M., & Ruiz, P. (2007). Racial disparities in diagnosis and treatment of depression: A literature review. *Psychiatric Quarterly, 78*(1), 3–14.
Smedley, A., & Smedley, B. D. (2005). Race as biology is fiction, racism as a social problem is real: Anthropological and historical perspectives on the social construction of race. *American Psychologist, 60*(1), 16–26.
Smith, L., Constantine, M. G., Graham, S. V., & Dize, C. B. (2008). The territory ahead for multicultural competence: The "spinning" of racism. *Professional Psychology: Research and Practice, 39*(3), 337–345.

Suchman, A. L. (2006). A new theoretical foundation for relationship-centered care. *Journal of General Internal Medicine, 21*(S1), S40–S44.

Sue, D. W., Bernier, Y., Durran, A., Feinberg, L., Pedersen, P. B., Smith, E. J., & Vasquez-Nuttall, E. (1982). Position paper: Cross-cultural counseling competencies. *The Counseling Psychologist, 10*, 45–52.

Sue, D. W., Capodilupo, C. M., & Holder, A. M. B. (2008). Racial microaggressions in the life experience of black Americans. *Professional Psychology: Research and Practice, 39*, 329–336.

Sue, D. W., Capodilupo, C. M., Torino, G. C., Bucceri, J. M., Holder, A. M., Nadal, K. L., & Esquilin, M. (2007). Racial microaggressions in everyday life: Implications for clinical practice. *American Psychologist, 62*, 271–286.

Sue, D. W., Ivey, A. E., & Pederson, P. B. (1996). *Theory of multicultural counseling and therapy*. Pacific Grove, CA: Brooks/Cole.

Sue, S., & Zane, N. (1987). The role of culture and cultural techniques in psychotherapy: A critique and reformulation. *American Psychologist, 42*(1), 37–45.

Tervalon, M., & Murray-Garcia, J. (1998). Cultural humility versus cultural competence: A critical distinction in defining physician training outcomes in multicultural education. *Journal of Health Care for the Poor and Underserved, 9*(2), 117–125.

US Department of Health and Human Services. (2001). *Mental health: Culture, race and ethnicity – A supplement fo mental health: A report of the Surgeon General*. Rockville, MD: US Department of Health and Human Services, Public Health Service, Office of the Surgeon General.

Van Ryn, M., & Fu, S. S. (2003). Paved with good intentions: Do public health and human service providers contribute to racial/ethnic disparities in health? *Am J Public Health, 93*(2), 248–255.

Von Foerster, H. (1981). *Observing Systems*. Seaside, CA: Intersystems Publications.

Von Hecker, U. (1997). How do logical inference rules help construct social mental models? *Journal of Experimental Social Psychology*, *33*, 367–400.

Vega, W. A. (2005). Higher stakes ahead for cultural competence. *General Hospital Psychiatry, 27*, 446–450.

Weinsheimer, J. C. (1985). *Gadamer's hermeneutics: A reading of Truth and Method*. New Haven, CT: Yale University Press.

Whaley, A. L. (1998). Racism in the provision of mental health services: A social-cognitive analysis. *American Journal of Orthopsychiatry, 68*(1), 47–57.

Yonteff, G. (2002). The relational attitude in Gestalt therapy theory and practice. *International Gestalt Journal, 25*(1), 15–34.

Adil Qureshi
Servei de Psiquiatria
Hospital Universitari Vall d'Hebron
CIBERSAM
Departament de Psiquiatria
Universitat Autònoma de Barcelona
Passeig de la Vall d'Hebron, 116
08035 Barcelona
Spain
E-mail: asfqureshi@gmail.com

Chapter 16

Integration of Immigrants in Psychiatry and Psychotherapy

Experiences and Concepts in Germany and Europe

Wielant Machleidt[1], Eckhardt Koch[2], Iris T. Calliess[1], Renate Schepker[3], Marc Ziegenbein[1], Marcel G. Sieberer[1], and Ramazan Salman[4]

[1] Department of Psychiatry, Social Psychiatry and Psychotherapy, Hanover Medical School, Germany
[2] Department of Psychiatry and Psychotherapy, Vitos Giessen-Marburg, Germany
[3] Department of Child and Aldolescent Psychiatry and Psychotherapy, ZfP Südwürtemberg, Ravensburg, Germany
[4] Ethno-Medical Center, Hannover, Germany

Abstract

Migration is a growing phenomenon throughout the world, including Germany and elsewhere in the EU. This massive movement of people has implications for health and consequently for health care professionals. Immigrants are not a homogenous group and their health is usually affected by the conditions under which they travel and the social conditions in which they live in the receiving country. In particular, the mental health care system in Europe is not sufficiently prepared for this challenge. In this chapter, we aim to give examples of good clinical practice and recommendations for preparing the mental health care services for immigrants in Germany and Europe.

Keywords: immigrants, mental health care, cultural competence, transcultural psychiatry

Introduction

Improving mental health care services and outcomes for immigrant and refugee groups is a common challenge for mental health systems in Europe. Various studies have consistently reported increased rates of mental disorders, underutilization of mental health care services, poorer care outcomes, and diminished satisfaction with services in these groups across Europe (see chapters 1 and 14). Germany is becoming more diverse every year as immigration is currently the key force in population growth. Although population size and rate of increase may differ between individual parts of the country, all of them will have to meet the challenge of providing mental health services to their multicultural population and develop mental health promotion strategies that improve the mental health status of these diverse groups.

Correspondingly, European immigration policy, German immigration law, and the policy for cross-cultural openness in the German health care system provide a general framework for the integration of immigrants with mental disorders. In a country such as Germany, with legally regulated migration, this is not a question of a one-sided adjustment on the part of the immigrant population to fit in with the existing health care system but, rather, of mental health care professionals also making a contribution to the opening up of and improvement in all areas of the care system, including the field of psychiatric/psychotherapeutic care, to help meet the needs of the immigrant population. This is to be achieved by a mutual process of growth in competence and increasing trust with the aim of providing immigrants with the same quality care and successful treatment as received by the native population (Machleidt, 2002; Machleidt, Salman, & Calliess, 2006).

Over the last decade in particular, there have been numerous encouraging initiatives toward more openness in the psychiatric/psychotherapeutic care system in Germany at local, state, and federal levels. Helpful groundwork for this has been provided by the services of the churches and those of charitable organizations particularly concerned with migration. The significance of care provision for mentally ill immigrants has become a topic for professional health organizations and academic institutions at scientific congresses and vocational training events. This has led to a considerable improvement in the intensity and quality of research concerning migration. As a result, awareness regarding the importance of psychiatric/psychotherapeutic care for immigrants has been raised among a wider range of professionals as well as the general public.

The Sonnenberg Guidelines

The 12 Sonnenberg Guidelines (see Table 16.1) form the basis of an initiative for the improvement in psychiatric/psychotherapeutic care provision for immigrants and for the integration of immigrants suffering from mental illness into the society of the German Federal Republic (Machleidt, 2002). The guidelines were formulated and adopted in November 2002 at a symposium on migration held by the international work group at Haus Sonnenberg/Oberharz, and aim to provide orientation for health professionals in the fields of psychiatry, psychosomatics, and psychotherapy.

These guidelines state the requirements for the psychological–medical care of immigrants, along with instructions for their application. They will be laid out in detail in the following sections.

Table 16.1. The 12 Sonnenberg Guidelines on requirements for psychiatric/psychotherapeutic care for immigrants

1. Integration of immigrants into the services of low-threshold regular psychiatric-psychotherapeutic care, including culture-sensitive and culture-competent treatment concepts.
2. Multicultural treatment teams in all professional groups in psychiatry, with a recruitment policy favoring persons with a migration background and additional language competencies.
3. Employment of trained interpreters as translators and cultural mediators to work both face-to-face and over the phone.
4. Community-based cooperation between regular psychiatric care services, general practitioners, and migration, social, and other expert services as well as key members of the various groups, organizations, and associations for immigrants. Special services for immigrants to meet particular regional requirements.
5. Participation of users and their relatives in the planning and organization of services.
6. Improved information for immigrants by means of handouts in their native language on regional, community-based psychiatric, clinical, and outpatient care services, and medical care providers.
7. Training and continuing education for various psychiatric/psychotherapeutic professionals concerning transcultural psychiatry (diagnostics, understanding of illness, and culture-based treatment approaches) and including language training.
8. Intensifying prevention programs for the mental health of children and adolescents from immigrant families.
9. Supporting the formation of self-help groups with or without professional assistance.
10. Ensuring quality standards for expert witnessing of immigrants in the context of criminal, civil (right of asylum), and social law.
11. Establishing transcultural psychiatry in the curricula of academic teaching.
12. Initiation of research projects on the mental health of immigrants and their treatment.

Guideline 1: Integration of Immigrants Into Care Services

The Attitude of the Therapist

A prerequisite for an open approach to immigrants is a positive social attitude and an accepting and interested attitude of a socially competent therapist working in the psychiatric/psychotherapeutic infrastructure. Above and beyond political and social development, comprehension of the psychology of migration and its processes concerning identity formation, acculturation, religiosity, racism, and so forth are helpful to this end (see chapter 15).

Commissioners for Integration and Migration in Institutions

A variety of working parties (working party for migration and public health of the representatives of the federal government responsible for migration, refugees, and integration; working party "psychiatry and migration" of the federation of chief physicians in psychiatry and psychotherapy) advocate the creation of special commissioners in hospitals to deal adequately with the specific requirements of immigrants. In doing so the following principles should be observed:

1. As a leadership role, cultural openness is a top-down procedure
2. Selected appointment of staff with a migration background
3. Cultural sensitivity during care is required from all members of staff, not just from those with a migration background
4. Ongoing advanced and further education

According to the national plan for integration (Bundesregierung, 2007) the improvement of health care for immigrants also requires:

1. Services oriented to requirements
2. Cross-cultural standard care
3. Interdisciplinary networking
4. Provision of appropriate points of access
5. Database security

Commissioners for integration appear to be well suited to implementing these requirements. Their responsibilities include the improvement of communication and the exchange of information with immigrant groups as well as the improvement of public relations, the impact on the organization of the concern, and the setting up of internal hospital statistics about patients with a migration background. Their further duties involve the establishment of a pool of interpreters, the translation of relevant documentation, special consultation hours, and information events. Thus, the responsibilities of a commissioner for integration include several of the demands formulated in the Sonnenberg Guidelines. Furthermore, Internet and intranet material should also reflect the interests of patients with a migration background. Internal vocational and further education should involve all professional groups and culturally sensitive nursing care should also be stressed in nursing schools (Gün, 2009).

Centers of Competence

Cross-cultural centers play an important role in the removal of barriers to access in the sense of providing "good practice."

Ethno-Medical Center Hanover

The role of the Ethno-Medical Center (EMZ) Hanover is to facilitate the integration of immigrants into the German health care system. The EMZ functions as a moderating, interlocked, and integrating health service. It contributes to the integration of immigrants into the health care system and offers support to professionals in the health and social services in their care work. Important areas of responsibility for the EMZ (see www.ethno-medizinisches-zentrum.de; website in German) are:

- Projects for illness prevention and health promotion "with immigrants for immigrants" (MIMI): Native-language health education campaigns with mediators, among other things, on topics in mental health (e.g., addiction and depression)
- Providing interpreters for the social and public health care sectors
- Further training for qualified personnel, training courses, conferences
- Projects for social-psychiatric, psychosomatic, and psychotherapeutic care
- EU health projects

Active networking has developed a tightly knit and sustainable system for culturally sensitive health promotion and prevention. Through its commitment, the EMZ is an "intermediary between the cultures."

Social-Psychiatric Competence Centers for Migration

The Social-Psychiatric Competence Centers for Migration (SPKoM) in the state of North Rhine-Westphalia (NRW) have developed a brief on culturally sensitive approaches for the treatment of ethnic minority patients intended to help overcome discrimination against those patient groups within the health care system. Above all, they should act as publicists of cross-cultural competence in the psychiatric care system. Some of their important tasks are:

- Grouping together previous experience, networking, and coordination of services, increasing the skills of staff in cross-cultural competence, supporting the formation of self-help groups
- Creating public awareness concerning the psychiatric problems of immigrants and formulation of guidelines and quality standards for their psychosocial care

So far, five of the seven Social-Psychiatric Competence Centers for Migration planned in NRW have taken up work (Landschaftsverband Rheinland, 2008).

Guideline 2: Multicultural Treatment Teams

Multicultural treatment teams predicate that therapeutic interventions require culturally competent care delivery for ethnic minority clients to protect their distinctive cultural orientations. Reflection on the "foreign view" is as indispensable as an inner readiness to practice multilingualism. For a good and effective therapist–patient relationship, the acquisition of cross-cultural competence and cultural sensitivity is just as useful as reflection on one's own cultural dependence in feeling, perception, and thought. Therefore, cultural diversity in multicultural therapy teams can be viewed as a characteristic of quality.

Guideline 3: Employment of Psychologically Trained Interpreters

The regional organization of interpretation services and the special training of translators as culture and language mediators (e.g., EMZ Hannover) have clearly proved their worth in the field of psychiatry and psychotherapy. Some large clinics have, for instance, established an in-house interpretation service, whereas telephone interpretation services are well suited for ad-hoc availability. However, such services are rarely available at present. As an alternative approach, some clinics have successfully introduced language training into their treatment options, mostly for native speakers of Russian or Turkish, aimed at improving their German language skills.

Guideline 4: Community-Based Cooperation

The social-psychiatric service of the local authority coordinates the institutions in the social-psychiatric network, which includes the regional psychiatric-psychotherapeutic clinics with their inpatient, partly residential, and aftercare facilities as well as general practitioners, psychiatrists, psychiatric neurologists, and special services provided by private bodies. This coordination ensures the cooperation of all participants, with the aim of providing mentally ill people – both native and immigrant – with the best possible options for participating in normal life through treatment, care, and rehabilitation. The general psychiatric network, as the organizing structure for the coordination and cooperation of the services provided in general psychiatric care, originally had the responsibility of integrating all patient groups, including those with a background of migration, in the standard care services. Virtual centers of competence, formed through networking between the locally based cooperation partners in the general psychiatric networks, are able to adapt the standard care services to the needs of the supported immigrant groups and thus improve both the clinical concept and individual treatment.

The must be to achieve increasing awareness and cultural sensitivity on the part of the services, which is mainly the responsibility of the regional psychiatric coordinators and the commissioners for integration or migration, respectively. In addition, focus group discussions with key members of the regional immigrant groups have been successful in taking on a mediator function between the psychiatric coordinators and regulated services and immigrant groups and the affected individuals. This concept envisages convincing influential opinion makers within the immigrant groups to take part in training on the structures and the points of access to the German health system, in particular, the psychiatric-psychotherapeutic treatment facilities (see also the EMZ project MIMI). By means of an annual health report, the regional psychosocial working groups (PSAG) can obtain an overview of the needs and actual care situation of immigrants in the social-psychiatric network, which can act as a basis for future planning.

In Germany, a one-of-a-kind study (Region Hannover, 2009; Sueße, 2010) carried out by the social-psychiatric network in the region around Hanover in the northern state of Lower Saxony (a region with approximately 1 million inhabitants) and the EMZ concerning the psychiatric care of 260,000 immigrants (23%) yielded the following results:

- The usage of general psychiatric inpatient care in specialist hospitals corresponded to the proportion of immigrants in the population as a whole (Koch, Hartkamp, Siefen, & Schouler-Ocak, 2008; Schouler-Ocak et al., 2008). In involuntary treatment, immigrants were overrepresented by almost 100%.
- Outpatient facilities such as social-psychiatric services (SPDi), suppliers of supervised accommodation, and psychiatric care services, as well as day care centers, contact centers, and rehabilitation facilities were underused by immigrants as compared to the native population.
- In almost all facilities, the proportion of immigrants among patients was two to three times greater than the proportion among staff, and this was particularly marked in those services where the proportion of patients with a migration background was higher, for example the SPDi, outpatient departments, emergency departments, day care clinics, and the wards.
- In immigrant counseling, service treatment was "immigrant to immigrant."
- In all services, the majority of migrant patients originated from the former Soviet Union and Turkey, followed by those from the former Yugoslavia, Poland, and the Mediterranean countries. Corresponding language skills in the team were desired.
- In order to improve the quality of work, all facilities supported staff members with a migration background and therapy skills in cross-cultural counseling, psycho- and family therapy, concepts for the treatment of immigrants, further education, and so forth.

The paramount desirables expressed were the employment of staff with a migration background and working on the "threshold" of the services, such as by providing immigrant communities with information concerning the services by means of mediators and intensification of cross-cultural further education. The danger of a "split in the system" due to the preponderant treatment "immigrant to immigrant" will solely affect the special migration services. A sustainable improvement in cross-cultural competence through the integration of immigrants into the psychiatric-psychotherapeutic standard care system can be regarded as a contribution to the integration of immigrants into the host society. The target of integration in standard care described in the fourth Sonnenberg guideline must be accompanied by the requirements raised in the fifth and sixth guidelines.

Guideline 5: User Participation in Service Planning

The founding of organizations for affected individuals and their families has led to an optimization of the health care system. Immigrant groups and their representatives should be involved in the planning of psychiatric-psychotherapeutic care. Thus, there will be a degree of social participation in practice – a requirement associated with social integration of immigrants into the health care system.

Guideline 6: Improved Information for Immigrants

Information can be transmitted by key figures in immigrant groups acting as mediators and disseminators to those affected, as well as by using media, such as multilingual handouts about the social-psychiatric network, multilingual Internet information (e.g., www.ethno-medizinisches-zentrum.de), and publicity in publications aimed specifically at immigrants (daily and local newspapers in native languages). Websites of associations for immigrants and therapists can also provide important information, such as, for example, the Ethno-Medical Center Hannover (EMZ – www.ethno-medizinisches-zentrum.de), the German-Turkish Society for Psychiatry, Psychotherapy and Psychosocial Health (DTGGP e.V – www.dtgpp.de; website in German and Turkish), the Association of Turkish-Language Psychotherapy and Psychosocial Counseling (GTP-AKTPT – www.aktpt-online.de; website in German), the Division of Cross-Cultural Psychiatry of the German Association for Psychiatry and Psychotherapy (DGPPN – www.dgppn.de ; website in German and partly also in English), the Working Group for Ethnic Medicine e.V (AGEM – www.agem-ethnomedizin.de), or the umbrella organization for cross-cultural psychiatry in German speaking countries (DTPPP e.V – www.transkulturellepsychiatrie.de; website in Germany, contains patient information in a number of languages), and others.

Guideline 7: Training and Continuing Education for Professionals

The further education toward qualification in general practice or becoming a consultant in psychiatry and psychotherapy, child and adolescent psychiatry and psychotherapy, or clinical psychology and all the other professions active in psychiatry and psychotherapy are essential further education modules for migration and cross-cultural psychiatry and psychotherapy. Specialist divisions of cross-cultural psychiatry in national and international professional bodies promote vocational and continuing education for all professional groups actively involved in the provision of mental health services, such as, for example, the Division of Cross-Cultural Psychiatry and Migration of the DGPPN and the Austrian Society for Psychiatry and Psychotherapy (OEGPP), the Section on Cultural Psychiatry of the European Psychiatric Association (EPA), and the World Psychiatric Association (TPS-WPA).

Guideline 8: Prevention Programs for Children and Adolescents

It is crucial that preventive strategies should involve family members due to the fact that the children of immigrant families cohabit with their nuclear families more often and exhibit more family cohesion than children in the native population (Hurrelmann and Andresen, 2007). Additionally, the family as a primary setting for socialization is particularly important for the children of immigrants because of its exclusivity. For instance, it has been reported that these children attend kindergarten less often and for a shorter period than native German children. From the relatively great importance of internal family socialization among immigrants it has been deduced that this socialization has a particularly clear effect on personal behavior. Moreover, it has been shown that use of the non-German native language within the family constitutes a risk factor for school achievement on the one hand but also aggregates a protective effect with regard to development of psychiatric symptoms on the other hand (Hurrelmann and Andresen, 2007). A bilingual–bicultural orientation is therefore highly recommended.

The significance of early learning, the promotion of independent exploration of the environment, the support of cognitive development, and the practice of basal cultural techniques in immigrant families were replicated by the HIPPY-programs in Switzerland and Austria for the children of Turkish immigrant families (Kağitçıbaşı, 1996). Intra-ethnic media campaigns have also shown positive effects with regard to ameliorating negative attitudes toward education and reducing family-internal violence.

However, there are still barriers to service use both in the area of help with child rearing, and with regard to outpatient psychological and psychiatric counseling for adolescents. Immigrants' continuing under-average participation in preventation and early diagnosis programs for children can be improved by strategically strengthening local presence and involving intra-ethnic mediators (summary in Schepker and Toker, 2008).

One of the major causes of concern is the lower level of educational achievement found in immigrant youths as compared to the native population, which may be partly due to discrimination they are exposed to. A vast body of research has reported higher rates of school dropout, failure in the transition from school to work, and youth unemployment among immigrant youths, which may all be seen as risk factors for developing psychopathology. In light of these circumstances, effective preventive strategies should involve political steps at the societal level and improvements in educational and economic policy as well as in public relations, and improved access pathways to educational and parental counseling services designed specifically for immigrants.

Guideline 9: Self-Help Groups

Points of contact in a number of large cities (SEKIS in Berlin, KISS in Cologne, or SHZ in Munich) are attempting to activate the self-help potential of immigrants through targeted self-help group initiatives. Through this, a number of individual self-help groups concerend with health-related issues, operating in the native language and ethnically homogenous, have been formed. Barriers to the utilization of such services, however, remain diverse – ranging from illiteracy and deficiencies in education and language, shame-related issues, and concerns over anonymity to concepts of external pathogenesis (Kofahl, Hollmann. & Möller-Beck, 2009). There are reports of rapid disbanding of and little consistency among such self-help groups. A number of recommendations have been made to support the continuation of such self-help efforts, including the creation of single-sex groups and group name changes turning a "self-help group" into a "solidarity group" or "health group"[1] in order to prevent stigmatization.

Guideline 10: Quality Standards for Expert Witnessing in Legal Contexts

Within the criminal justice system there is a culturally appropriate diagnosis level for the legal culpability of mentally ill immigrants under §§ 20, 21 of the German criminal code (StGB), and with regard to the indication for involuntary commitment under §§ 63, 64 StGB. However, high levels of diagnostic misinterpretation and underdiagnosis of personality disorders, an inappropriate use of psychological testing tools, and skepticism in prognosis remain current. In the area of civil law, the assessment of traumatized asylum-seeking refugees, in particular, requires compliance with higher and well-defined quality standards. In social law, the assessment of immigrants in the area of social medicine requires the consideration of the overall situation of the affected person. Ambiguity in questions of visa status often leads to stress disorders and obstructs successful approaches to rehabilitation. The identification of culture-bound components in mental disorders by means of taking a thorough biographical case history together with the appropriate psychological tests is crucial for the clinical assessment of the affected individual, successful rehabilitation measures, and the reinforcement of coping strategies.

Guideline 11: Transcultural Psychiatry in Academic Curricula

In a nation open to immigration it is essential for schools and universities to foster knowledge and understanding of other cultures in order to promote social competence and thereby reduce the potential for social and cultural conflict within society. The curricula for university courses in social sciences and sociology, as well as in psychology and medicine, now contain lectures on migration, social integration, mental health, and so forth, and these are well received by the students. Such cross-cultural curriculum additions have already been introduced successfully in social work and social education as well as in further qualifications for nursing staff and other professional groups active in psychiatry.

---

1 S. Straßheim (personal communication, 2009).

Guideline 12: Research on Immigrant Mental Health

Financial support from the German Research Foundation (DFG), the European Union, and other foundations has led to an improvement in the academic situation related to migration studies in Germany. The international migration movements in central Europe have been studied extensively. Meaningful data exists on the epidemiology of mental disorders, even though representative data on the prevalence and comorbidity of mental disorders in immigrants in Germany have yet to be provided (Bundesamt für Migration und Flüchtlinge, 2005). New results (Balkir, Arens & Barnow, 2012; Sieberer et al., 2011; Walter et al., 2007) are available concerning addiction and depression (for instance, via the European Alliance Against Depression). Such studies are necessary, along with similar studies that allow evaluation of the type and extent of assistance for mentally ill immigrants and examine the ways in which the access points can be improved and better accessibility to psychiatric services and facilities can be achieved. Numerous studies have provided information about the causes of mental disturbances in immigrants and their psychopathological form. Trials are under way for cross-cultural treatment concepts under inpatient conditions and in individual and group psychotherapy.

Conclusions: Take-Home Message

- The Sonnenberg Guidelines (Machleidt, 2002) arose from a cooperative initiative of cross-cultural professional societies and institutions with the aim of sustainable improvement in psychiatric–psychotherapeutic care for immigrants. They have become the recognized standard for modern cross-cultural psychological medicine.
- The 12 programmatic requirements deal with areas of integration in standard care; cultural sensitivity and competence in treatment; communication and information in immigrants' native languages; inclusion of affected individuals and self-help groups; cross-cultural vocational, advanced, and further education; legal questions and health care research projects.
- Improved accessibility of general psychiatric services and facilities can be promoted through centers of competence, commissioners for integration and migration within institutions, multicultural teams, mediator activity in immigrant communities, and the dispersal of information.
- The social-psychiatric networks can best obtain an overview of the situation regarding regional cross-cultural care by investigating the facilities and services involved in immigrant care in the framework of a health care report. This serves as a foundation for planning the construction, development, and optimization of immigrant care, in particular for the prevention and treatment of children and adolescents with a migration background.
- Cross-cultural curricula in university courses in social sciences and sociology, as well as psychology and medicine, are an essential building block in teaching

and not less important for educationalists and nursing staff. A society such as the German one, containing an increasing proportion of immigrants, is well advised to make "cultural competence" a quality feature of education.

References

Balkir, N., Arens, E. A., & Barnow S. (2012). Exploring the relevance of autonomy and relatedness for mental health in healthy and depressed women from two different cultures: When does culture matter? *International Journal of Social Psychiatry.* Advance online publication. doi: 10.1177/0020764012441428

Bundesamt für Migration und Flüchtlinge. (2005). *Migrationsbericht 2005* [Migration report 2005 of the German Federal Office for Migration and Refugees]. Retrieved from http://www.bundesregierung.de/Content/DE/Publikationen/IB/migrationsbericht-2005,property=publicationFile.pdf

Bundesregierung. (2007). *Der Nationale Integrationsplan: Neue Wege – Neue Chancen* [The national integration strategy: New directions – new opportunities]. Retrieved from http://www.bundesregierung.de/Content/DE/Publikation/IB/Anlagen/nationaler-integrationsplan,property=publicationFile.pdf

Gün, A. K. (2009). Erfordernis und Aufgaben von Integrationsbeauftragten in der stationären Versorgung [Requirements and responsibilities of integration commissioners in inpatient settings]. In C. Falge, & G. Zimmermann (Eds.), *Interkulturelle Öffnung des Gesundheitssystems. Schriftenreihe des ZERP, Band 51.* (pp. 157–170). Baden-Baden, Germany: Nomos.

Hurrelmann, K., & Andresen, S. (2007). *TNS Infratest Sozialforschung: Kinder in Deutschland 2007. 1. World Vision Kinderstudie* [TNS Infratest Social studies: Children in Germany, 2007. 1st world vision child study]. Frankfurt am Main, Germany: Fischer.

Kağitçıbaşı, Ç. (1996). *Family and human development across cultures. A view from the other side.* Mahwah, NJ: Erlbaum.

Koch, E., Hartkamp, N., Siefen, R. G., & Schouler-Ocak, M. (2008). Patienten mit Migrationshintergrund in stationär-psychiatrischen Einrichtungen – Pilotstudie der Arbeitsgruppe „Psychiatrie und Migration" der Bundesdirektorenkonferenz [Patients with a migration background in psychiatric inpatient settings – pilot study of the federal directors' conference's working group on „psychiatry and medicine"]. *Nervenarzt, 79*, 328–339.

Kofahl, C., Hollmann, J., & Möller-Bock, B. (2009). Gesundheitsbezogene Selbsthilfe bei Menschen mit Migrationshintergrund [Health-related self-help in individuals with a migration background]. *Bundesgesundheitsblatt-Gesundheitsforschung-Gesundheitsschutz, 52*, 55–63.

Landschaftsverband Rheinland. (2008). *Interkulturalität in der Gemeindepsychiatrie* [Intercultural approaches in community psychiatry]. Cologne, Germany: Landschaftsverband Rheinland.

Machleidt, W. (2002). Die 12 Sonnenberger Leitlinien zur psychiatrisch-psychotherapeutischen Versorgung von MigrantInnen in Deutschland [The 12 Sonnenberg Guidelines on psychiatric-psychotherapeutic services for migrants in Germany]. *Nervenarzt, 73*, 1208–1209.

Machleidt, W., Salman, R., & Calliess, I. T. (Eds.) (2006). *Sonnenberger Leitlinien. Integration von Migranten in Psychiatrie und Psychotherapie. Erfahrungen und Konzepte in Deutschland und Europa* [Sonnenberg Guidelines. The integration of migrants in psychiatry and psychotherapy. Experience and concepts in Germany and Europe]. Berlin, Germany: VWB.

Region Hannover. (2009). Sozialpsychiatrische Versorgungssituation von Migranten in der Region Hannover [The social-psychiatric care situation for migrants in the Hanover region]. Retrieved from http://www.hannover.de/data/download/RH/Ges_Soz/sozpsych/sozpsych_Versorgung_Migranten_RH.pdf

Schepker, R., & Toker, M. (2008). *Transkulturelle Kinder- und Jugendpsychiatrie. Grundlagen und Praxis* [Transcultural child and adolescent psychiatry. Foundations and practical application]. Berlin, Germany: Medizinisch-wissenschaftliche Verlagsgesellschaft.

Schouler-Ocak, M., Bretz, H. J., Penka, S., Koch, E., Hartkamp, N., Siefen, R. G., … Heinz, A. (2008). Patients of immigrant origin in inpatient psychiatric facilities. *European Psychiatry, 23*, 21–27.

Sieberer, M., Maksimovic, S., Ersöz, B., Machleidt, W., Ziegenbein, M., & Calliess, I. T. (2011). Depressive symptoms in first-and second-generation migrants: A cross-sectional study of a multi-ethnic working population. *International Journal of Social Psychiatry.* Advance online publication. doi: 10.1177/0020764011418418

Sueße, T. (2010). Zur sozialpsychiatrischen Versorgung von Migranten in der Region Hannover [On the provision of social-psychiatric care for migrants in the Hanover region]. In H. Elgeti (Ed.), *Psychiatrie in Niedersachsen* (pp. 167-170). Bonn, Germany: Psychiatrie-Verlag.

Walter, U., Krauth, C., Kurtz, V., Salman, R., & Machleidt, W. (2007). Health and health care of migrants with particular regard to addiction. *Nervenarzt, 78,* 1058–1061.

Wielant Machleidt
Department of Psychiatry, Social Psychiatry and Psychotherapy
Hanover Medical School
Carl-Neuberg-Str. 1
30625 Hannover
Germany
E-mail: machleidt.wielant@mhhannover.de

Keyword Index

Contributors

Elisabeth A. Arens
Department of Clinical Psychology and Psychotherapy
Institute of Psychology
University of Heidelberg
Heidelberg, Germany
E-mail: elisabeth.arens@psychologie.uni-heidelberg.de

Hans-Jörg Assion
LWL-Hospital Dortmund
Dortmund, Germany
E-mail: Hans-joerg.assion@wkp-lwl.org

Sofie Bäärnhielm
Transcultural Centre
Stockholm County Council
S:t Görans' Hospital
Stockholm, Sweden
E-mail: sofie.baarnhielm@sll.se

Nazli Balkir
Department of Clinical Psychology and Psychotherapy
Institute of Psychology
University of Heidelberg
Heidelberg, Germany
E-mail: nazli.balkir@psychologie.uni-heidelberg.de, nazlibalkir@gmail.com

Sven Barnow
Department of Clinical Psychology and Psychotherapy
Institute of Psychology
University of Heidelberg
Heidelberg, Germany
E-mail: sven.barnow@psychologie.uni-heidelberg.de

Emily A. Butler
Norton School Family and Consumer Sciences
Family Studies & Human Development
University of Arizona
Tucson, AZ, USA
E-Mail: eabutler@u.arizona.edu

Iris T. Calliess
Department of Psychiatry, Social Psychiatry and Psychotherapy
Hanover Medical School
Hanover, Germany
E-mail: Calliess.Iris@mhhannover.de

Kenneth R. Conner
University of Rochester Medical Center
Rochester, NY, USA
E-mail: kenneth_conner@urmc.rochester.edu

Francisco José Eiroa-Orosa
Servei de Psiquiatria
Hospital Universitari Vall d'Hebron
CIBERSAM
Departament de Psiquiatria
Universitat Autònoma de Barcelona
Barcelona, Spain
E-mail: franciscojose.eiroa@uab.cat

Herta Flor
Department of Cognitive and Clinical Neuroscience
Central Institute of Mental Health
Medical Faculty Mannheim
Heidelberg University
Mannheim, Germany
E-mail: herta.flor@zi-mannheim.de

Shihui Han
Department of Psychology
Peking University
Beijing, China
E-mail: shan@pku.edu.cn

Tobias Heikamp
Department of Psychology
University of Konstanz
Konstanz, Germany
E-mail: tobias.heikamp@uni-konstanz.de

Eckhardt Koch
Vitos Hospital for Psychiatry and Psychotherapy
Marburg, Germany
E-mail: Eckhardt.Koch@vitos-giessen-marburg.de

Michael Linden
Charité Research Group Psychosomatic Rehabilitation
Berlin, Germany
E-mail: michael.linden@charite.de

Wielant Machleidt
Department of Psychiatry, Social Psychiatry and Psychotherapy
Hanover Medical School
Hanover, Germany
E-mail: machleidt.wielant@mhhannover.de

Juan Mezzich
Department of Psychiatry
Mount Sinai School of Medicine
New York University
New York, NY, USA
E-mail: juanmezzich@aol.com, juan.mezzich@mssm.edu

Georg Northoff
Institute of Mental Health Research
University of Ottawa
Ottawa, ON, Canada
E-mail: georg.northoff@theroyal.ca

Jaak Panksepp
Department of VCAPP
Washington State University
Pullman, WA, USA
E-mail: jpanksepp@vetmed.wsu.edu

Adil Qureshi
Servei de Psiquiatria
Hospital Universitari Vall d'Hebron
CIBERSAM
Departament de Psiquiatria
Universitat Autònoma de Barcelona
Barcelona, Spain
E-mail: aqureshi@vhebron.net

Ramazan Salman
Ethno-Medical Center Hanover
Hanover, Germany
E-mail: ethno@salman.info

Renate Schepker
ZfP Südwürttemberg Weissenau
Abt. Kinder- und Jugendpsychiatrie
Ravensburg, Germany
E-mail: renate.schepker@zfp-weissenau.de

Meryam Schouler-Ocak
Charité Psychiatric University Clinic at St. Hedwig's Hospital
Berlin, Germany
E-mail: meryam.schouler-ocak@charite.de

Marcel G. Sieberer
Department of Psychiatry, Social Psychiatry and Psychotherapy
Hanover Medical School
Hanover, Germany
E-mail: Sieberer.Marcel@mh-hannover.de

Gisela Trommsdorff
Department of Psychology
University of Konstanz
Konstanz, Germany
E-mail: Gisela.Trommsdorff@uni-konstanz.de

Tekleh Zandi
UGGZ-Centraal
Institute for Mental Health Care
Amersfoort, The Netherlands
E-mail: t.zandi@ggzcentraal.nl

Liang Zhou
School of Public Health
Central South University
Changsha, Hunan, China
E-mail: Zhouliang1976@gmail.com

Marc Ziegenbein
Department of Psychiatry, Social Psychiatry and Psychotherapy
Hanover Medical School
Hanover, Germany
E-mail: Ziegenbein.Marc@mh-hannover.de